AN ATLAS OF
RADIOLOGICAL
ANATOMY

AN ATLAS OF RADIOLOGICAL ANATOMY

JAMIE WEIR

MBBS, FRCP (Ed), DMRD, FRCR

Consultant Radiologist Aberdeen Teaching Hospitals,
Honorary Senior Lecturer to the University of Aberdeen,
Examiner to the Part I Examination of the Royal College of Radiologists, London

PETER ABRAHAMS

MBBS

Senior Lecturer in Anatomy The Middlesex Hospital Medical School
University of London,
Examiner in Anatomy to the Royal College of Surgeons of England

Churchill Livingstone
EDINBURGH LONDON MELBOURNE AND NEW YORK 1986

CHURCHILL LIVINGSTONE
Medical Division of Longman Group UK Limited

Distributed in the United States of America by Churchill
Livingstone Inc., 1560 Broadway, New York, N.Y. 10036, and by
associated companies, branches and representatives throughout
the world.

First edition 1978 (Pitman Publishing Ltd)
Second edition 1986

ISBN 0 443 037027

British Library Cataloguing in Publication Data
  Weir, Jamie
    An atlas of radiological anatomy.
    1. Anatomy, Human – Atlases   2. Diagnosis,
    Radioscopic – Atlases
    I. Title   II. Abrahams, Peter, b. 1947
    611'.002'4616   QM25

    ISBN 0-272-79393-0

Printed in Great Britain by Butler & Tanner Ltd,
Frome and London

Dedicated
to Meg and Lucy

CONTENTS

ACKNOWLEDGEMENTS

We wish to thank the following for providing radiograms for this publication.

Aberdeen Teaching Hospitals, Scotland
Drs S N Allison, A P Bayliss, L A Gillanders, A F MacDonald, F W Smith, P R Ward;
Department and Schools of Radiography

Institute of Neurological Studies, Glasgow, Scotland
Dr M D M Hadley

The Middlesex Hospital, London, England
Drs M Chapman, S Colenso, J Dougal, B Kendall, the late R Lodge, H W Loose, J N Pattison, R Speller, C G Whiteside;
Department and Schools of Radiography

Royal Melbourne Hospital, Victoria, Australia
Dr B Tress

Institute of Orthopaedics, London, England
Dr D Stoker

Moorfields Eye Hospital, London, England
Dr G A S Lloyd

Royal Free Hospital, London, England
Dr R Dick

St. Thomas's Hospital, London, England
Professor N L Browse and the late Professor J B Kinmonth

University of Cambridge
Professor T Sherwood

Harefield Hospital, Middlesex, England
Dr R B Pridie

Technical assistance
Mr M J Foster, Ohio Nuclear Inc.
Mr A J Pope, The Middlesex Hospital
Miss Vicky Sparks, Graphics

To the following young ladies we would like to extend our special thanks for their secretarial skills:

Aberdeen	Miss Jean Bell
Iowa City	Mrs Margie Rinehart
	Mrs Karen Tower
The Middlesex Hospital	Mrs Lynda Dibble
	Miss Joan Lewis
	Miss Elaine Samuels

PREFACE TO FIRST EDITION

Radiographs are an essential element in clinical diagnosis and doctors need to be proficient in their interpretation. However, few are given comprehensive instruction in the anatomy of the normal radiograph, let alone in the complexities of pathology. We have designed this book with the intention of encompassing the full range of normal radiological anatomy for the use of radiologists, radiographers, medical students and clinicians. It will be of particular value to those involved in postgraduate radiology examinations.

Most radiographs in this atlas are in the standard form of negatives, and, for ease of understanding, a negative line drawing with anatomical labels is included facing each plate. Radiographs are often difficult to interpret due to their complexity. We have traced accurate line drawings which stress the important features, to aid interpretation. The unique presentation of using negative lines should simplify the process. Beneath each radiograph are set out a number of clinical points which will help in understanding that projection or technique; for example, hazards of a particular procedure, hidden zones, common fracture sites or practical points of interpretation. Where several pages cover the same anatomy (e.g. carotid arteriography) the clinical notes on each page relate to the whole group.

For easy reference, the book is divided into sections on plain radiographs, contrast examinations and miscellaneous radiographs. The plain radiographs are subdivided into anatomical regions, and those using contrast media into the major body systems. We have tried to cover completely the standard radiological anatomy of the body using normal radiographs taken during routine examinations on adults. No post-mortem specimens have been used and no paediatric or developmental studies have been included as these deserve a separate atlas. Certain radiographic projections are deliberately omitted as they do not contribute further to the normal anatomy. These projections are, of course, often of considerable value in pathological states. For further reading in anatomy, clinical medicine and radiology, a section on 'Further reading' is included.

Wherever possible, anatomical terms used are those laid down in *Nomina Anatomica* (3rd edn., by G A G Mitchell, Excerpta Medica Foundation, 1968) but also included are the well established, more popular radiological terms. The shape and size of radiographs illustrated vary according to projection and technique employed: cones and diaphragms have been used to enhance the quality of some projections. The physical principles of radiographic techniques such as tomography, subtraction, macroradiography and xeroradiography, are not covered, and the reader is advised to consult basic radiology texts. The contrast media used are mentioned briefly in the text but no attempt has been made to cover possible alternatives.

We trust this book will link the science of pure anatomy with that of clinical radiology, for both are variations on a theme.

Aberdeen   J W
London   P A

PREFACE TO SECOND EDITION

Basic human anatomy does not change; however, the means of demonstrating it has altered considerably since the first edition in 1978. X-ray computed tomography (CT) scanners were only in their infancy for sections outside the brain, and nuclear magnetic resonance (NMR; or magnetic resonance imaging, MRI) was only a research project. These two imaging modalities, together with ultrasound, have added enormously to the diagnosis of disease and have proved excellent in demonstrating normal anatomy.

We have thus increased the scope of this Atlas to include CT, NMR and ultrasound *only* to allow better definition of anatomical structures and we have tried to avoid unnecessary duplication. For example, only a limited number of sagittal ultrasound scans of the abdomen are included to supplement the anatomy demonstrated on CT and 'plain' radiography. We have therefore deliberately omitted large numbers of repetitive scans, of different imaging techniques, in order to keep the atlas to a reasonable size. Those readers who wish to study either the detailed anatomy of one imaging technique only or the physical principles of the new sections included should consult the 'Further reading' section at the end of this Atlas.

The three sections new to the second edition are: CT of the body, from the base of the skull, through the neck, chest, abdomen and pelvis, and including the arm and the leg; ultrasonic anatomy of the abdomen, pelvis, heart and eye, with a special section on the neonatal brain; and NMR imaging of the adult brain and spinal cord, with additional views of the female pelvis and the heart.

In view of the better definition of certain anatomical structures in these new sections, we have removed, where appropriate, a few of the original radiographs.

Aberdeen   J W
London   P A

ABBREVIATIONS

a.	artery		m.	muscle
ant.	anterior		med.	medial
brev.	brevis		n.	nerve
ext.	extensor		post.	posterior
fl.	flexor		r.	right
inf.	inferior		sup.	superior
l.	left		t.	tendon
lat.	lateral		v.	vein
lig.	ligament		vs.	vessel
long.	longus			

HEAD AND NECK

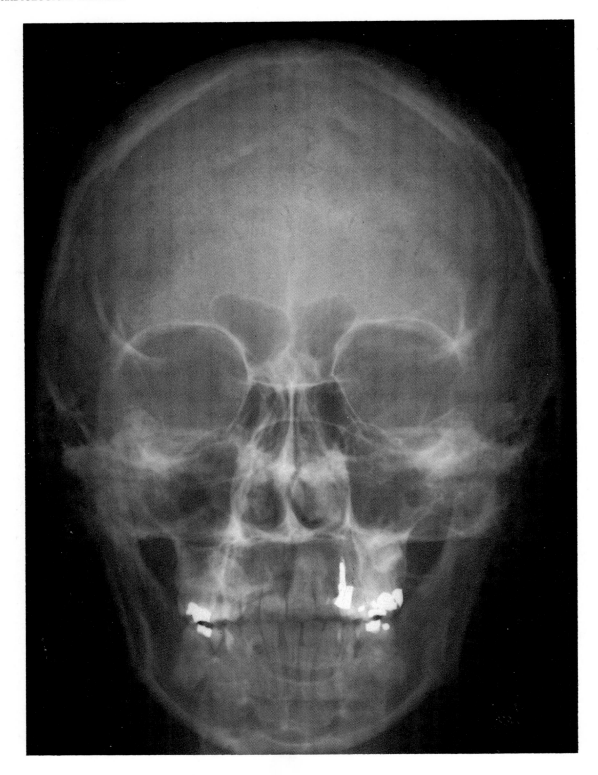

20° OCCIPITOFRONTAL VIEW OF SKULL

This projection allows the orbits to be checked for their equality of size, which is important in patients with proptosis. The floor of the hypophyseal fossa can be seen through the nasal cavity and this should be looked at closely if a pituitary tumour is suspected. Check the supraorbital fissure and the greater and lesser wings of sphenoid for any abnormality. Exclude vault fractures in the frontal region and blowout fractures through the floor of the orbit. The nasal cavity, the medial wall of the maxillary antrum and the ethmoid air cells are well seen in this projection.

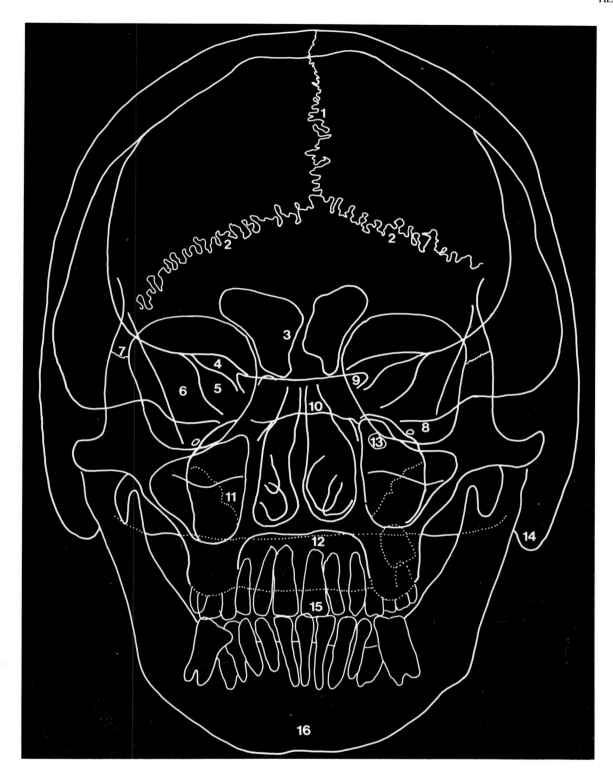

1   Sagittal suture

2   Lambdoid suture

3   Frontal sinus

4   Lesser wing of sphenoid

5   Supraorbital fissure

6   Greater wing of sphenoid

7   Frontozygomatic suture

8   Petrous ridge

9   Ant. clinoid process

10   Floor of hypophyseal fossa

11   Lat. pterygoid plate

12   Base of skull

13   Foramen rotundum

14   Tip of mastoid

15   Upper central incisor tooth

16   Mandible

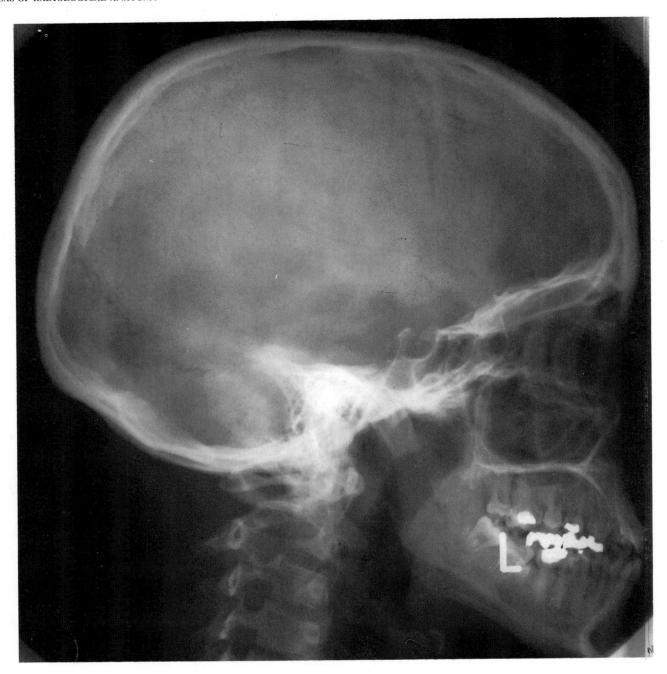

LATERAL VIEW OF SKULL

This is probably the most important of the skull views. There are several features which must be checked on this projection: the hypophyseal fossa, both for pituitary tumours and for the effects of raised intracranial pressure; the position of the pineal, if calcified; the width of the soft tissue shadow on the posterior aspect of the nasopharynx and oropharynx, and the posterior walls of the maxillary antra. Do not confuse vault fractures with vascular markings and suture lines. Look for other physiological calcification sites; for example, habenular calcification (reverse C-shape), petroclinoid and interclinoid ligament calcification. The frontal, sphenoid and maxillary air sinuses are clearly visualized on this projection.

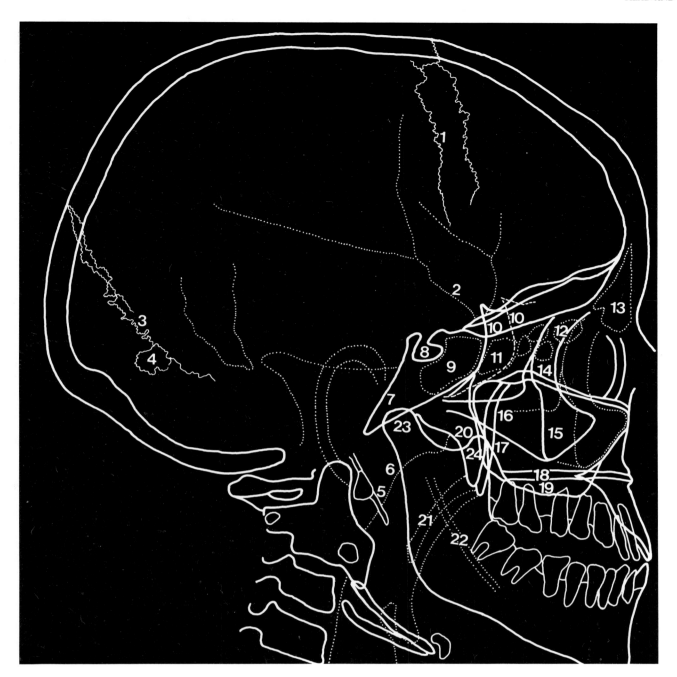

1 Coronal suture	**9** Sphenoid sinus	**17** Post. boundary of maxillary sinus
2 Middle meningeal a. impression	**10** Greater wing of sphenoid	**18** Hard palate
3 Lambdoid suture	**11** Post. ethmoid cells	**19** Alveolar process of maxilla
4 Wormian bone	**12** Ant. ethmoid cells	**20** Pterygoid plates
5 Styloid process	**13** Frontal sinus	**21** Soft palate and uvula
6 Post. wall of nasopharynx	**14** Frontal process of zygomatic bone	**22** Mandibular canal
7 Clivus (basilar parts of sphenoid and occipital bones)	**15** Malar process of maxilla	**23** Head of mandible
8 Hypophyseal fossa	**16** Zygomatic arch	**24** Coronoid process

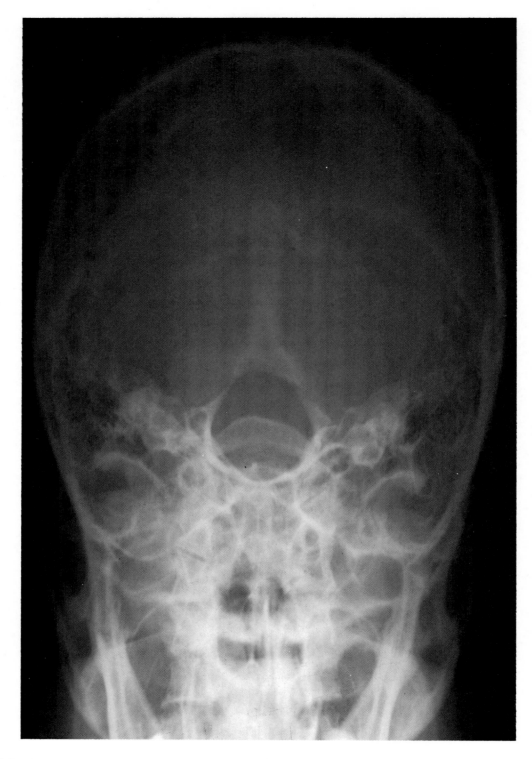

30° FRONTO-OCCIPITAL VIEW OF SKULL (TOWNE'S PROJECTION)

This view shows the region of the foramen magnum, the occipital bone and the petrous ridges, which should be checked for any abnormality. Check for posterior vault fractures. See if the pineal or the choroid plexuses of the lateral ventricles are calcified and, if they are, check that there is no midline shift. This view also demonstrates the zygomatic arch clearly. The dorsum sellae is best seen on this view.

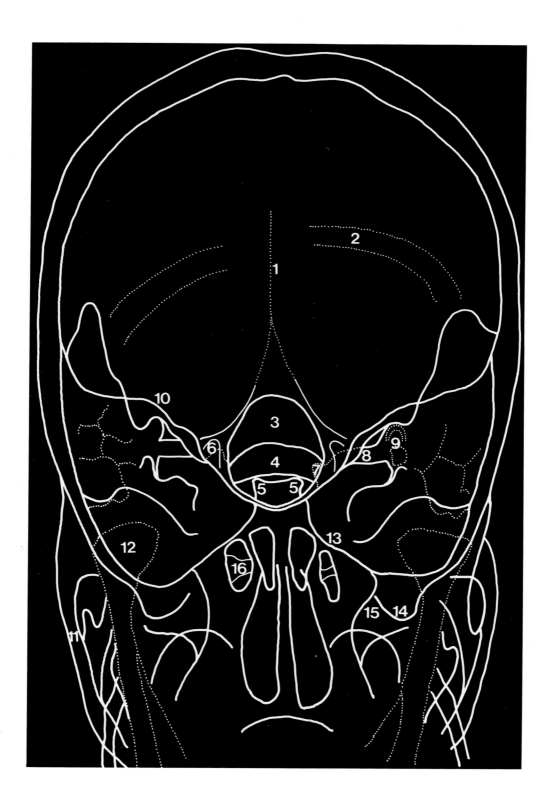

1   Internal occipital crest

2   Impression of lateral sinus

3   Foramen magnum

4   Arch of atlas

5   Post. clinoid processes

6   Occipital condyles

7   Ant. clinoid processes

8   Internal auditory meatus

9   Inner ear

10 Arcuate eminence of petrous temporal bone

11 Zygomatic arch

12 Condylar process of mandible

13 Floor of middle cranial fossa

14 Infratemporal tubercle of greater wing of sphenoid

15 Infraorbital fissure

16 Ethmoid sinus

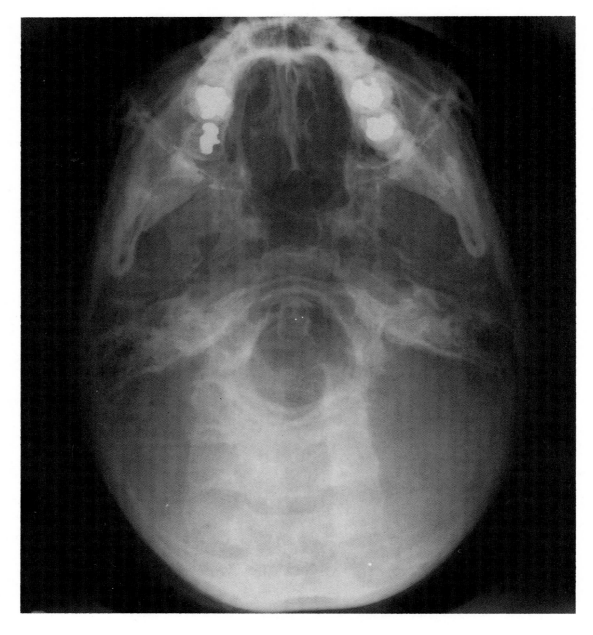

SUBMENTOVERTICAL VIEW OF SKULL

This projection is of the base of the skull. The sphenoid air sinus is well shown. The numerous exit foramina from the skull are easily identified. Look for enlargement of the foramen spinosum, which can occur in vascular vault meningiomas with a large external carotid arterial supply. Check the petrous apex and the region of the jugular foramen. Check the middle ear and its ossicles. Identify the three bony lines which overlap anteriorly: the greater wing of the sphenoid, the posterior wall of the orbit and the posterior wall of the maxillary antrum.

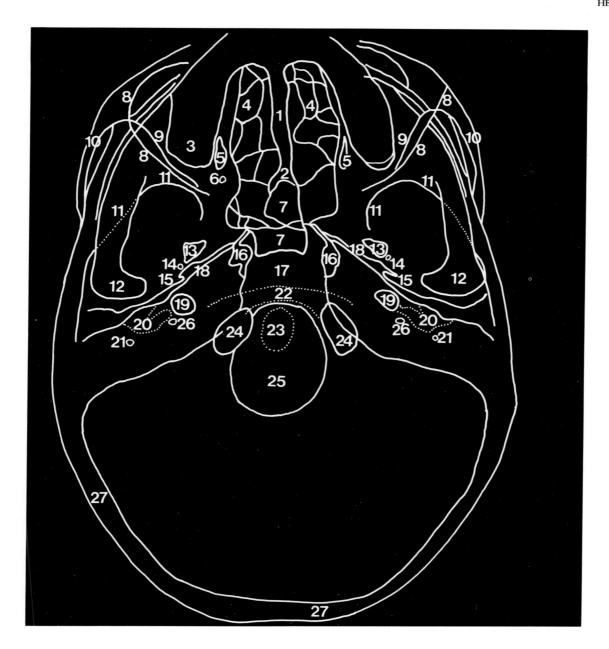

1   Nasal septum (vomer and perpendicular plate of ethmoid)

2   Post. border of vomer

3   Maxillary sinus

4   Ethmoid sinuses

5   Greater palatine foramen

6   Lesser palatine foramen

7   Sphenoid sinus

8   Post. orbital margin (greater wing of sphenoid)

9   Post. boundary of maxillary sinus

10   Zygomatic arch

11   Lesser wing of sphenoid

12   Head of mandible (condylar process)

13   Foramen ovale

14   Foramen spinosum

15   Spine of sphenoid

16   Foramen lacerum

17   Basilar parts of occipital and sphenoid bones (clivus)

18   Pharyngotympanic tube (eustachian tube)

19   Carotid canal

20   Jugular foramen

21   Stylomastoid foramen

22   Ant. arch of atlas

23   Odontoid process of axis (dens)

24   Occipital condyles

25   Foramen magnum

26   Canaliculus for tympanic nerve

27   Inner and outer tables of skull

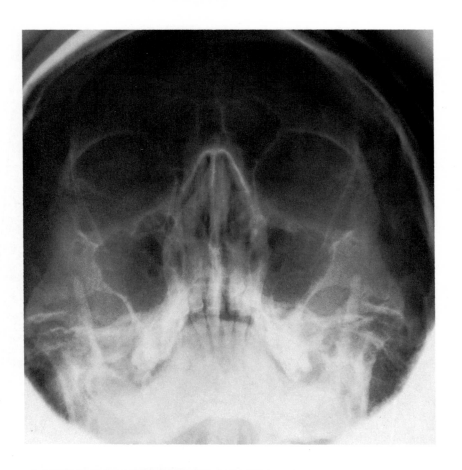

OCCIPITOMENTAL AND OCCIPITOFRONTAL VIEWS OF SKULL

These two projections show the frontal and maxillary sinuses to their best advantage. The maxillary antrum is seen on the occipitomental view; in particular, the roof of the antrum, the floor of the orbit, is clearly visualized. The frontal sinus is seen on both views. Look for sinus abnormalities such as mucosal thickening and fluid levels. Also check for facial fractures. The infraorbital foramen and the foramen rotundum can be seen on these projections.

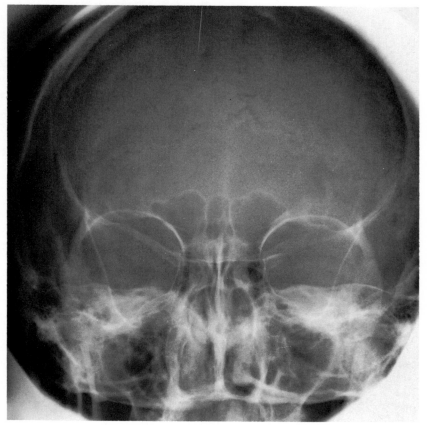

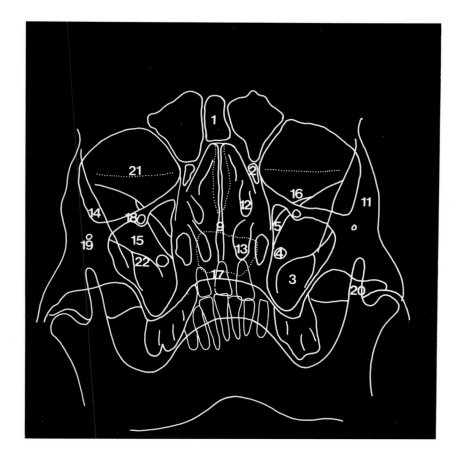

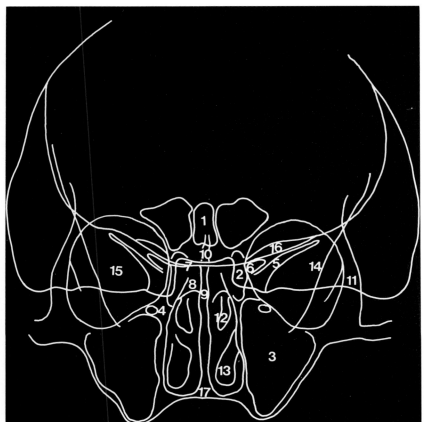

1   Frontal sinus

2   Ethmoid sinus

3   Maxillary sinus

4   Foramen rotundum

5   Supraorbital fissure

6   Ant. clinoid process

7   Post. clinoid process

8   Floor of hypophyseal fossa

9   Nasal septum

10   Crista galli

11   Frontal process of zygomatic bone

12   Middle concha (turbinate)

13   Inf. concha (turbinate)

14   Lat. border of greater wing of sphenoid

15   Greater wing of sphenoid

16   Lesser wing of sphenoid

17   Hard palate

18   Infraorbital foramen

19   Zygomaticofacial foramen

20   Coronoid process of mandible

21   Soft tissue lower lid

22   Pterygoid plates of sphenoid

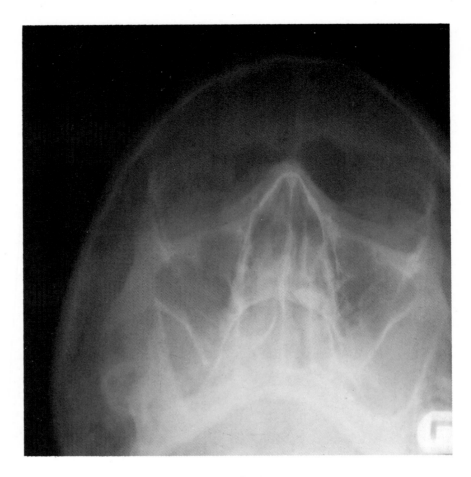

20° OCCIPITOMENTAL VIEW OF SKULL AND OBLIQUE VIEW OF OPTIC FORAMEN

This extra overtilted view of the facial bones is useful for assessing facial fractures involving the maxillary antrum, particularly the lateral wall. The coronoid process, the ramus of the mandible and the zygomatic arch are also obvious in this projection.

The oblique view of the orbit shows the optic canal. To obtain this view, tilt the orbitomeatal baseline 30° upwards from the occipitofrontal position and rotate the head 39° away from the affected side. Both optic canals should be visualized so that enlargement can be detected. One cause for this is an optic nerve glioma.

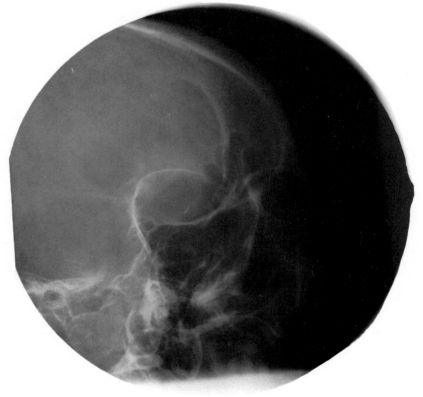

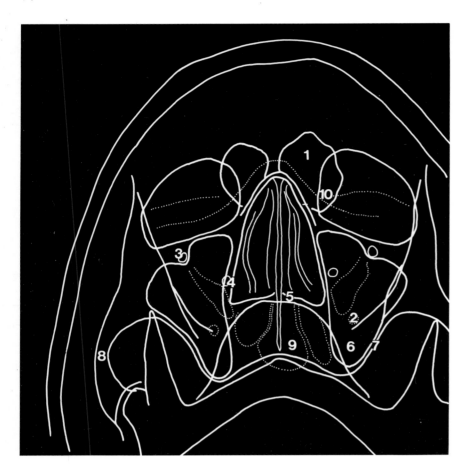

20° Occipitomental View of Skull

1 Frontal sinus

2 Foramen ovale

3 Infraorbital foramen

4 Foramen rotundum

5 Hard palate

6 Maxillary antrum

7 Lat. wall of maxillary antrum

8 Zygomatic arch

9 Sphenoid sinus

10 Soft tissue lines of nose and lower lid

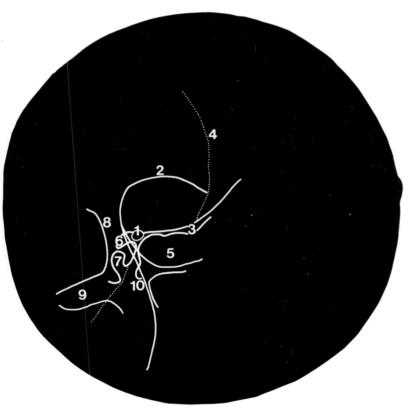

Oblique View of Optic Foramen

1 Optic foramen

2 Supraorbital ridge

3 Sphenoid ridge

4 Frontal bone

5 Sphenoid air sinus

6 Ant. clinoid process

7 Post. clinoid process

8 Frontal process of zygomatic bone

9 Zygomatic arch

10 Lat. border of greater wing of sphenoid

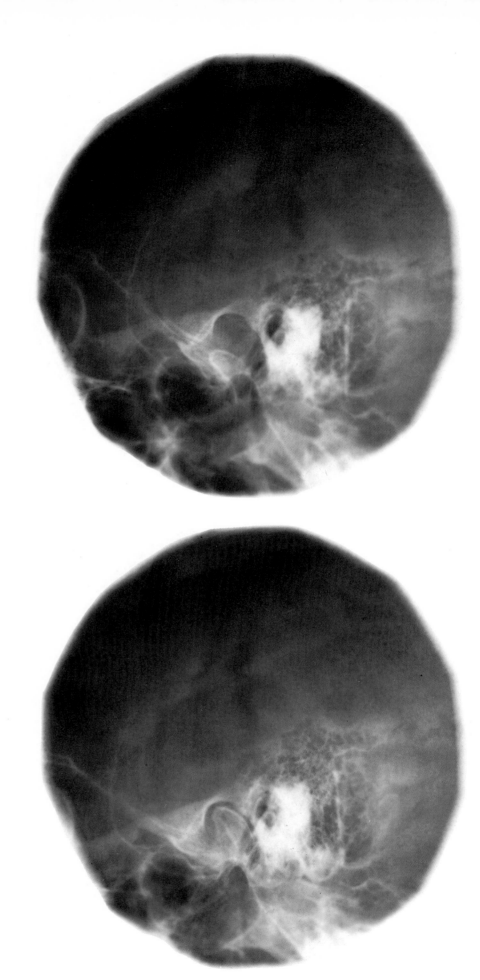

TEMPOROMANDIBULAR JOINT— MOUTH OPEN AND CLOSED

These projections are taken so that the temporomandibular joints are projected clear of the skull base. They are performed with the mouth open and closed to show the forward movement of the mandibular head as far as the articular tubercle. The joint itself is two separate synovial cavities separated by a plate of fibrocartilage and, being synovial, it can be affected by the erosive arthropathies (e.g. rheumatoid arthritis) as well as osteoarthritis. Both sides should be x-rayed to show any difference in the range of movement.

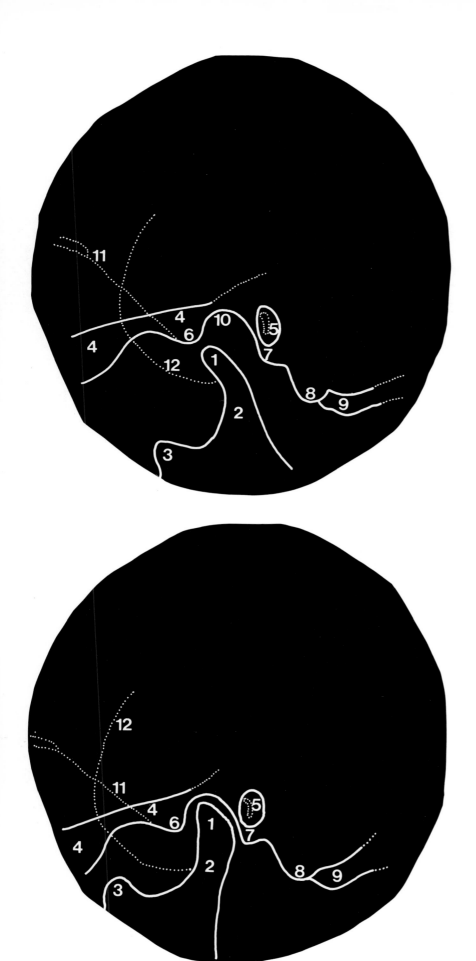

1 Head of mandible (condyloid process)

2 Neck of mandible

3 Coronoid process

4 Zygomatic arch

5 External auditory meatus and handle of malleus

6 Articular tubercle

7 Tympanic plate

8 Mastoid process

9 Groove for post. belly digastric muscle

10 Mandibular fossa

11 Greater wing of sphenoid (basal surface)

12 Lesser wing of sphenoid

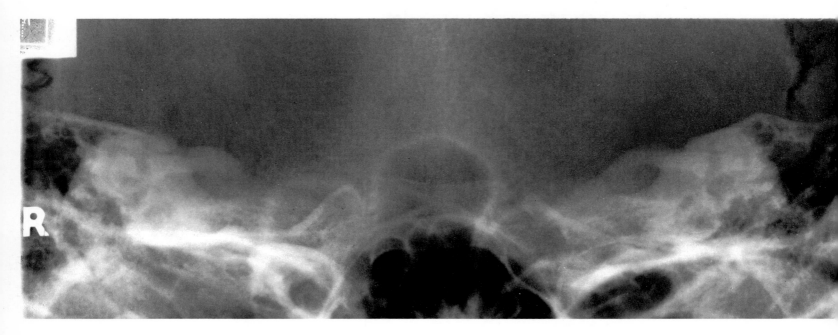

SLIT TOWNE'S PROJECTION OF TEMPORAL BONE

This macroradiogram shows the middle and internal ears. Look for the changes caused by eighth nerve tumours; for example, enlargement of the internal auditory canal, erosion of the roof and posterior rim, and disappearance of the crista transversalis. Look for congenital anomalies of the middle and inner ears. Note the high position of the head of the malleus and incus, in the epitympanic recess. Look for evidence of infection, either acute or chronic.

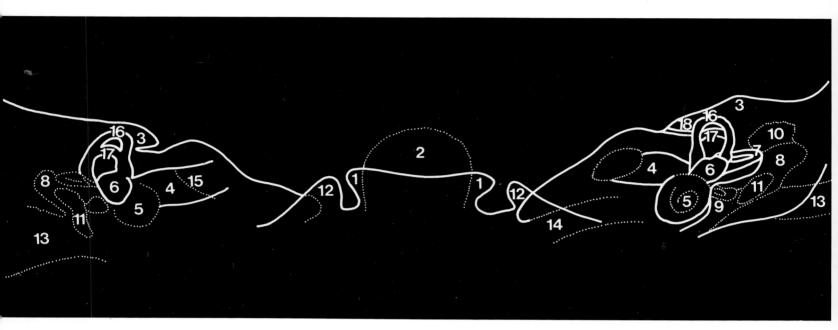

1	Post. clinoid process	7	Lat. semicircular canal	13	External auditory meatus (acoustic)
2	Foramen magnum	8	Epitympanic space (attic)	14	Carotid canal
3	Arcuate eminence of petrous temporal bone	9	Stapes	15	Post. wall of internal auditory meatus
4	Internal auditory meatus	10	Mastoid antrum	16	Sup. semicircular canal
5	Cochlea	11	Malleus and incus	17	Post. semicircular canal
6	Vestibule	12	Ant. clinoid process	18	Vein of subarcuate fossa

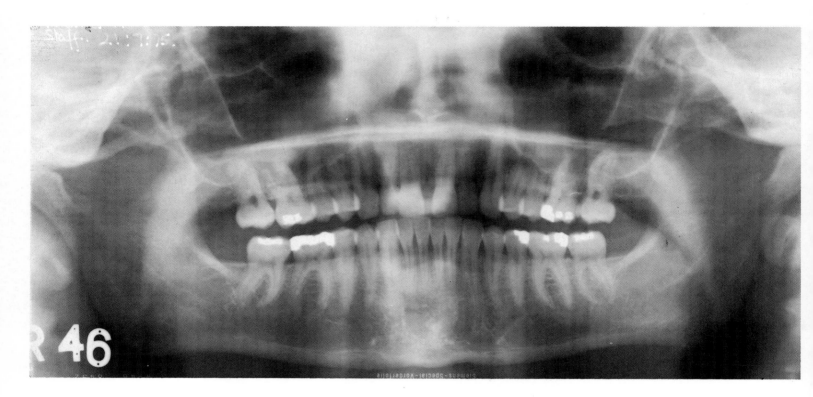

ORTHOPANTOMOGRAM

This special tomogram is taken to show the full set of upper and lower teeth. The position of all 32 adult teeth is instantly visible (this patient is missing the four third molar teeth or wisdoms). Note the difference in the root sockets of the incisors, canines, premolars and molars. Also note the protrusion of some roots of the upper teeth into the floor of the maxillary antrum, the alveolar portion of the maxilla. This view is useful for mandibular fractures, both before and after reduction. The lamina dura or periodontal membrane is seen as a thin dark line adjacent to the roots. This disappears in cases of hyperparathyroidism.

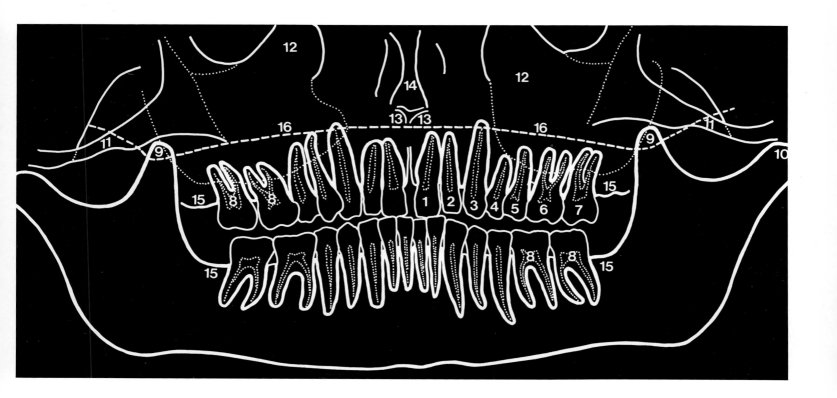

1 Central incisor	7 Second molar	13 Ant. nasal spine of maxilla
2 Lateral incisor	8 Pulp chamber	14 Vomer (nasal septum)
3 Canine	9 Coronoid process	15 Sites for third molars
4 First premolar	10 Head of mandible	16 Hard palate
5 Second premolar	11 Zygoma	
6 First molar	12 Maxillary sinus	

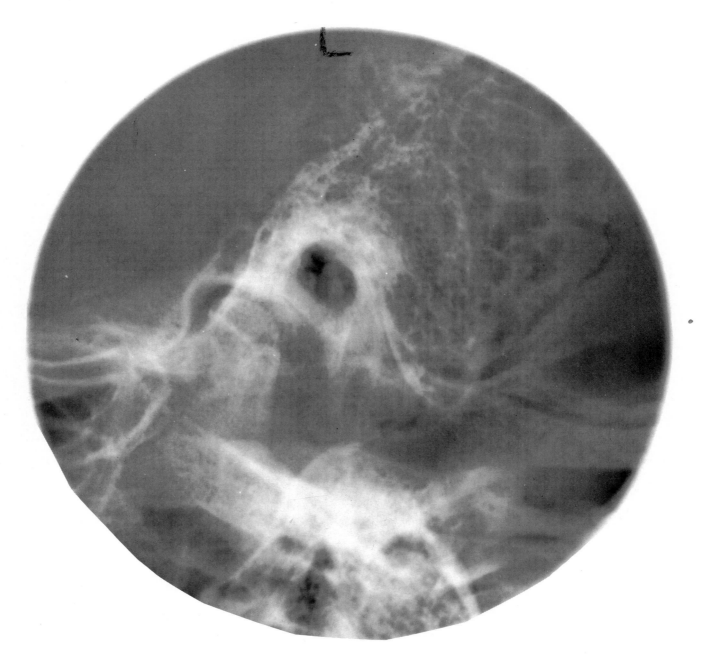

LATERAL OBLIQUE PROJECTION OF MASTOID PROCESS

This view shows the external auditory meatus projected over the internal auditory meatus and the handle of the malleus. The mastoid air cells are again seen and the lateral sinus plate shows clearly. Note that this view also gives a good view of the tempo-romandibular joint. See again the cellularity of the normal mastoid, which tends to rule out a cholesteatoma as in these cases the mastoid is usually but not invariably sclerotic.

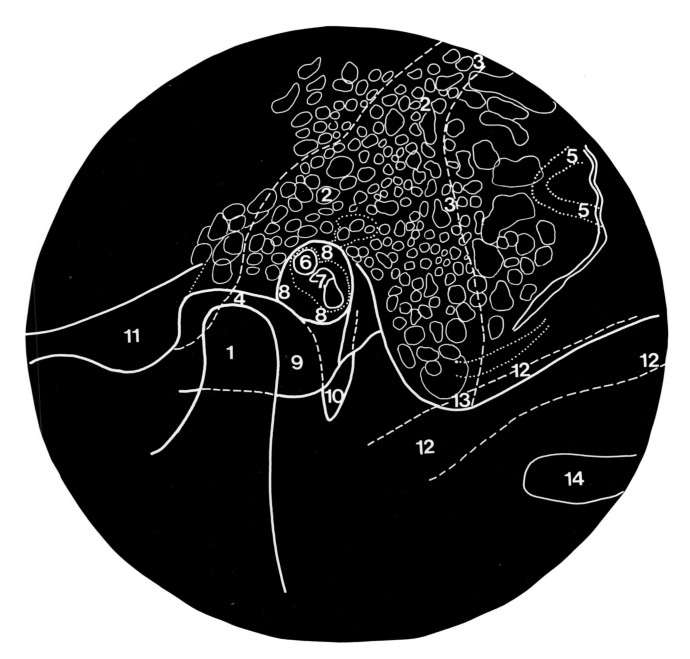

1	Head of mandible (condylar process)	6	Internal auditory meatus	11	Zygomatic process
2	Mastoid air cells	7	Auditory ossicles (malleus, incus)	12	Lat. sinus impression—opposite side
3	Lat. sinus plate	8	External auditory meatus (acoustic meatus)	13	Tip of mastoid process
4	Temporomandibular joint			14	Foramen magnum
5	Mastoid emissary v.	9	Tympanic part of temporal bone		
		10	Styloid process		

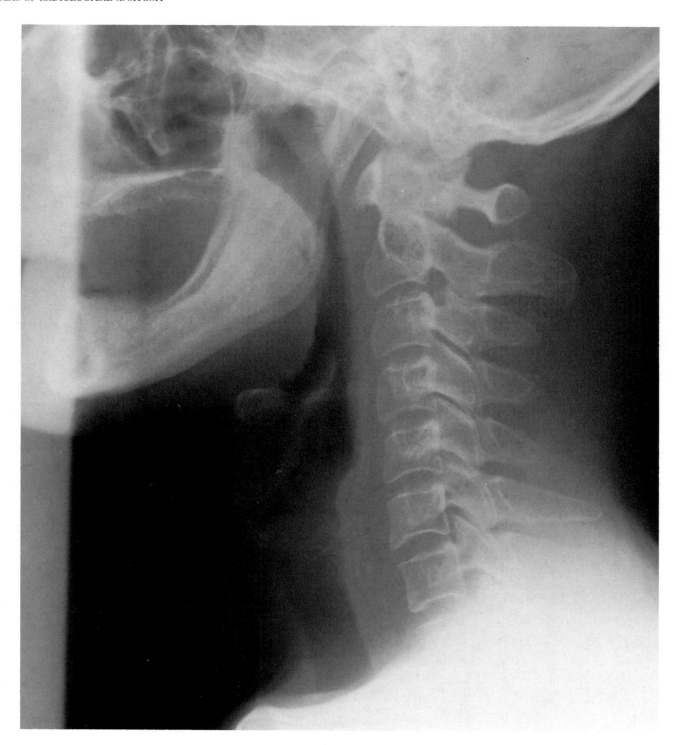

LATERAL SOFT TISSUE FILM OF THE NECK

This film uses the natural air of the pharynx and larynx as contrast medium. The cartilages of the larynx are seen and undergo true ossification rather than calcification. The retropharyngeal space between the posterior wall of the trachea and the anterior border of the cervical spine should not exceed the AP diameter of one vertebral body. Note the following: the articulation of the thyroid and cricoid cartilages; the air in the ventricle of the larynx between the true and false cords, and the position of the larynx extending from C3 to C6. The pharynx can also be seen in its anatomical divisions of nasopharynx above the soft palate, oropharynx between soft palate and base of tongue, and hypopharynx from base of tongue inferiorly.

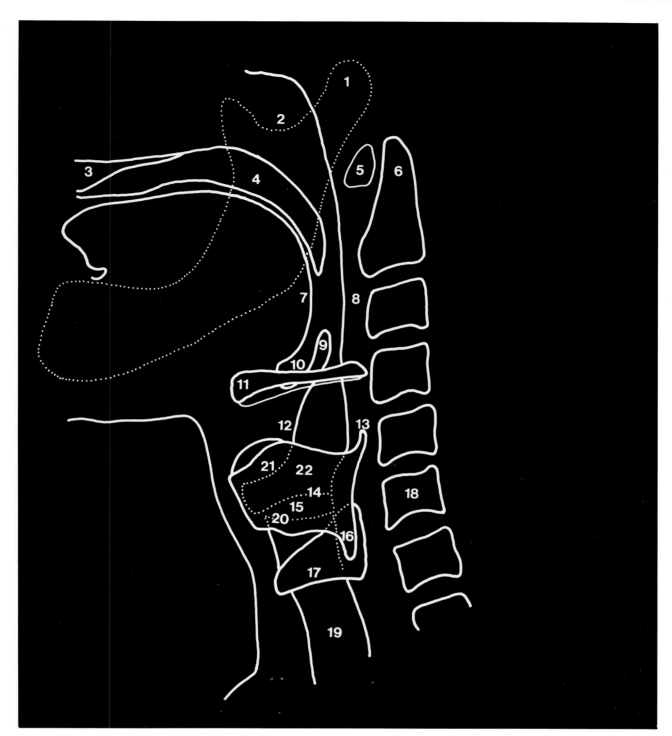

1 Head of mandible	9 Tip of epiglottis	17 Cricoid cartilage
2 Air in nasopharynx	10 Vallecula	18 C6 vertebra
3 Hard palate	11 Body of hyoid bone	19 Air in trachea
4 Soft palate	12 Epiglottis	20 Vocal folds (true cords)
5 Ant. arch of atlas	13 Sup. cornu of thyroid cartilage	21 Lamina of thyroid cartilage
6 Odontoid process of axis (dens)	14 Vestibular folds (false cords)	22 Vestibule of larynx
7 Post. aspect of tongue	15 Ventricle	
8 Retropharyngeal space	16 Inf. cornu of thyroid cartilage	

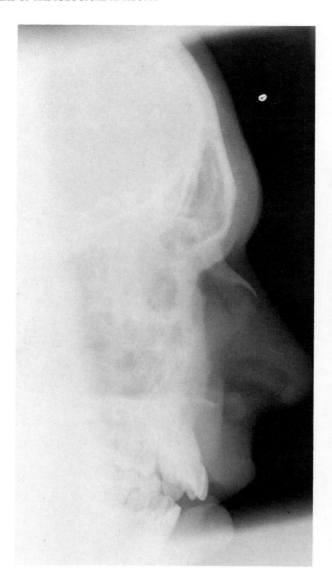
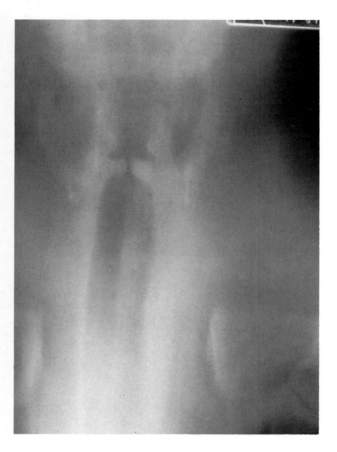

LATERAL SOFT TISSUE FILM OF THE FACE AND ANTEROPOSTERIOR TOMOGRAM OF THE LARYNX

The soft tissue projection of the face is taken mainly for nasal spine and nasal bone fractures; however, nasal fracture displacement is best visualized on an axial projection (not included). This soft tissue view is also useful for the assessment of dental occlusion or bite.

The tomogram of the larynx is taken in phonation 'EE' to show the stretching and adduction of the vocal cords. If one or both cords are paralysed, abduction will not take place. The commonest site for a laryngeal carcinoma is the anterior part of the vocal cords and most small lesions here should be readily visible. Look for upward and downward extension of the tumour.

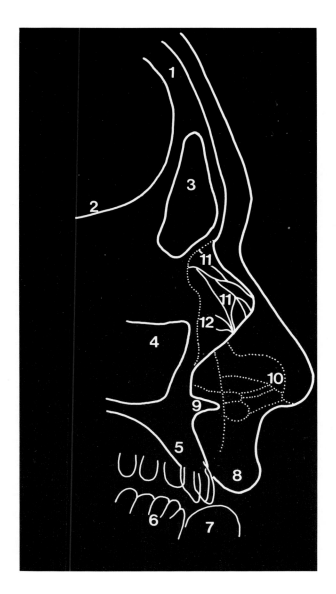

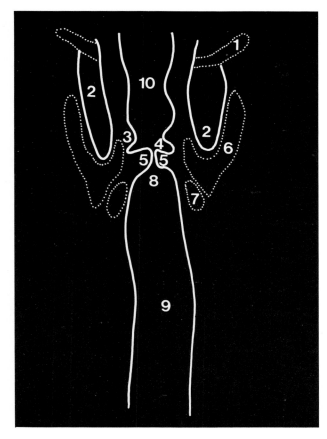

Lateral Soft Tissue of the Face

1 Frontal bone

2 Orbital plate of frontal bone

3 Frontal sinus

4 Maxillary sinus

5 Maxilla

6 Mandible with teeth

7 Lower lip

8 Upper lip

9 Ant. nasal spine of maxilla

10 Vestibule

11 Nasal bone

12 Frontal process of maxilla

Anteroposterior Tomogram of Larynx

1 Greater cornu of hyoid

2 Piriform fossae

3 Vestibular folds (false cords)

4 Ventricle

5 Vocal folds in 'EE' phonation (true cords)

6 Thyroid cartilage

7 Cricoid cartilage

8 Infraglottic portion of larynx

9 Trachea

10 Vestibule

UPPER LIMB

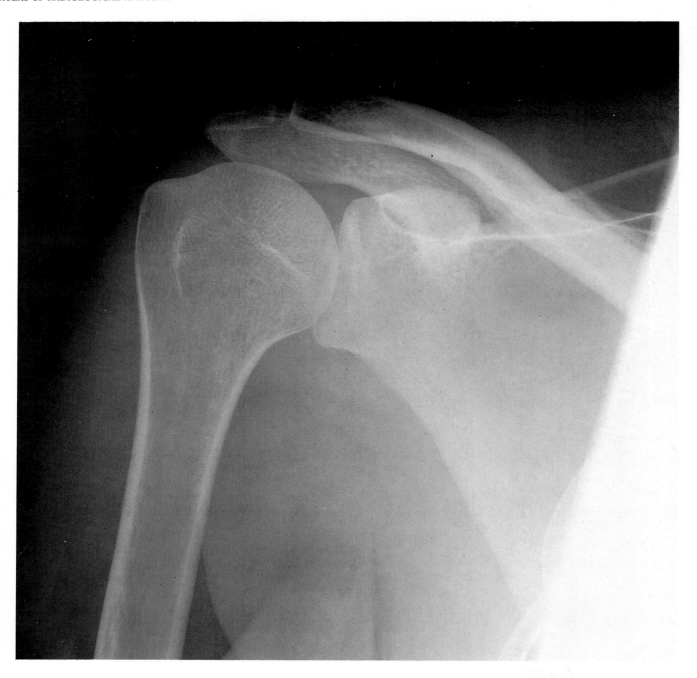

ANTEROPOSTERIOR VIEW OF SHOULDER

The middle and outer parts of the clavicle are well seen and are common fracture sites. Check the acromioclavicular joint to see if there is any subluxation or dislocation present. This should be confirmed by a weight-bearing view if suspected. Look for fractures and dislocations of the humeral head. Both anterior and posterior dislocations can be missed on this view unless another radiogram at a different angle is performed. Look for supraspinatus tendon calcification. Look for deformities of the rotator cuff, evidence of recurrent dislocation or occasional congenital foramina of the scapula.

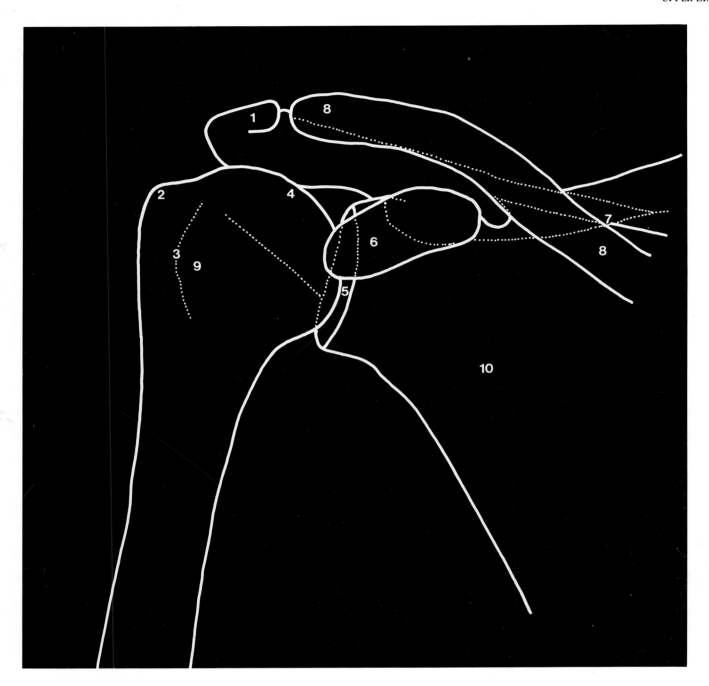

1	Acromion	4	Head of humerus	8	Clavicle
2	Greater tuberosity	5	Glenoid fossa	9	Lesser tuberosity
3	Intertubercular sulcus (bicipital groove)	6	Coracoid process	10	Subscapular fossa
		7	Spine of scapula		

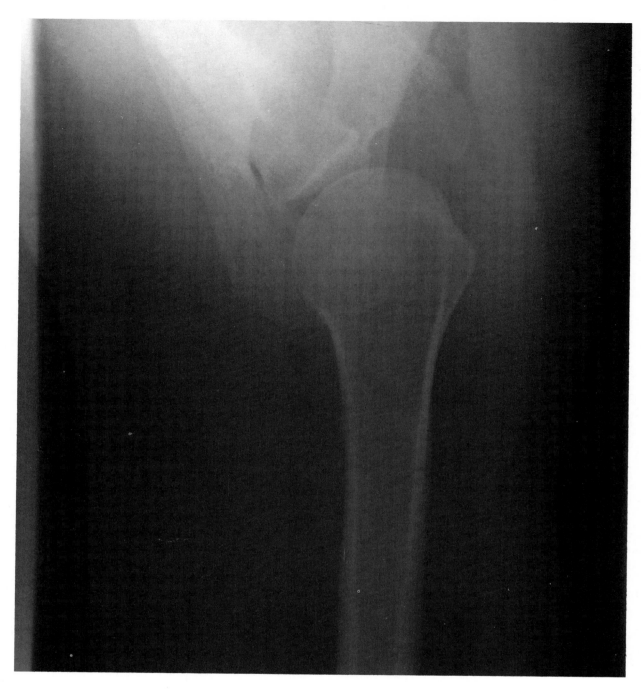

SUPEROINFERIOR VIEW OF SHOULDER (AXIAL WITH ABDUCTION)

This projection shows the position of the head of the humerus in relation to the glenoid cavity. It also shows, on this normal radiograph, that there is no dislocation. In patients with suspected dislocation this radiograph may not be possible to obtain and a lateral shoot-through is a further method of evaluating displace-ment. Fractures of the coracoid process and acromion, although uncommon, can be visualized on this film. Fracture of the greater tuberosity, which may be missed on the anteroposterior projection, can again be seen.

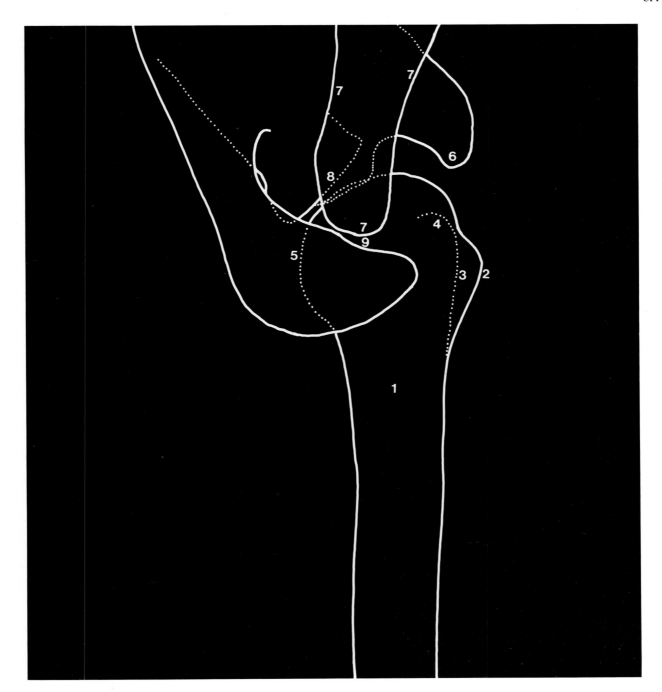

1	Humerus	4	Greater tuberosity	7 Borders of clavicle
2	Lesser tuberosity	5	Acromion	8 Glenoid
3	Intertubercular sulcus	6	Coracoid process	9 Acromioclavicular joint

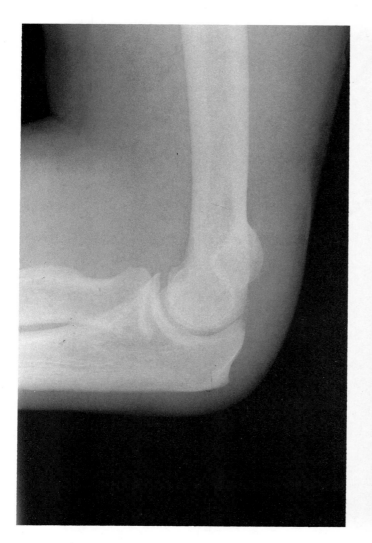
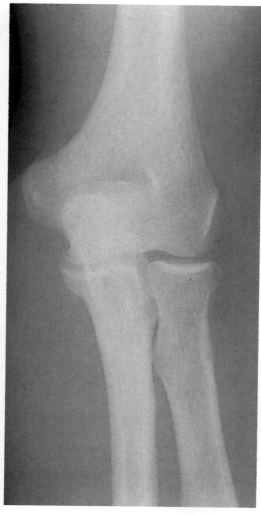

ANTEROPOSTERIOR AND LATERAL VIEWS OF ELBOW

Effusions into the elbow joint are commonly associated with un-displaced fractures of the radial head due to trauma. These radial head fractures may be difficult to see unless full projections are taken. The anterior and posterior fat pads are a particularly useful guide in assessing an effusion, as both will be elevated from their resting position against the distal end of the humerus. The two views are again needed in trauma cases to show any dislocation with or without associated fractures. A supracondylar fracture in children is particularly important because of the risk of a Volk-mann's contracture due to ischaemic fibrosis.

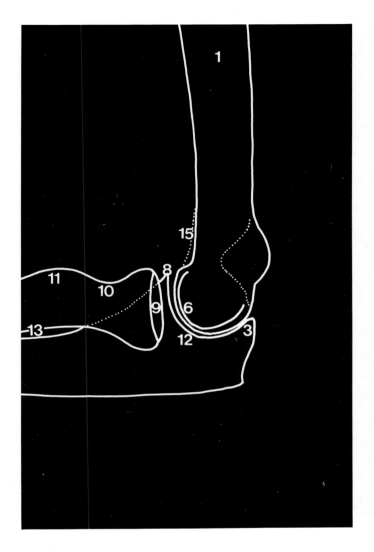
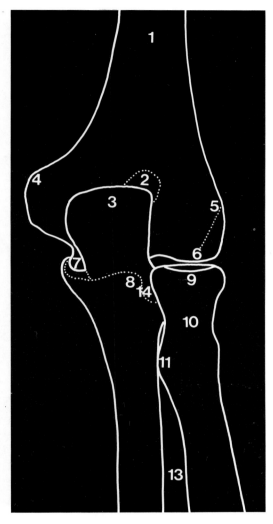

1 Humerus	6 Capitulum	11 Radial tuberosity
2 Olecranon fossa	7 Trochlea	12 Trochlear notch
3 Olecranon process	8 Coronoid process of ulna	13 Site of interosseus membrane
4 Med. epicondyle	9 Head of radius	14 Radial notch
5 Lat. epicondyle	10 Neck of radius	15 Ant. fat pad

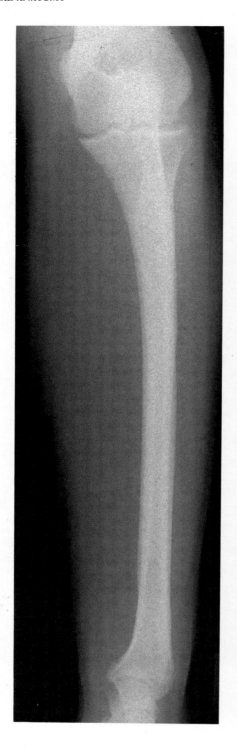
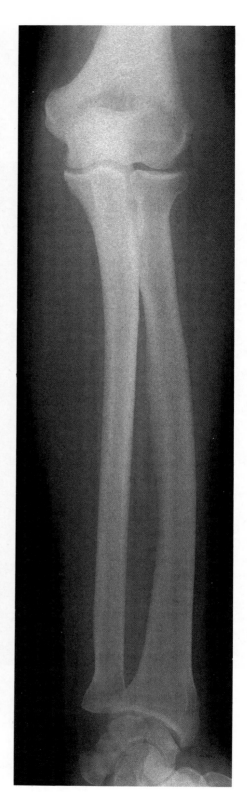

LATERAL AND ANTEROPOSTERIOR VIEWS OF FOREARM

When the forearm bones are x-rayed for trauma it is essential to have views of the joints at either end. This applies to any long bone examination. Fractures of the forearm bones are often paired, and if single fractures with displacement occur then either wrist or elbow dislocation of the other bone must be looked for. Examples of this are fracture of the ulna with forward dislocation of the radial head (Monteggia) and fracture of the radial shaft with distal radioulnar dislocation (Galeazzi).

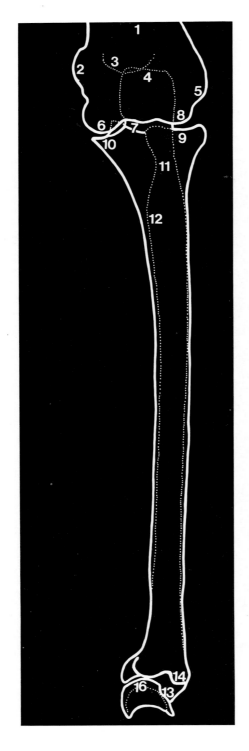
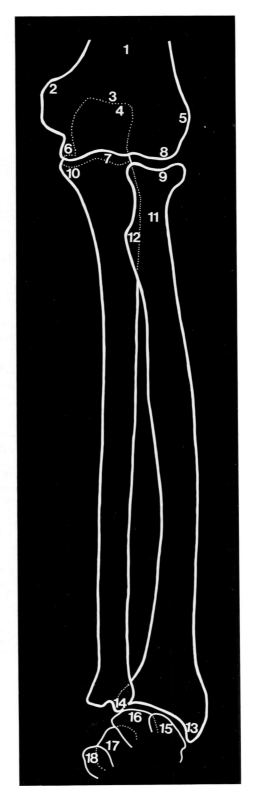

1	Humerus	7	Trochlear notch	13	Styloid process of radius
2	Med. epicondyle	8	Capitulum	14	Styloid process of ulna
3	Olecranon fossa	9	Head of radius	15	Scaphoid
4	Olecranon process	10	Coronoid process of ulna	16	Lunate
5	Lat. epicondyle	11	Neck of radius	17	Triquetral
6	Trochlea	12	Radial tuberosity	18	Pisiform

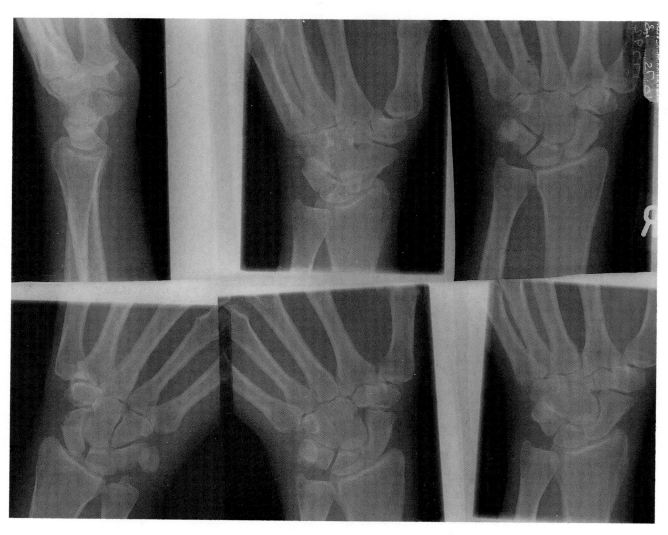

ROUTINE VIEWS OF SCAPHOID

These six projections show all the carpal bones with their normal relationships. Fractures and dislocations are particularly important in the wrist, as considerable incapacitation with osteoarthritis can result from delayed treatment. Note that fractures of the scaphoid may not show for 10 days following the injury. If a fracture of the waist of the scaphoid is mistreated, ischaemic necrosis of the distal fragment may result. It is important to learn the normal appearance of the positions of the carpal bones so that dislocations are not overlooked. These six views will also show distal radial and ulnar fractures.

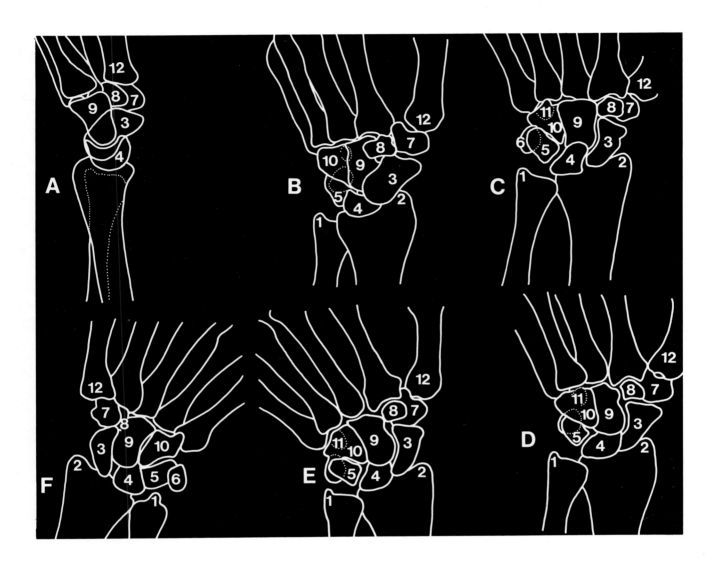

A Lateral

F Reverse oblique

B Oblique

E Posteroanterior in ulnar deviation

C Posteroanterior

D Oblique in ulnar deviation

1   Ulna, styloid process

2   Radius, styloid process

3   Scaphoid

4   Lunate

5   Triquetral

6   Pisiform

7   Trapezium

8   Trapezoid

9   Capitate

10   Hamate

11   Hook of hamate

12   First metacarpal

ANTEROPOSTERIOR VIEW OF HAND AND AXIAL VIEW OF CARPAL TUNNEL

Common fracture sites include the following: fracture of the distal radius and ulna with backward displacement (Colles' fracture); forward displacement of this fracture may occur which is relatively rare (Smith's fracture); fracture of the base of the first metacarpal (Bennett's fracture); spiral fractures of the metacarpals and distal shaft fractures of the fourth and fifth metacarpal bones may follow a punch!

Note that many systemic diseases have bony and soft tissue abnormalities which can be seen on a hand radiograph, e.g. hyperparathyroidism, scleroderma and rheumatoid arthritis.

The axial view is taken to assess the size and shape of the carpal tunnel.

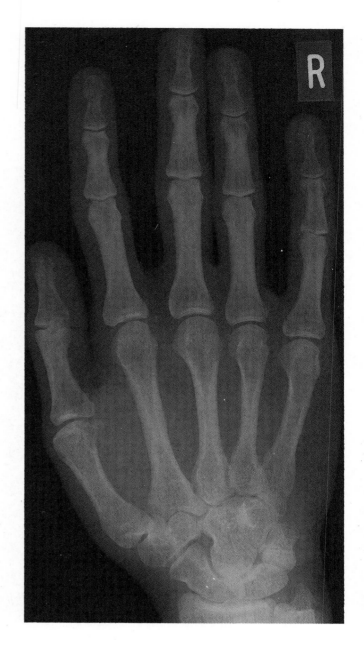

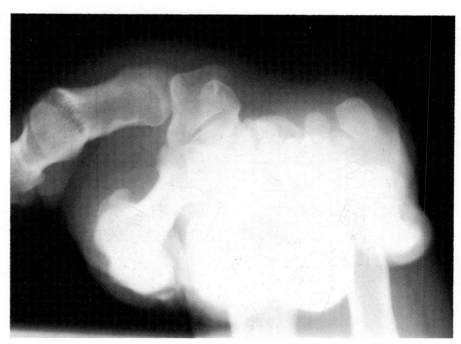

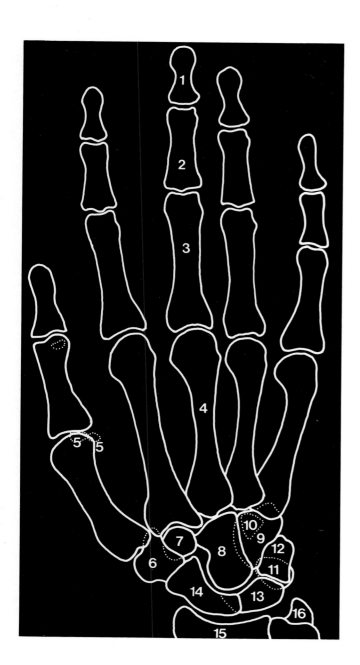

1 Distal phalanx

2 Middle phalanx

3 Proximal phalanx

4 Metacarpal

5 Sesamoid bones in flexor pollicis brevis and adductor pollicis

6 Trapezium

7 Trapezoid

8 Capitate

9 Hamate

10 Hook of hamate

11 Pisiform

12 Triquetral

13 Lunate

14 Scaphoid

15 Radius

16 Styloid process of ulna

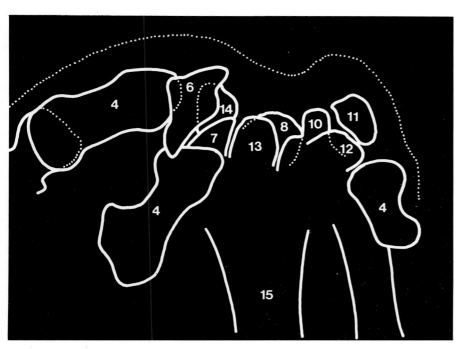

THORAX

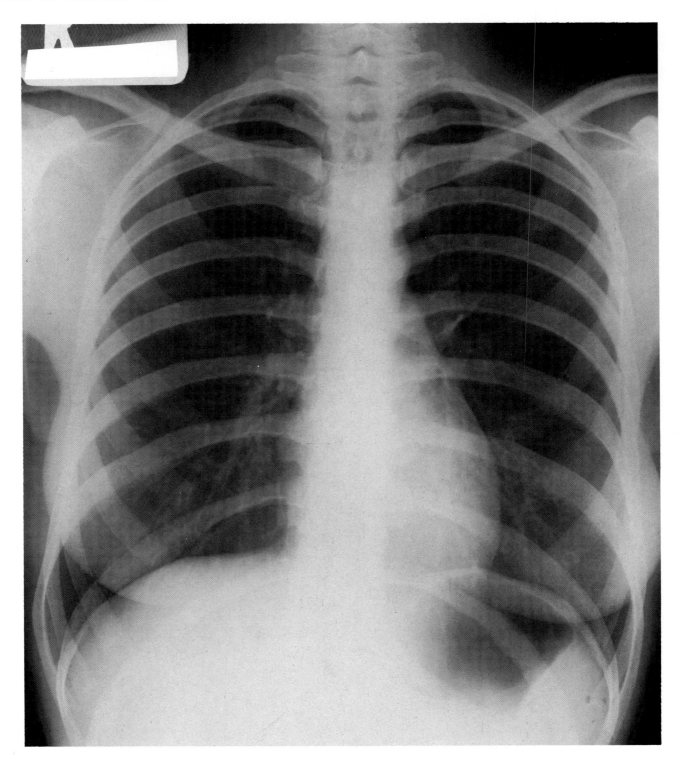

POSTEROANTERIOR VIEW OF THORAX

This is the commonest radiogram taken and thus it is important that the normal anatomy is known thoroughly. As with any radiograph, a system must be devised so that all the film is looked at in turn. However, certain hidden areas on a chest film warrant special attention and these include: behind the first ribs, behind the heart shadow, the posterior costophrenic angles which are obliterated on this view by the diaphragmatic shadows, and the hilar regions. Note the air in the trachea and main extrapulmonary bronchi. Note that the hilar shadows are composed only of vessels and the normal intrapulmonary bronchi cannot be visualized. The right heart border is formed from the superior vena cava, right atrium and inferior vena cava. The left heart border is formed from the aortic knuckle, the pulmonary conus, the left atrial appendage and the left ventricle.

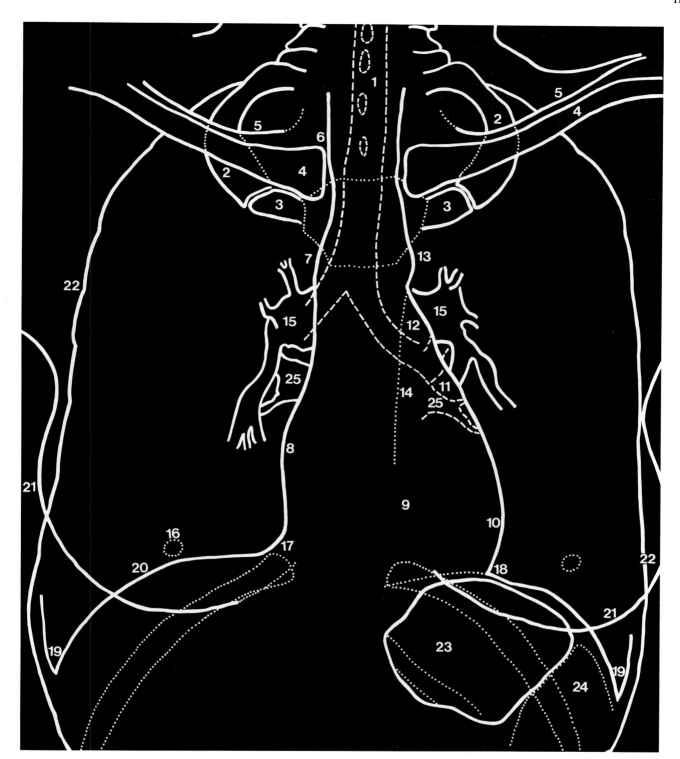

1	Air in trachea	9	R. ventricle	17	Inf. vena cava
2	First rib	10	L. ventricle	18	L. cardiophrenic angle
3	First costal cartilage	11	L. auricle (auricular appendage of l. atrium)	19	Lat. costophrenic angles
4	Clavicles			20	R. cupola of diaphragm
5	Skin line over clavicles	12	Pulmonary trunk (conus)	21	Breast shadow
6	R. brachiocephalic v. (innominate v.)	13	Aortic knuckle or knob	22	Lat. border of thoracic cage
		14	Lat. border of descending thoracic aorta	23	Fundal air bubble
7	Sup. vena cava	15	Pulmonary artery	24	Spleen
8	R. atrium	16	R. nipple	25	Pulmonary veins

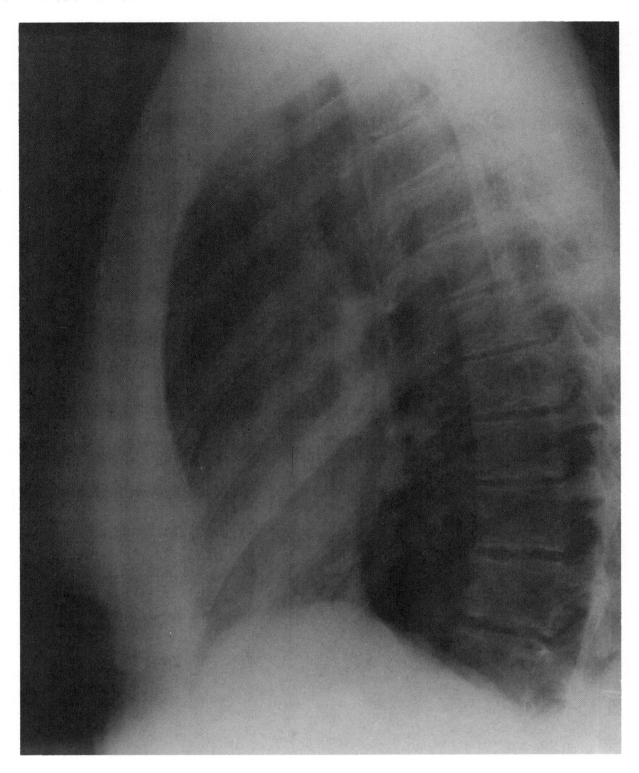

LEFT LATERAL VIEW OF THORAX

This projection demonstrates mediastinal divisions into the superior, anterior, middle and posterior. Note the backwards slant of the trachea from the thoracic inlet to the carina. This slant should be borne in mind when tracheal tomograms are performed. Note the position of the outflow tract of the right ventricle and the high position of the left atrium. Note the position of the lung fissures, the left oblique fissure reaching its inferior limit about 5 cm behind the sternum. The right oblique fissure travels more anteriorly at its lower limit. Note also the apparently radiolucent anterior mediastinum in the normal.

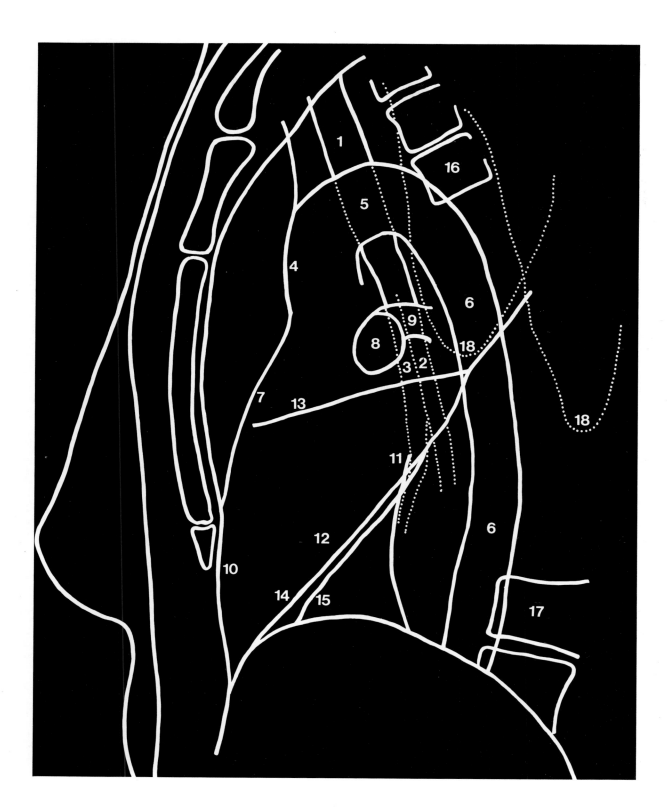

1 Trachea	7 Pulmonary outflow tract	13 Horizontal fissure
2 L. main bronchus	8 R. main pulmonary a.	14 R. oblique fissure
3 R. main bronchus	9 L. main pulmonary a.	15 L. oblique fissure
4 Ascending thoracic aorta	10 Site of r. ventricle	16 Vertebral body of T4
5 Aortic arch	11 Site of l. atrium	17 Vertebral body of T11
6 Descending thoracic aorta	12 Site of l. ventricle	18 Inf. angle of scapula

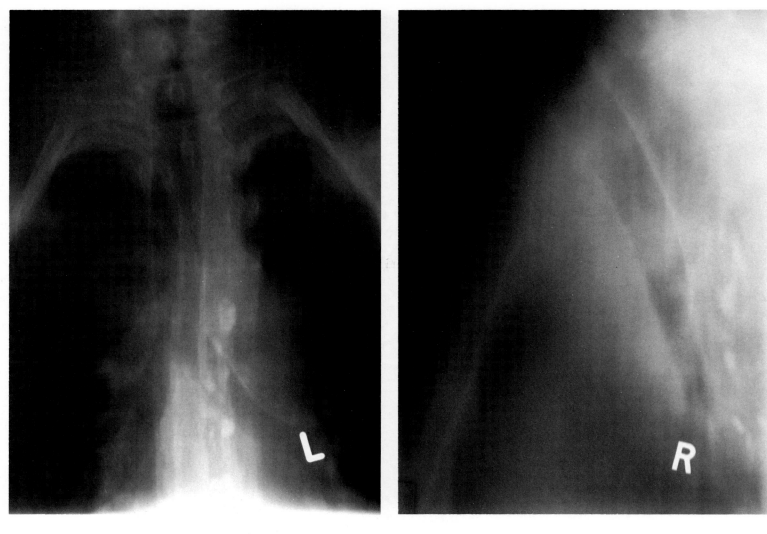

ANTEROPOSTERIOR AND LATERAL TOMOGRAMS OF MEDIASTINUM

These tomograms demonstrate the trachea and major bronchi, and show lesions which may be obscured on routine chest films. Note that to see the whole of the trachea on the AP projection, inclined plane tomography is necessary because of the backwards angulation of the trachea from its origin to the carina. Note that the left main bronchus is more horizontal than the right because of the position of the left atrium. Note also the position of the carina at the level of T4 posteriorly or the manubriosternal angle anteriorly. The pleural reflections of the upper lobes can be visualized lying posteriorly on the AP view.

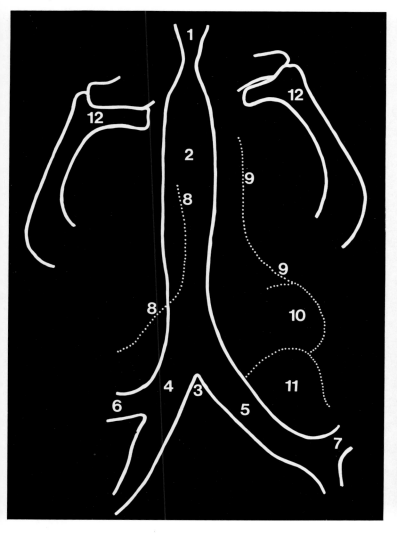
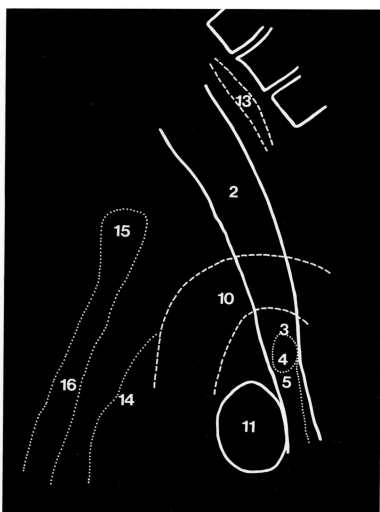

1	Larynx	6	R. upper lobe bronchus (sup. lobe)	12	First rib
2	Trachea	7	L. upper lobe bronchus (sup. lobe)	13	Air within oesophagus
3	Carina (bifurcation of main bronchi)	8	Pleural reflection of r. upper lobe	14	Outflow of r. ventricle
4	R. main bronchus	9	L. pleural reflection	15	Manubrium sterni
5	L. main bronchus	10	Aorta	16	Body of sternum
		11	Pulmonary artery		

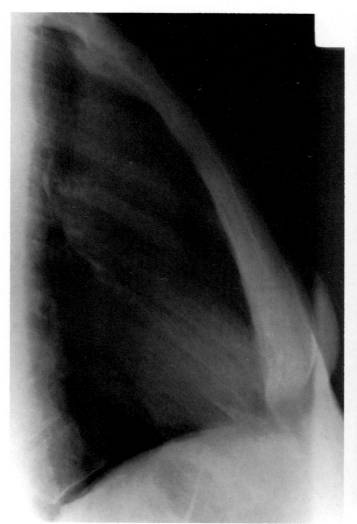
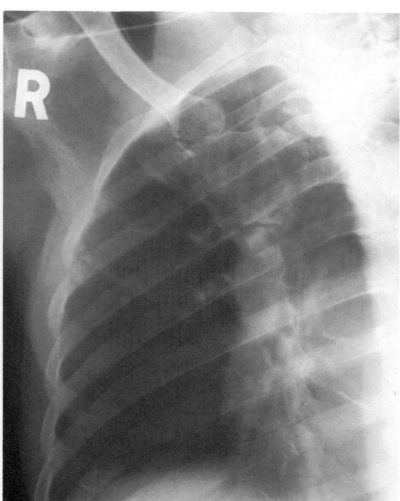

LATERAL AND OBLIQUE VIEWS OF STERNUM

These projections visualize clearly the manubrium, the sternum and the xyphoid process. Note the articulation of the manubrium with the clavicle. Note that the second costochondral junction joins at the manubriosternal joint. Originally, the sternum consists of four segments, which begin to fuse around puberty. Note that only ribs one to seven (true ribs) have direct attachment to the sternum and manubrium via their costal cartilages. The sternum may be fractured, due often to steering wheel injuries in road traffic accidents. It may also be eroded posteriorly by an aneurysm of the ascending aorta.

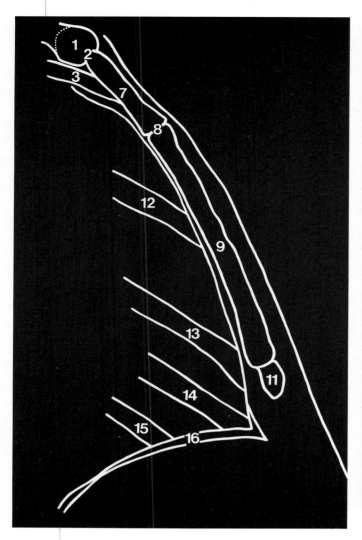
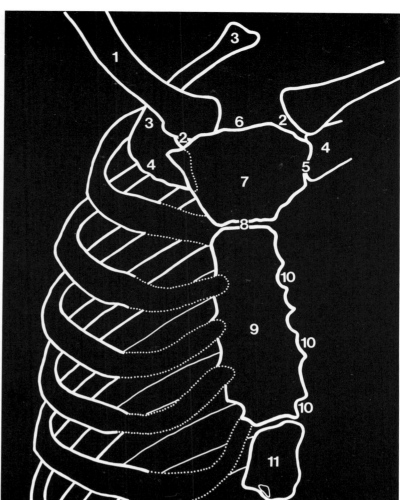

1	Clavicle	7	Manubrium sterni	12	Third rib
2	Sternoclavicular joints	8	Manubriosternal joint (sternal angle, angle of Louis)	13	Fifth rib
3	First rib			14	Seventh rib
4	First costal cartilage	9	Body of sternum	15	Ninth rib
5	Facet for first rib	10	Facets for costal cartilages	16	Diaphragm
6	Jugular notch (suprasternal notch)	11	Xiphisternum		

ABDOMEN AND PELVIS

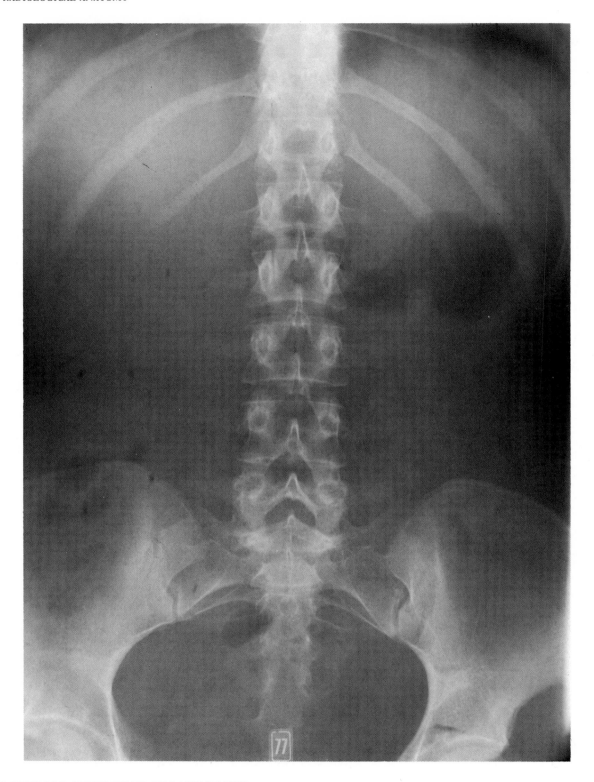

ANTEROPOSTERIOR VIEW OF PLAIN ABDOMEN

This a supine view to show the general layout of abdominal viscera. Note the slightly lower position of the right kidney compared to the left, due to the liver mass. Note the position of the spleen and liver edge. Note also the normal gas shadow in the antrum of the stomach. When considering abdominal films in patients with abdominal pathology, it is often essential to have an erect film in addition to the one shown. These two films are complementary in showing abnormalities. Look for bowel gas patterns, renal and gall bladder calculi, the psoas outlines, the normality of the bone structure, and check also the hernial orifices.

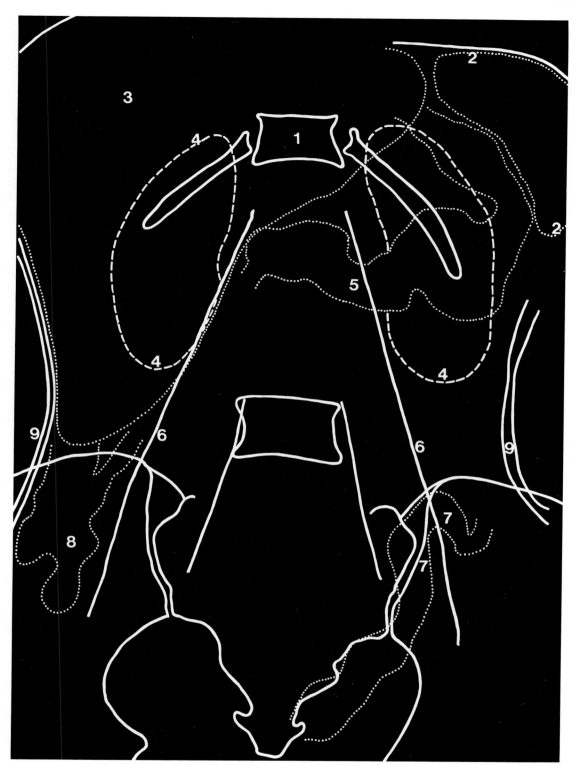

1 T12 vertebra

2 Splenic shadow

3 Liver shadow

4 Renal outlines

5 Gas in antrum of stomach

6 Psoas shadow (line)

7 Gas in sigmoid colon

8 Air in caecum and ascending colon

9 Abdominal wall

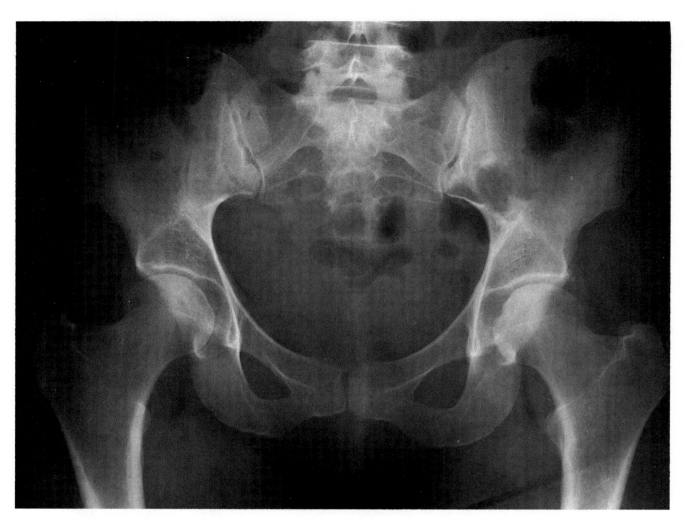

ANTEROPOSTERIOR VIEW OF PELVIS

The bones and soft tissues of the pelvis should be studied in this view. We have not included AP sacrum and specialized sacroiliac joint views as they do not add significantly to the normal anatomy demonstrated here. Fractures and dislocations occurring in the pelvic bones are particularly important in relation to their effects on the pelvic contents. As with any fixed bony ring, fractures and dislocations must be checked to make sure there is no further breach of the ring, as commonly occurs. Ramus fractures of the obturator ring are often multiple because of this. Look for dislocation of the femoral head in relation to the acetabular fossa and check the relationship of the sacroiliac joint. If there is suspected instability of the pubic symphysis, as occurs in professional sportsmen, particularly footballers, then films should be taken with the patient weight-bearing on one leg and then the other to see if there is any movement of the joint.

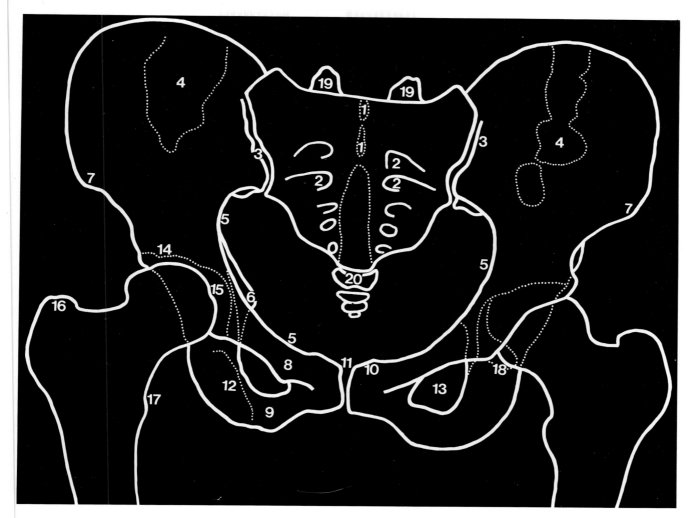

1	Sacral spinous crest	8	Sup. ramus of pubis	15	Fovea of femoral head
2	Ant. sacral foramina	9	Inf. ramus of pubis	16	Greater trochanter
3	Sacroiliac joint	10	Pubic tubercle	17	Lesser trochanter
4	Gas in bowel overlying iliac fossae	11	Pubic symphysis	18	Acetabular fossa (teardrop)
5	Pelvic brim	12	Ischial tuberosity	19	Articular facets of S1
6	Ischial spine	13	Obturator foramen	20	Four coccygeal segments
7	Ant. sup. iliac spine	14	Acetabular rim		

LOWER LIMB

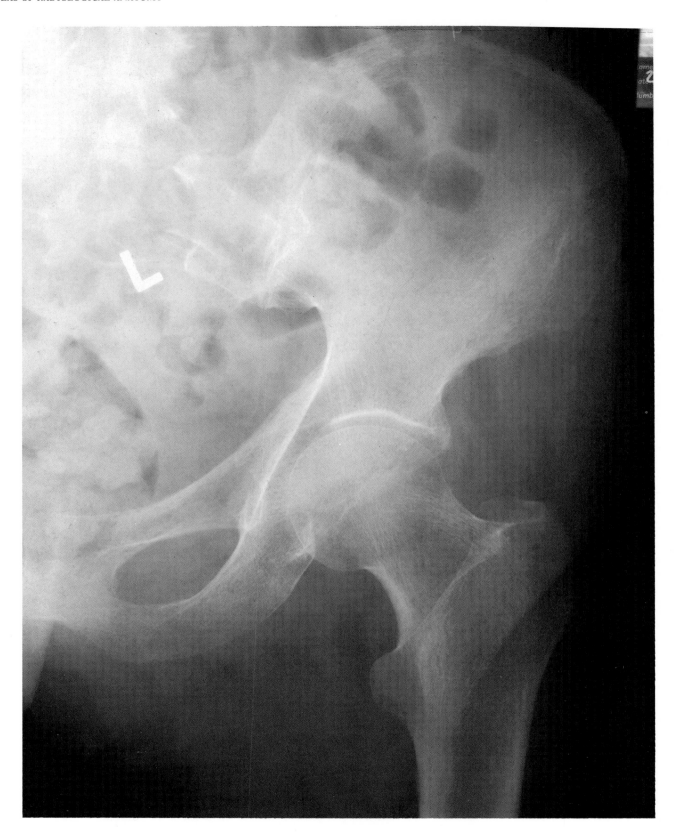

ANTEROPOSTERIOR VIEW OF HIP

Shenton's line is formed from the continuity of the inferior aspect of the femoral neck through to the inferior aspect of the superior pubic ramus. This gives a good guide to the normal relationship of the head of the femur to the pelvis. Synovial membrane is very extensive around the hip joint and, like the capsule, comes well down the femoral neck, especially anteriorly. Note the normal pattern of the bone trabeculae in the femoral neck, indicating the lines of stress. Fractures of the femoral neck are common, especially in the old, and as they may be impacted they are sometimes difficult to visualize. If severe separation of the femoral head occurs then the possibility of avascular necrosis exists and it must therefore be checked on follow-up films.

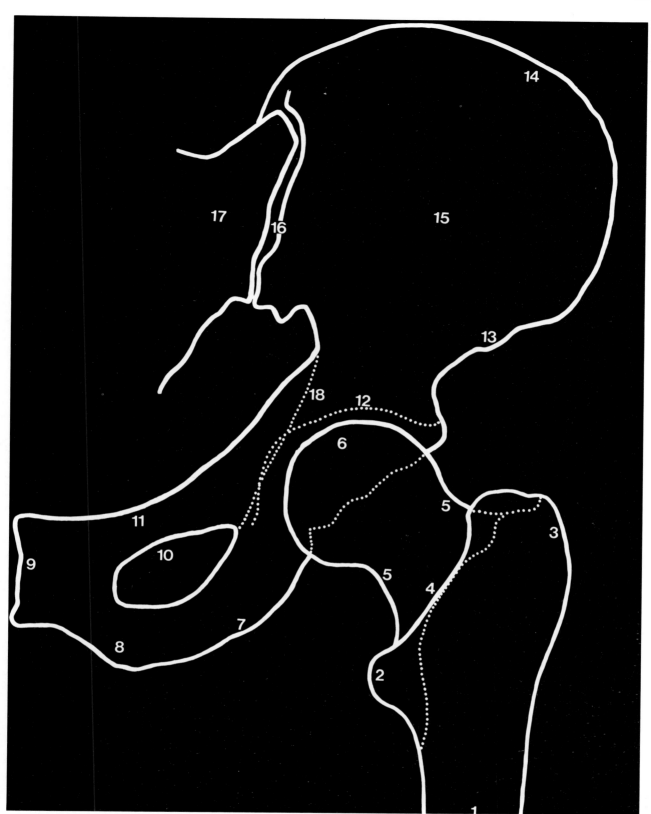

1	Shaft of femur	7	Ischial tuberosity	13	Ant. inf. iliac spine
2	Lesser trochanter	8	Ischiopubic ramus	14	Iliac crest
3	Greater trochanter	9	Pubis	15	Iliac fossa
4	Intertrochanteric crest	10	Obturator foramen	16	Sacroiliac joint
5	Neck of femur	11	Sup. ramus of pubis	17	Ala or lateral mass of sacrum
6	Head of femur	12	Acetabular rim	18	Iliopectineal line

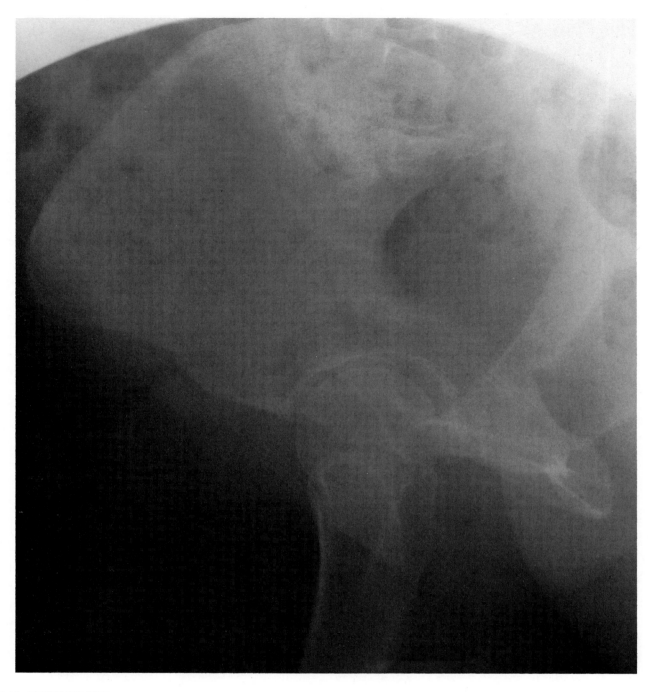

LATERAL VIEW OF HIP

This view demonstrates the femoral neck and the relationship of the femoral head to the acetabulum. Fractures of the femoral neck can again be visualized on this film and, in particular, the degree of angulation can be assessed. Dislocations around the hip are not infrequent in road traffic accidents. In most cases the displace-ment is posterior due to the impact a patient receives whilst in the sitting position. Dislocations in an anterior direction are much less common. Associated fracture dislocations must be checked for.

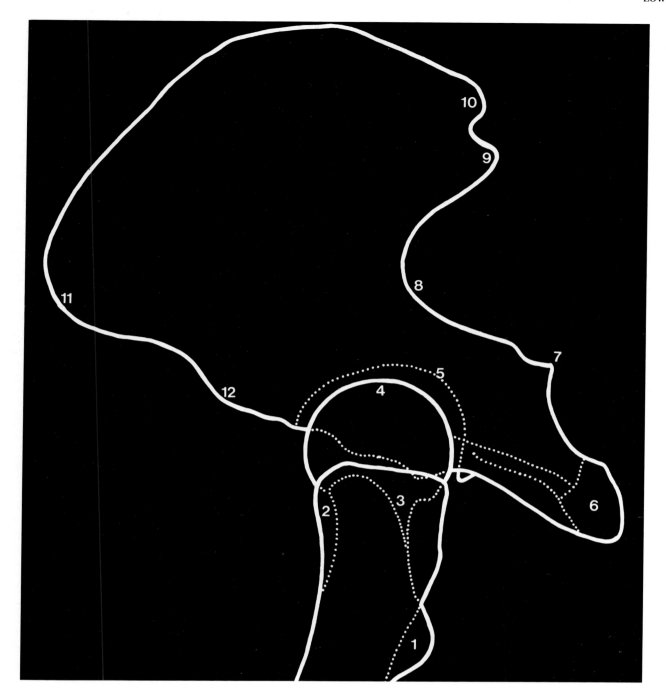

1	Lesser trochanter	5	Acetabular rim	9	Post. inf. iliac spine
2	Greater trochanter	6	Ischial tuberosity	10	Post. sup. iliac spine
3	Intertrochanteric line	7	Ischial spine	11	Ant. sup. iliac spine
4	Head of femur	8	Greater sciatic notch	12	Ant. inf. iliac spine

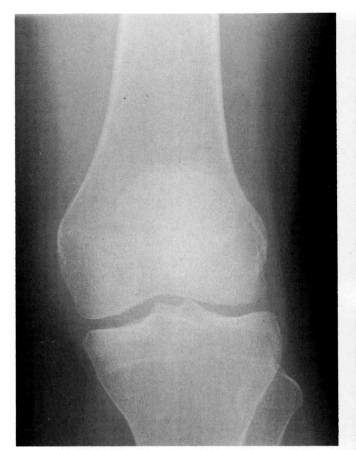
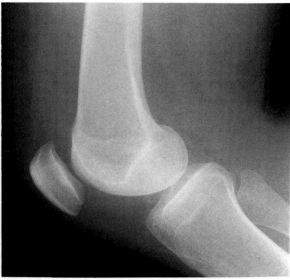
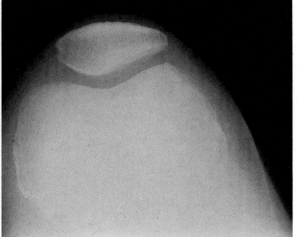

ANTEROPOSTERIOR, LATERAL AND SKYLINE VIEWS OF KNEE

The knee joint is complicated anatomically and consists of three articulations: two between the condyles of the femur and the tibia, and the third between the femur and the patella. The synovial cavity is common to all three joints but is indented by the two menisci between the femur and the tibia. These menisci are best seen in the contrast arthrograms in the 'Miscellaneous' section. Fractures of all three bones can occur and can be visualized on these views. A fracture of the patella may only be visible on the skyline view. It should not be confused with a congenital bipartite patella, which is often present bilaterally. To assess whether there is free fat within the joint space, radiography with a horizontal beam should be performed and, if positive, is a fair indication of bone damage. A tunnel view has not been included but is of use when looking for a loose body or evidence of osteochondritis dissecans. Note also on the skyline view that the lateral femoral condyle projects higher than the medial condyle to resist lateral dislocation of the patella.

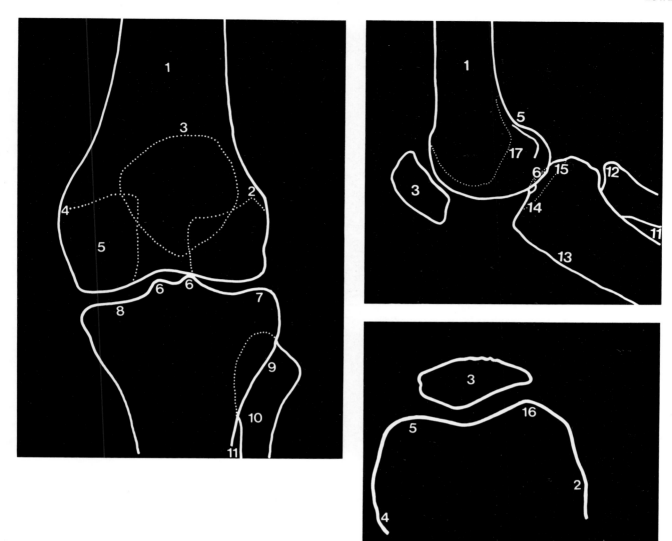

1	Femur	7	Lat. condyle of tibia
2	Lat. epicondyle	8	Med. condyle of tibia
3	Patella	9	Head of fibula
4	Med. epicondyle	10	Neck of fibula
5	Med. condyle	11	Interosseous membrane
6	Intercondylar eminences (tibial spines)	12	Styloid process of fibula

13	Tibial tuberosity
14	Ant. intercondylar area
15	Post. intercondylar area
16	Lat. condyle
17	Intercondylar notch

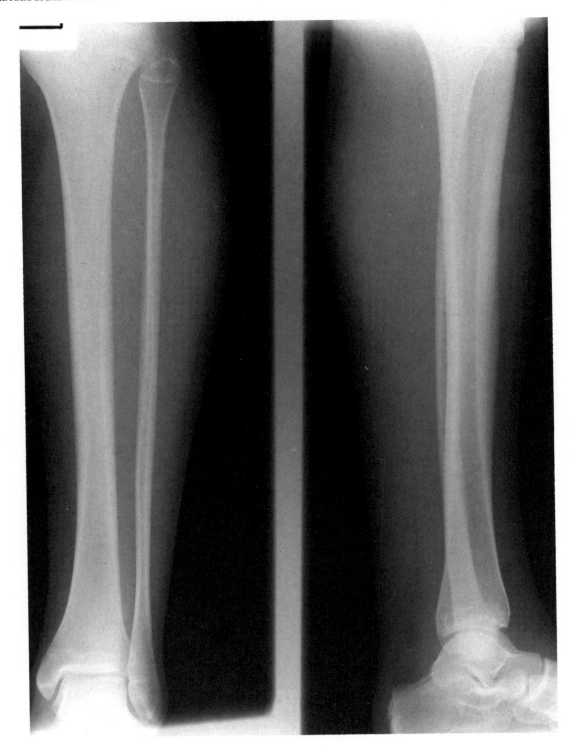

ANTEROPOSTERIOR AND LATERAL VIEWS OF TIBIA AND FIBULA

This tibia and fibula are connected by an interosseous membrane similar to that of the forearm. Again with paired long bones, fracture of one bone is often accompanied by a fracture of the other. As mentioned before with the forearm radiograph, if one bone is fractured with considerable displacement then both proximal and distal joints should be checked for dislocation of the other bone. Note that the head of the fibula does not form part of the knee joint but has a separate synovial joint with the tibia. Fractures of the tibia and fibula are often compound because of the lack of soft tissues anteriorly. Fractures of the mid tibial shaft are prone to non-union because of the apparent poor vascularity. Paget's disease and syphilis are causes of 'sabre tibia'.

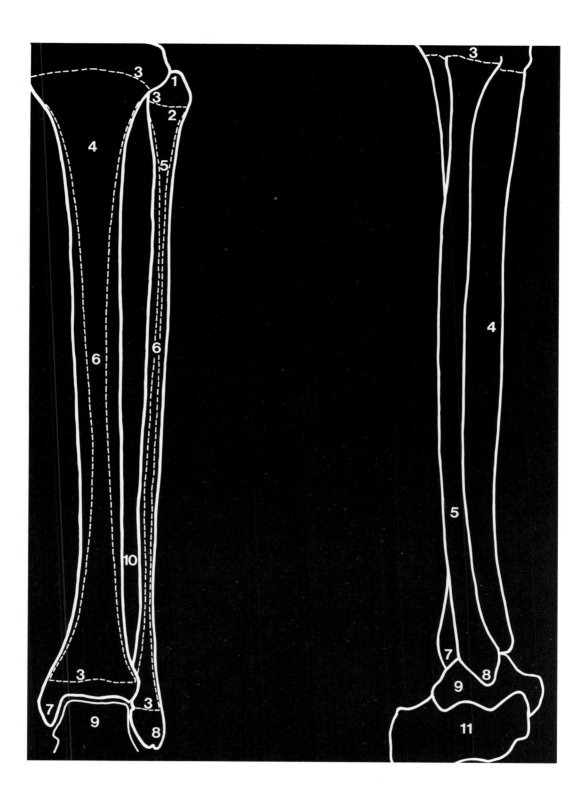

1 Head of fibula

2 Neck of fibula

3 Epiphyseal plates

4 Tibia

5 Fibula

6 Marrow cavity

7 Med. malleolus

8 Lat. malleolus

9 Talus

10 Site of interosseus membrane

11 Calcaneus

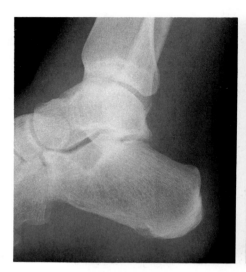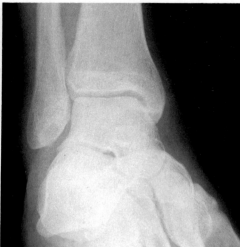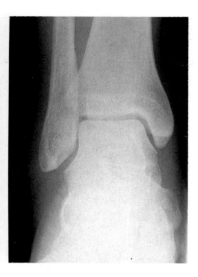

LATERAL, OBLIQUE-ANTEROPOSTERIOR AND ANTEROPOSTERIOR VIEWS OF ANKLE

Numerous sesamoid bones and supernumerary bones occur around the foot and ankle. The os trigonum appears in about 8% of adults as an extra bone posterior to the ankle joint adjacent to the talus. Fractures and dislocations are common at the ankle joint, due in part to the thin fibrous capsule. Pott's fractures are of three types: first degree, fracture of one malleolus; second degree, fracture of both malleoli often with subluxation of the talus; third degree, associated backwards displacement of the talus and disruption of the ankle mortise. Talar and calcaneal fractures also occur. Crush fractures of the calcaneus through the body often occur when patients fall from a height onto their heels; occupations such as parachuting, window-cleaning and cat-burglary have an especially high incidence! These calcaneal fractures are often bilateral. Medial and lateral ligament tears may be visualized radiographically by strain views to show movement of the talus in relation to the distal tibia in the AP projection.

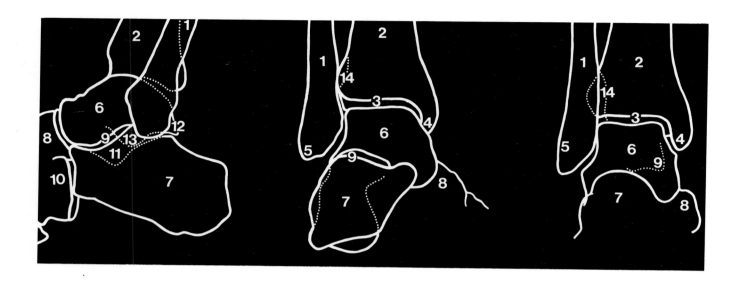

1	Fibula	6	Talus	11 Sustentaculum tali
2	Tibia	7	Calcaneus	12 Post. process of talus
3	Ankle joint	8	Navicular	13 Lat. process of talus
4	Med. malleolus	9	Talocalcaneal joint	14 Inf. tibiofibular joint
5	Lat. malleolus	10	Cuboid	

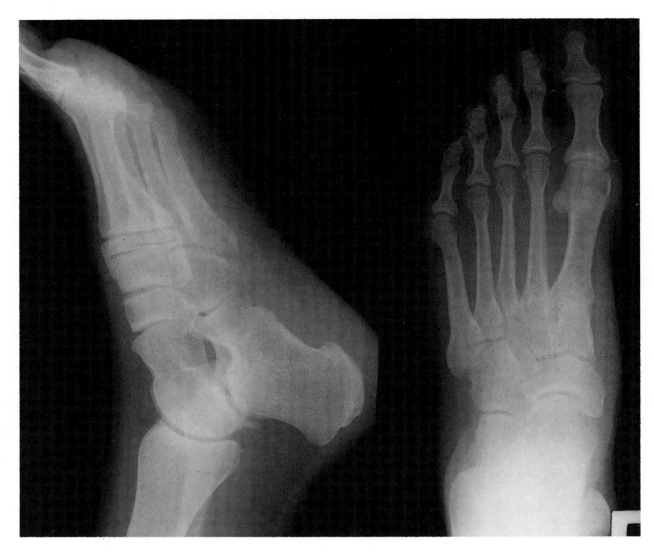

DORSIPLANTAR AND LATERAL VIEWS OF FOOT

In the lateral projection the longitudinal arch of the foot can be seen and it should be noted that the weight-bearing parts of the foot are the inferior aspect of the calcaneus and the heads of the metatarsals. Note the position of the tarsal bones forming the transverse arch. Common fracture sites include the base of the fifth metatarsal, which should not be confused with an epiphysis frequently present on the tubercle of the base of this bone. A stress fracture (march fracture) is often seen along the distal shaft of the second and third metatarsals. There is a strong incidence of such fractures in occupations such as new army recruits on route marches and long distance walkers. The foot is also the site of two special forms of osteochondritis seen before epiphyseal fusion: the first in the metatarsal head (Freiberg), and the second in the tarsal navicular (Köhler).

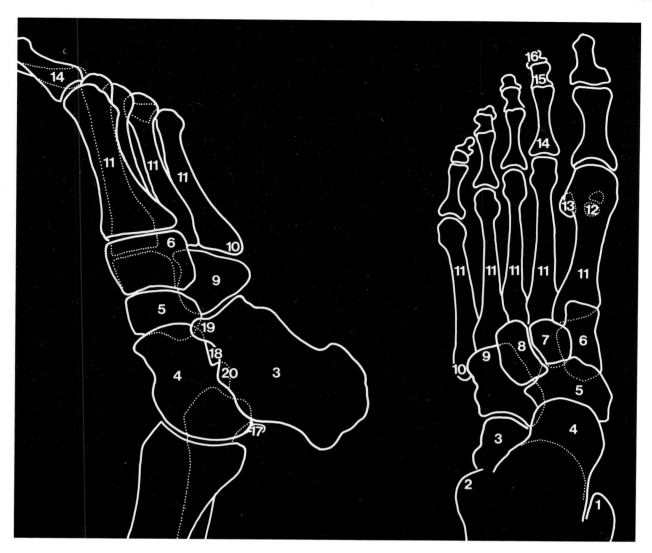

1 Med. malleolus	8 Lat. cuneiform	14 Proximal phalanx
2 Lat. malleolus	9 Cuboid	15 Middle phalanx
3 Calcaneus	10 Styloid process of fifth metatarsal	16 Distal phalanx
4 Talus	11 Metatarsal shafts	17 Os trigonum
5 Navicular	12 Bipartite sesamoid bone	18 Sinus tarsi
6 Med. cuneiform	13 Sesamoid bone in t. of flexor hallucis brevis	19 Ant. process of calcaneus
7 Intermediate cuneiform		20 Sustentaculum tali

VERTEBRAL COLUMN

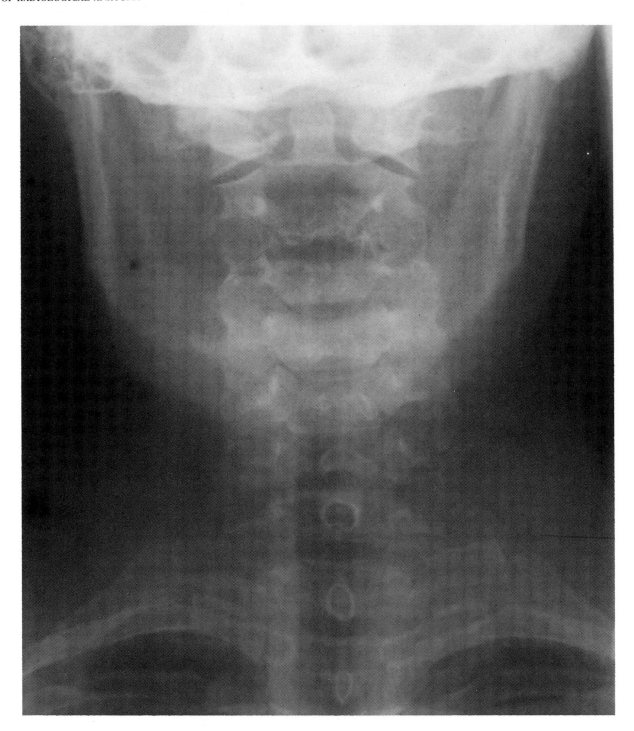

ANTEROPOSTERIOR VIEW OF CERVICAL SPINE

This projection is taken with the jaw moving but with the head and cervical spine firmly fixed. This allows C1 and C2 to be visualized and not be obscured by the mandibular shadow. The odontoid process of the axis is formed embryologically from the centrum of the atlas. The spinous processes should be in line and are often bifid in the cervical region. Tomography of the odontoid process in this plane may be needed to show fractures, avascular necrosis and involvement by rheumatoid arthritis. Look for cervical ribs from C7; though rare (0.5–1%), they may have important clinical manifestations. Air in the trachea and larynx can be seen to overlie the lower cervical spine, and ossification in the thyroid cartilage can occasionally cause confusion in identifying the normal anatomy.

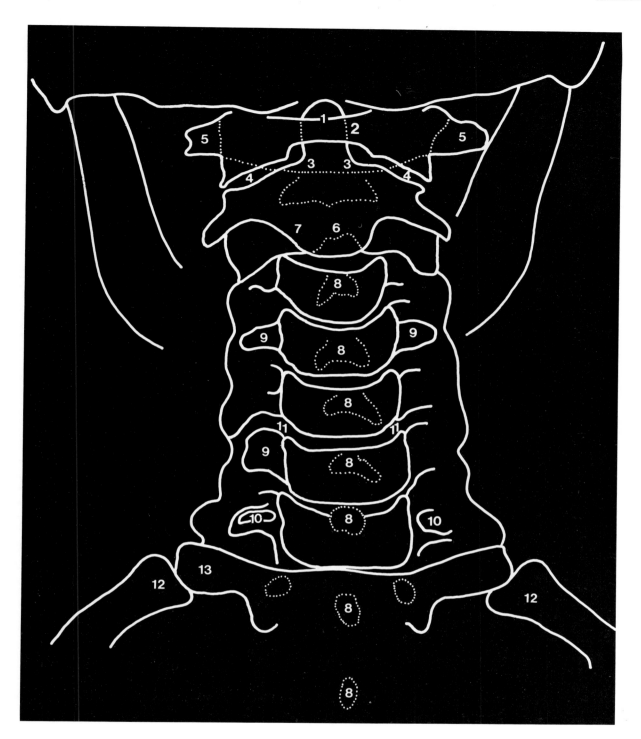

1   Odontoid process of axis (dens)

2   Ant. arch of atlas

3   Post. arch of atlas

4   Atlantoaxial joint

5   Transverse process of atlas

6   Spinous process of axis (C2)

7   Lamina of axis

8   Spinous processes (C3–T1)

9   Transverse processes

10 Foramen transversarium of C7

11 Synovial joint between arches of
    C5 and C6

12 First rib

13 Transverse process of T1

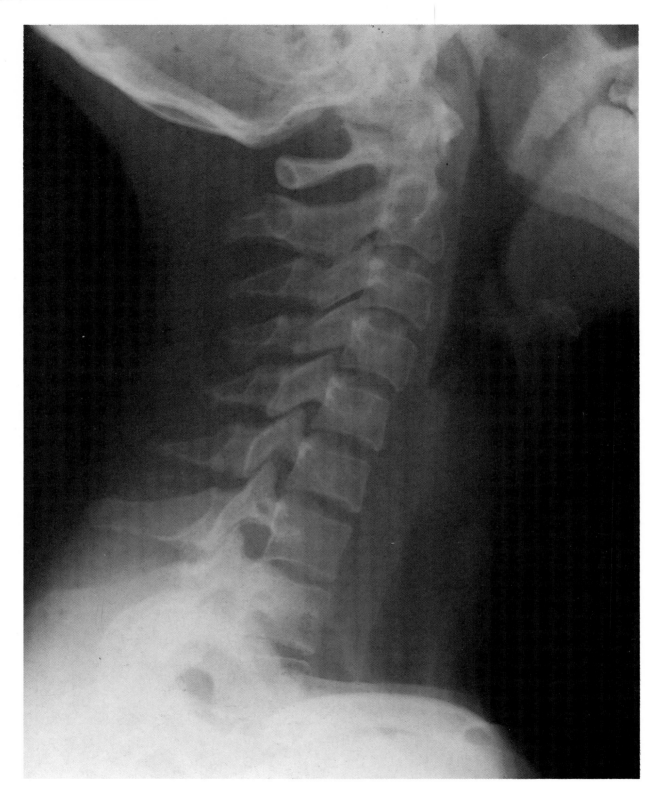

LATERAL VIEW OF CERVICAL SPINE

This is a very important view and should include from the base of the occiput to at least the level of T1. The C7/T1 disc space must be visible on a lateral film, particularly in cases of injury so that a fracture or dislocation is not missed. Note that two important lines are visible, formed by the posterior margins of the bodies of the cervical vertebrae and the posterior limit of the cervical spinal canal. Both of these should be continuous lines and any irregularity may be due to an unsuspected dislocation. Often views in hyperextension and flexion may be needed to show vertebral subluxation or atlantoaxial subluxation. The anteroposterior sagittal diameter of the cervical spinal canal should not be less than 10 mm and is normally between 14 and 21 mm. If less than 10 mm, there is likely to be spinal cord compression.

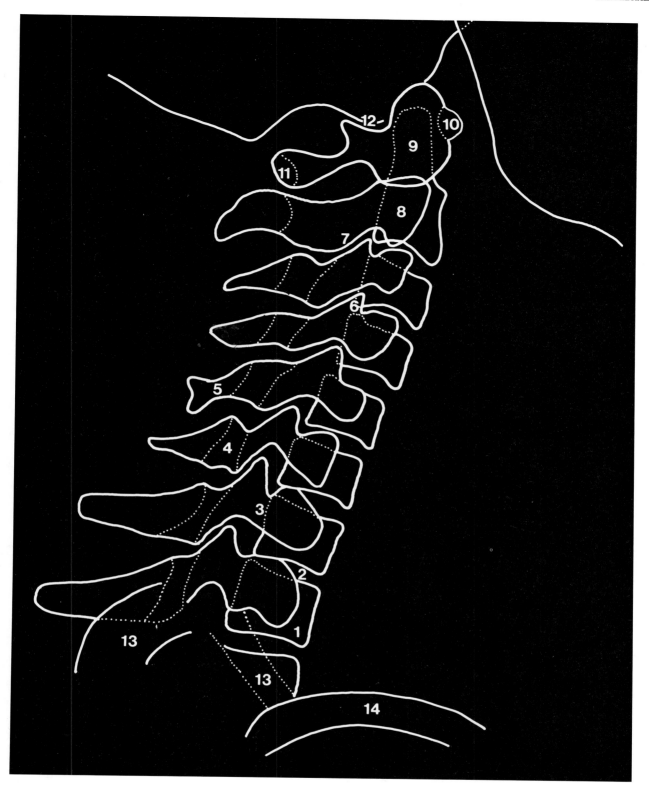

1	Body of T1	6	Sup. articular process of C4	11	Post. tubercle of C1 (atlas)
2	Intervertebral space	7	Inf. articular process of C2 (axis)	12	Atlanto-occipital joint
3	Pedicle of C7	8	Transverse process of C2 (axis)	13	First rib
4	Lamina of C6	9	Odontoid process of axis (dens)	14	Clavicle
5	Spinous process of C5	10	Arch of C1 (atlas)		

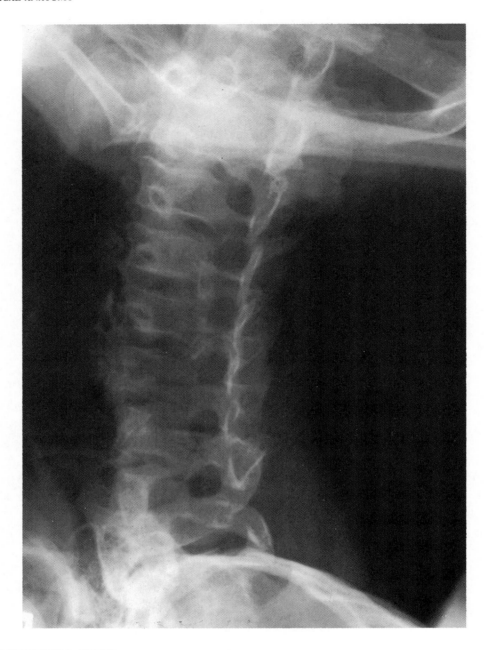

OBLIQUE VIEW OF CERVICAL SPINE

This view shows the exit foramina for the spinal nerves and the articular facet joints. Fractures involving the laminae can be seen. Disruption of the normal facet articulation may only be visible on this view. Any degenerative disease which occurs in the cervical spine may cause osteophyte formation, between the vertebral bod-ies, which may impinge on the cervical spinal nerves. This projection allows the foramina to be screened for these osteophytes. The foramen transversarium of C3 is visualized—this contains the vertebral vein and artery. Note that there are eight cervical spinal nerves but only seven cervical vertebrae.

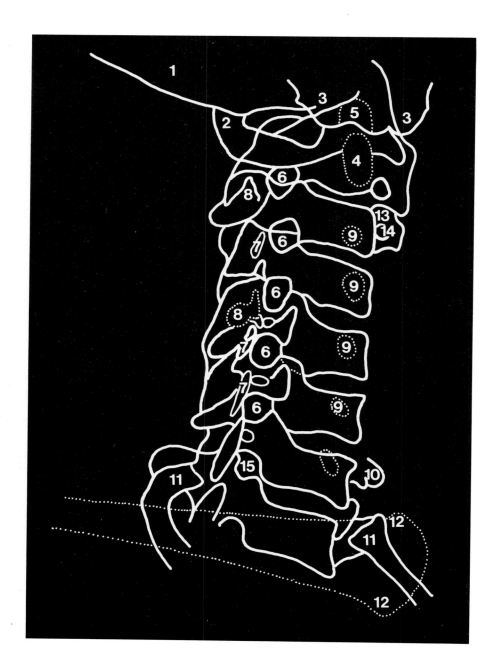

1	Occipital bone	6	Intervertebral foramina	11	First rib
2	Post. arch of atlas	7	Laminae	12	Sternal end of clavicle
3	Mastoid air cells	8	Bifid spinous processes	13	Transverse process of opposite side
4	Transverse process of axis (C2)	9	Transverse processes	14	Foramen transversarium of C3
5	Odontoid process of axis (dens)	10	Ant. tubercle of transverse process of C7	15	Site of spinal nerve C8

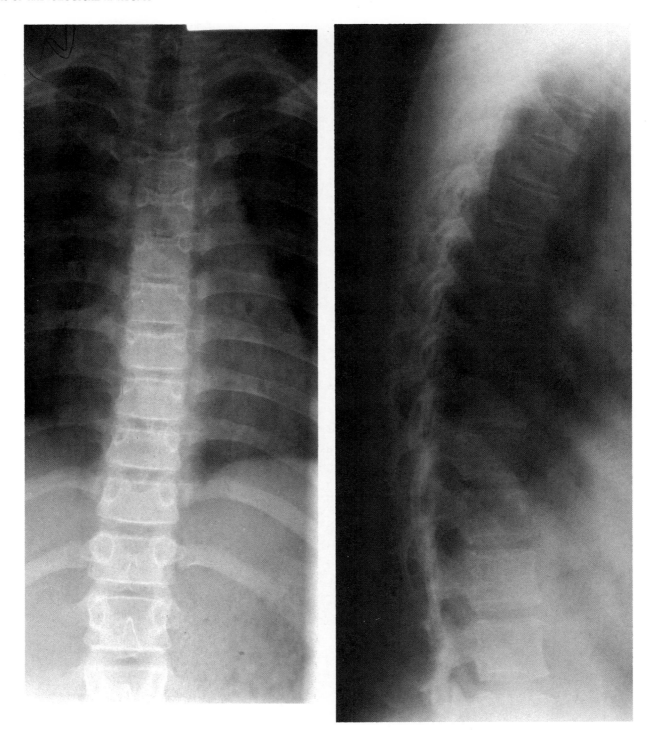

ANTEROPOSTERIOR AND LATERAL VIEWS OF THORACIC SPINE

The lateral view shows the normal thoracic kyphosis. It may also reveal many systemic disorders; for example, renal osteodystrophy, ankylosing spondylitis, osteoporosis, osteomalacia and some haemopoietic disorders. Note that the upper few thoracic vertebrae are not visible on the ordinary lateral film and often a special lateral thoracic inlet view has to be taken in order to demonstrate this area. The anteroposterior view shows the prominence of the pedicles, which should be checked thoroughly if secondary deposits are suspected. This projection also shows any paravertebral shadow which may occur in such conditions as tuberculosis, osteomyelitis, Hodgkin's reticulosis or extramedullary haemopoiesis.

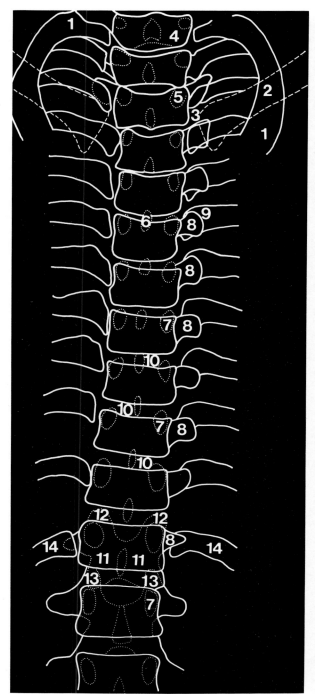
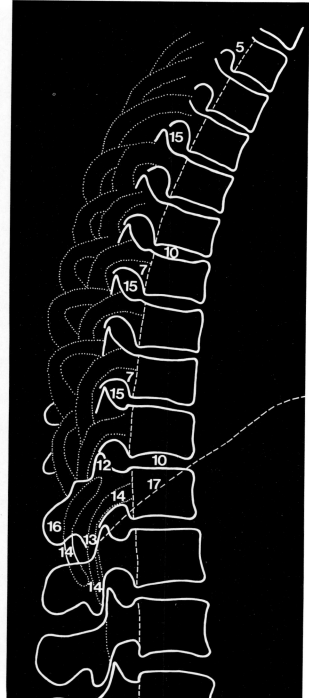

1	First rib	7	Pedicles	12	Sup. articular process of T12
2	Clavicle	8	Transverse processes	13	Inf. articular process of T12
3	Sternoclavicular joint	9	Costovertebral joint of sixth thoracic vertebra (T6)	14	Twelfth rib
4	First thoracic vertebra			15	Intervertebral foramen
5	Pedicle of third thoracic vertebra (T3)	10	Sites of intervertebral discs	16	Spinous process of T12
6	Spinous process of fifth thoracic vertebra (T5)	11	Laminae of twelfth thoracic vertebra (T12)	17	Diaphragm

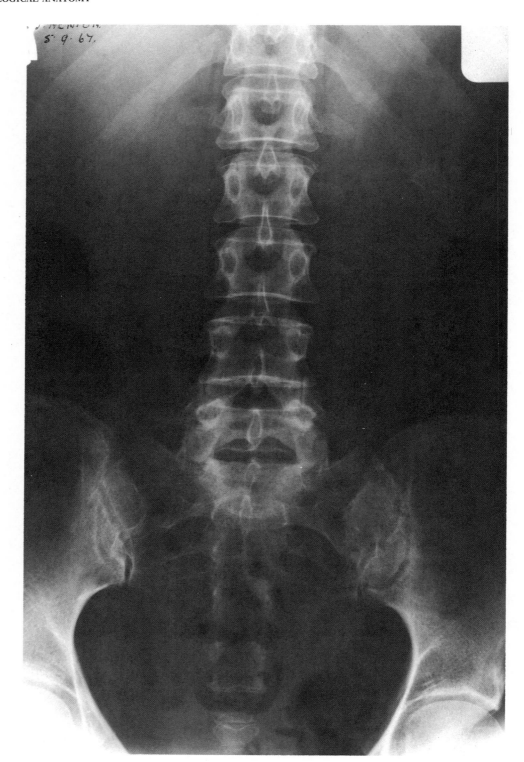

ANTEROPOSTERIOR VIEW OF LUMBOSACRAL SPINE

The interpedicular distance should increase from L1 to L5 in the normal. The distance can decrease in Down's syndrome. The accessory process seen here in L1 is a congenital variant which arises at the tip of the true transverse process but fails to fuse. This is a common anomaly. Note the position of the spinous processes of the lumbar vertebrae. Another common congenital variant is sacralization or partial sacralization of L5. Note the position of the psoas major borders.

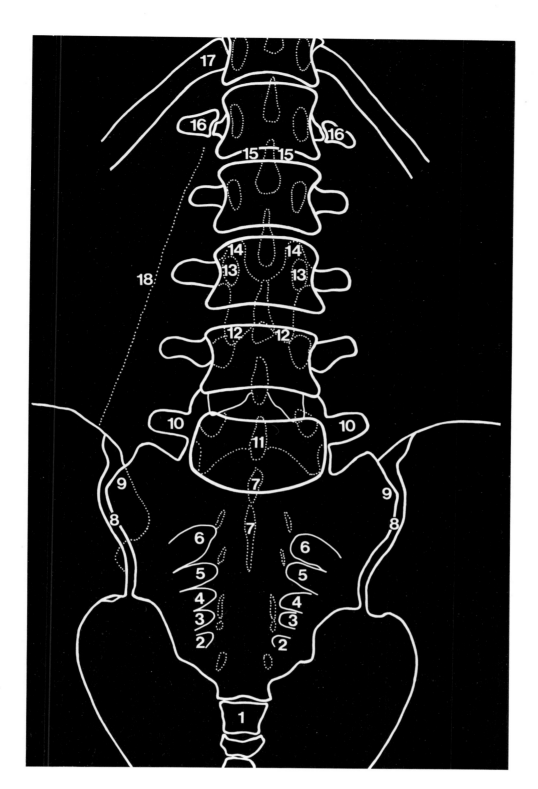

1   Coccyx

2   Fifth sacral foramina

3   Fourth sacral foramina

4   Third sacral foramina

5   Second sacral foramina

6   First sacral foramina

7   Sacral spinous tubercles (median crest)

8   Sacroiliac joint

9   Ala of sacrum

10   Transverse process of L5

11   Spine of L5

12   Inf. articular process of L3

13   Pedicle of L3

14   Sup. articular process of L3

15   Intervertebral space

16   Accessory process of transverse process

17   Twelfth rib

18   Psoas major border

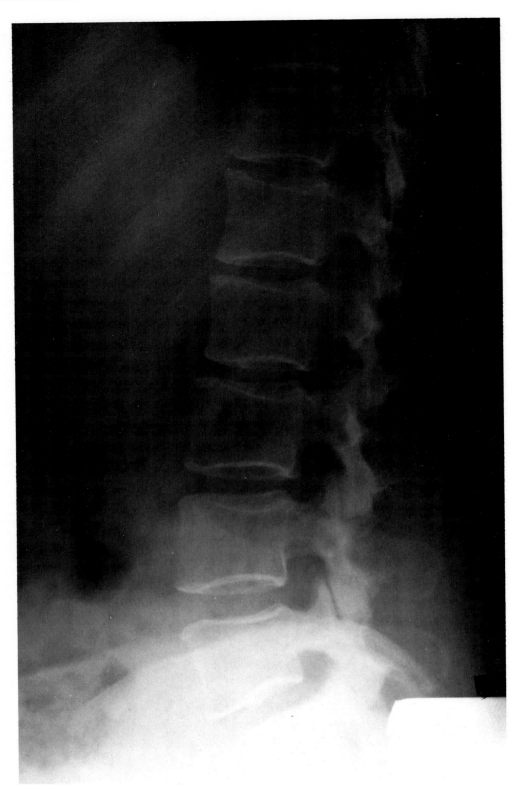

LATERAL VIEW OF LUMBAR SPINE

The normal lumbar lordosis is clearly shown. Note the width of the disc spaces from L1 to L5. Note also that the disc space between L5 and S1 is narrower than those above, but to be considered pathologically narrow, it should be less than one-half of the height of the L4/5 disc space. In these patients other signs of degenerative changes are usually present. As in the lateral view of the cervical spine, this view allows the AP sagittal diameter of the lumbar spinal canal to be measured, and this should not be less than 15 mm or more than 25 mm.

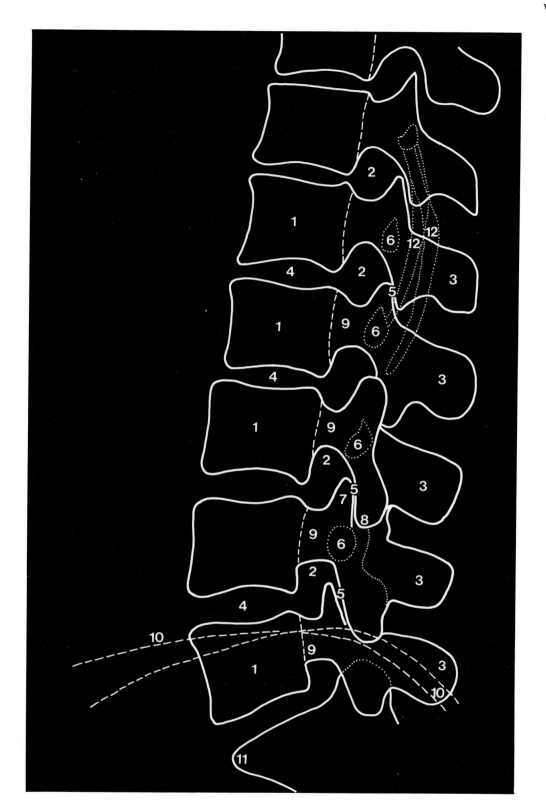

1	Lumbar vertebral body	5	Synovial joint between articular processes
2	Intervertebral foramen	6	Transverse process
3	Spinous process	7	Sup. articular process of L4
4	Site of intervertebral disc	8	Inf. articular process of L3
		9	Pedicle
		10	Iliac crest
		11	Sacral promontory
		12	Twelfth rib

OBLIQUE VIEW OF LUMBAR SPINE

This view is particularly useful to show the pars interarticularis region and the apophyseal joints. Note that the pars interarticularis is a purely radiological term; its equivalent anatomically being the anterior part of the lamina. The oblique view causes a certain well known appearance of a Scottie dog: the dog's collar is the pars interarticularis, the eye is the pedicle, the nose is the transverse process and the ear is the superior articular facet. Defects of ossification of the pars may lead to spondylolisthesis. Again, as in the cervical spine, facet articulation disorders can be seen.

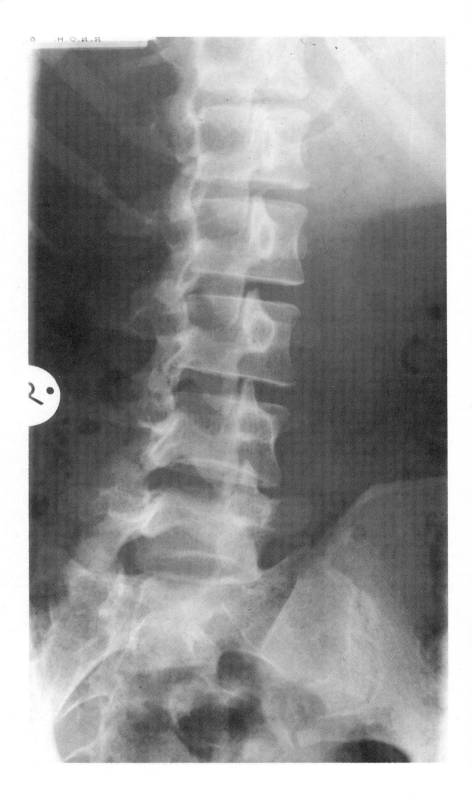

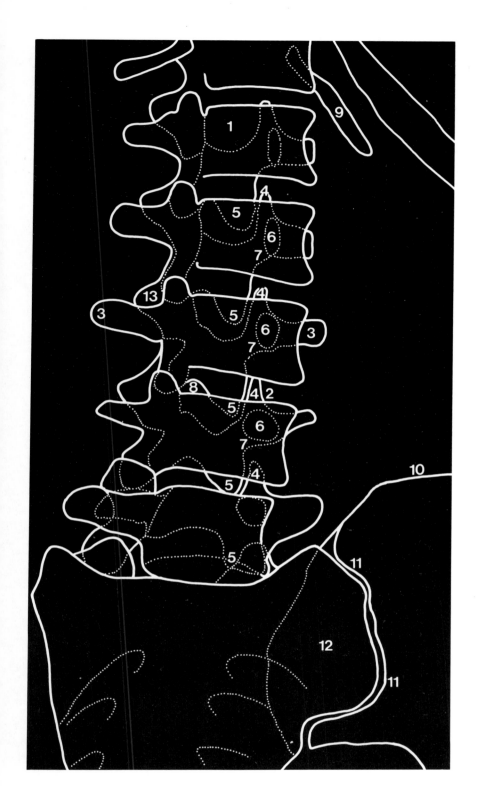

1   Body of first lumbar vertebra (L1)

2   Site of intervertebral disc L3/4

3   Transverse process of L3

4   Sup. articular process

5   Inf. articular process

6   Pedicle

7   Pars interarticularis

8   Intervertebral foramen

9   Twelfth rib

10   Iliac crest

11   Sacroiliac joint

12   Ala of sacrum

13   Spinous process

CENTRAL NERVOUS SYSTEM

CERVICAL MYELOGRAM— POSTEROANTERIOR VIEW

The contrast medium (iophendylate) has been introduced into the subarachnoid space via the lumbar route. The patient is positioned to give the radiograph shown. In this projection the margins of the spinal cord can be seen as well as the exit sites of the cervical spinal nerves. Cervical disc lesions can be located by indentation of the theca and, if severe, may cause obstruction to the flow of cerebrospinal fluid (c.s.f.) and contrast medium. In some cases the disc protrusion may compress the spinal cord itself. Subdural and extradural secondary deposits may also be seen. Note that the contrast medium used is heavier than the c.s.f., does not mix with it and has a tendency to droplet formation.

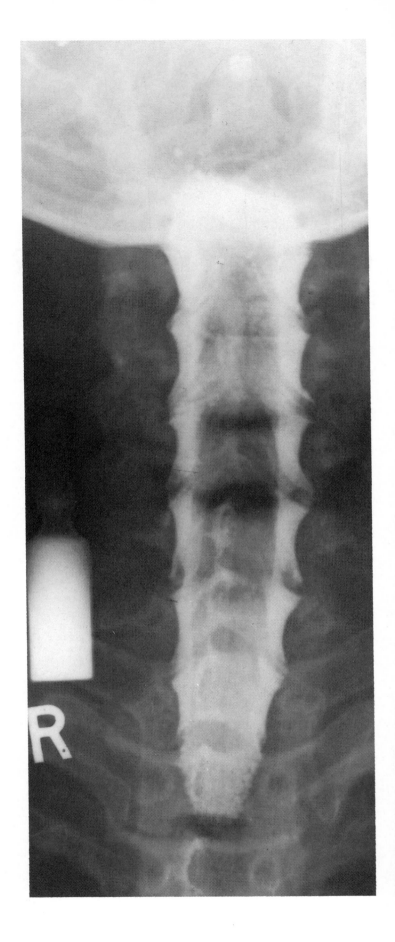

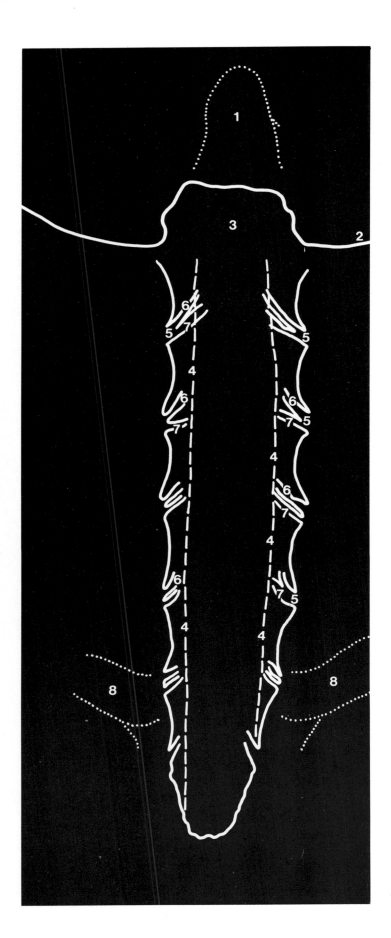

1 Odontoid process of axis (dens)

2 Occiput

3 Contrast medium in subarachnoid space

4 Lat. margin of spinal cord

5 Sites of exit of cervical spinal nn.

6 Dorsal root of spinal n.

7 Ventral root of spinal n.

8 First rib

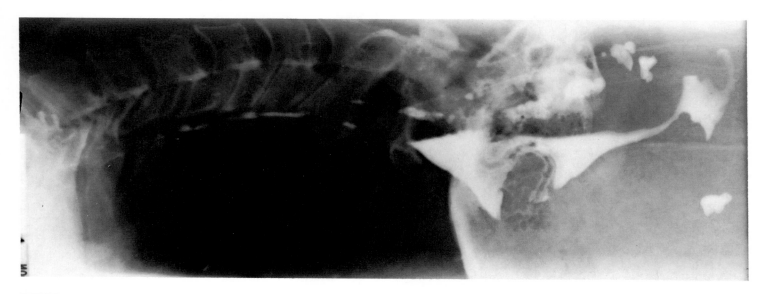

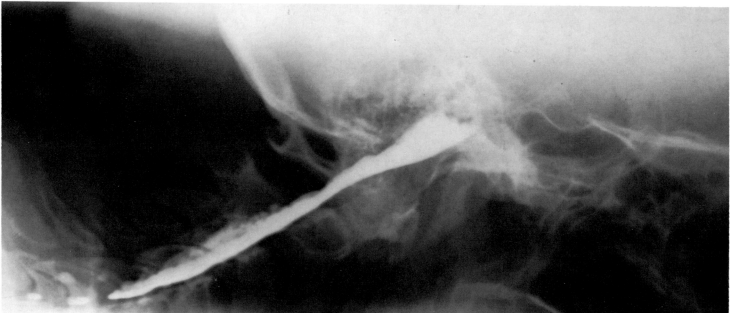

CERVICAL MYELOGRAM—SUPINE AND PRONE, LATERAL FORAMEN MAGNUM

These two decubitus views, using the horizontal x-ray beam, demonstrate the region of the foramen magnum and the basal subarachnoid cisterns. The cerebellar tonsils can be seen on the supine view and their normal position should be noted. They may become displaced inferiorly in the Arnold–Chiari malformation (cerebellar ectopia). Other vertebral anomalies may well exist in this malformation. Contrast is also seen to run into the fourth ventricle and cerebral aqueduct. It is also possible, by careful tilting of the patient, to show the internal auditory meatus. Intrathecal and extrathecal lesions of the cervical spine will also be demonstrated in these two views.

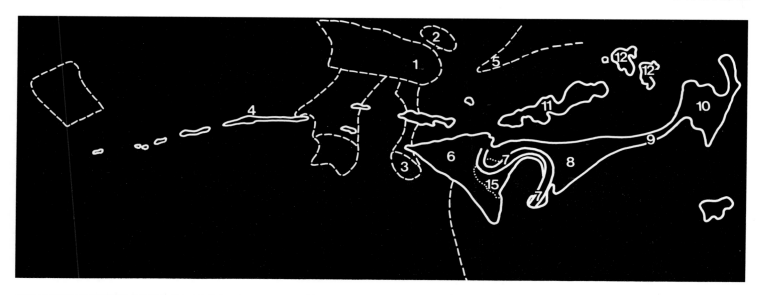

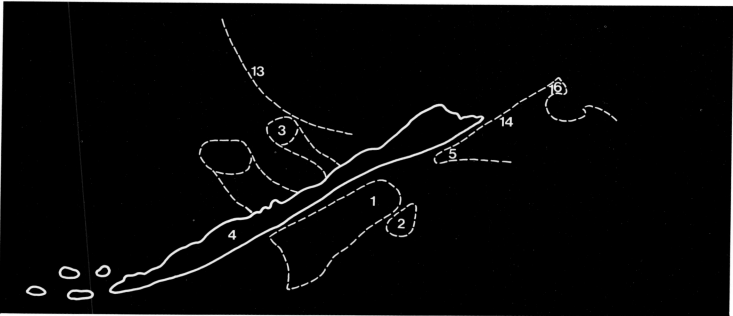

1	Odontoid process of axis (dens)	6	Cerebellomedullary cistern (cisterna magna)
2	Ant. arch of atlas	7	Post. inf. cerebellar artery
3	Post. tubercle of atlas	8	Fourth ventricle
4	Contrast medium within cervical subarachnoid space	9	Cerebral aqueduct
5	Foramen magnum, ant. rim	10	Third ventricle

11	Pontine cistern
12	Interpeduncular cistern
13	Occiput
14	Clivus (basilar parts of sphenoid and occipital bones)
15	Cerebellar tonsils
16	Post. clinoid process

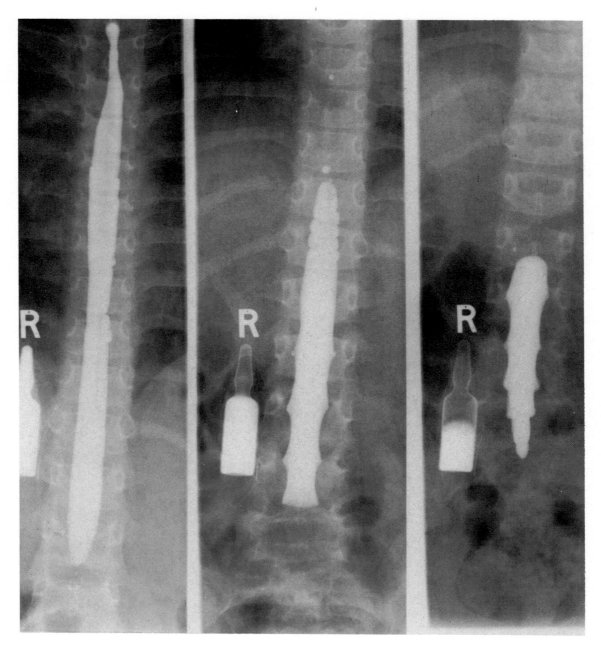

MYELOGRAM—POSTEROANTERIOR VIEWS OF THORACIC AND LUMBAR REGIONS

These three views again show the position of the spinal cord and the meningeal extensions around the spinal nerve roots. Note in this case that the lumbar puncture needle has been removed to allow the patient to proceed to supine views (not shown). The small bottles containing contrast medium are strapped to the patient's back and indicate the patient's position on each of the three films. Again, any interruption to contrast flow can be detected and nerve root impression by disc lesions can also be seen.

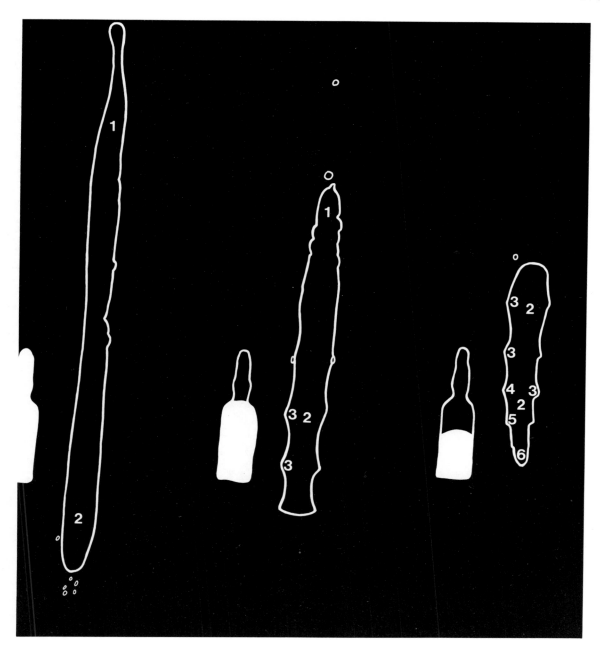

1 Contrast medium in thoracic subarachnoid space

2 Contrast medium in lumbar subarachnoid space

3 Extensions of subarachnoid space around n. roots

4 Extension around fourth lumbar n. root

5 Extension around fifth lumbar n. root

6 Terminal thecal sac

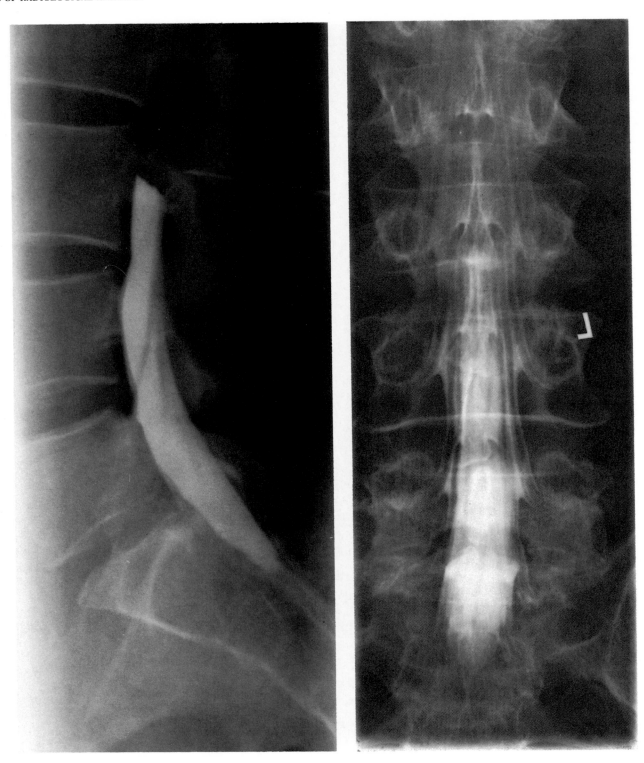

LUMBAR MYELOGRAM—ERECT LATERAL VIEW AND WATER-SOLUBLE RADICULOGRAM

These two views show the differences between the oil-based contrast (iophendylate) and the water-soluble contrast (meglumine iocarmate). The water-soluble contrast mixes freely with the cerebrospinal fluid and, therefore, penetrates the recesses of the subarachnoid space much better than the oil-based contrast. The nerve roots and exiting spinal nerves can be seen most clearly. The erect lateral view shows the usual needle puncture site at the L2/3 space. Remember that the spinal cord usually terminates in the adult at approximately the L1/2 level. Beware using this level in children as the cord may extend to L2/3. Note the normal slight indentations on the anterior thecal margin due to the normal discs. Note also that the subarachnoid space ends at S1/2 in this patient but this level is variable.

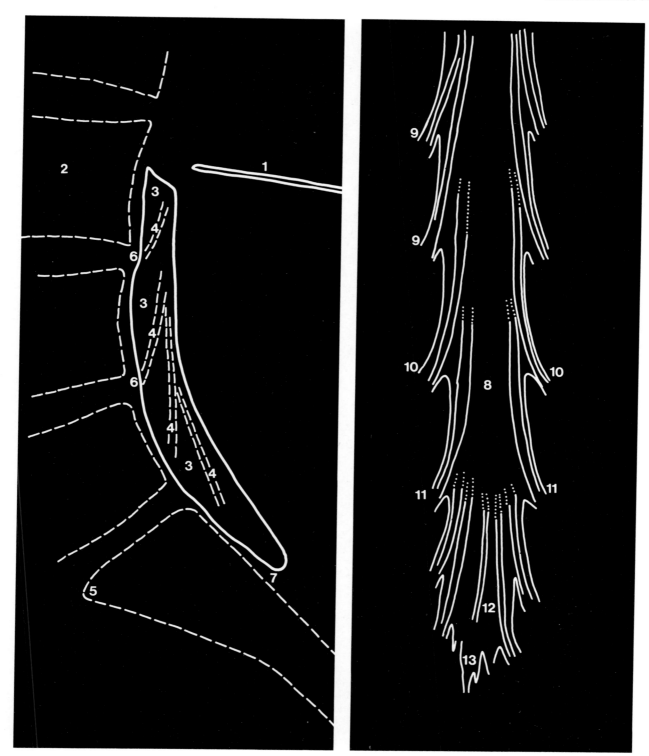

1 Lumbar puncture needle in the L2/3 space

2 Third lumbar vertebral body

3 Contrast medium in subarachnoid space

4 Spinal nn. within subarachnoid space (cauda equina)

5 Sacral promontory

6 Normal intervertebral disc indentations on ant. thecal margin

7 Terminal thecal sac at S1/2

8 Subarachnoid space at the level of L4

9 Lat. extensions of subarachnoid space around spinal n. roots

10 Third lumbar spinal n.

11 Fourth lumbar spinal n.

12 Cauda equina

13 Caudal thecal sac

PNEUMOENCEPHALOGRAMS— FOURTH VENTRICLE

The pneumoencephalograms shown on this and the next seven pages demonstrate the normal anatomy of the ventricular system and the subarachnoid cisterns. This procedure is performed by injecting air into the subarachnoid space, usually via the lumbar route. It can also be performed by direct injection into the ventricles through burr holes. As with any lumbar puncture examination, raised intracranial pressure is a major contraindication as it may cause herniation of the brain stem. The technique itself can be performed under either local or general anaesthesia but necessitates complicated manoeuvres to ensure that air penetrates all the spaces requiring examination. The films illustrated are mostly tomograms so that there is optimum demonstration of the anatomy. The fourth ventricle has five openings: cranially, the aqueduct leading from the third ventricle, a midline foramen of Magendie, two lateral foramina of Luschka and a small communication caudally with the central canal of the spinal cord.

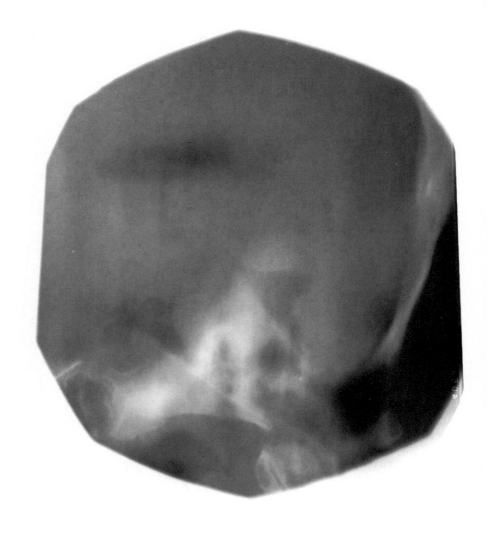

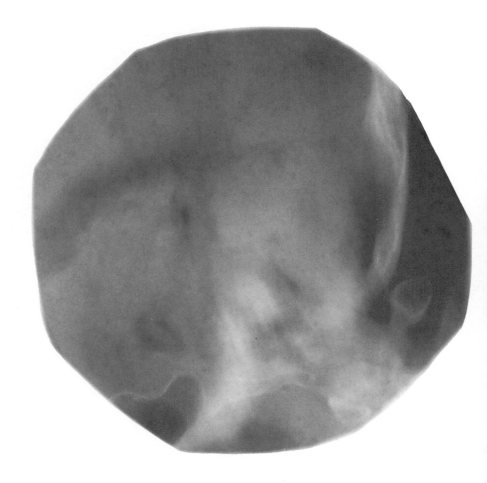

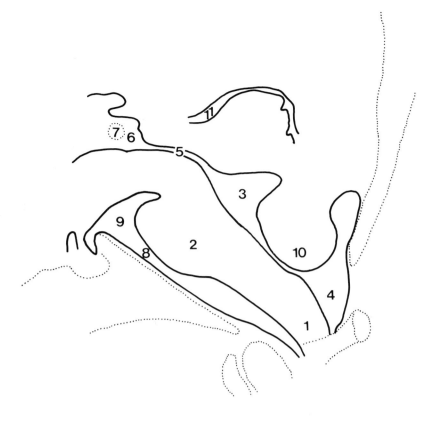

1 Medulla

2 Pons

3 Fourth ventricle

4 Cerebellomedullary cistern
   (cisterna magna)

5 Cerebral aqueduct (Sylvius)

6 Third ventricle

7 Interthalamic adhesion (massa
   intermedia, middle commissure)

8 Pontine cistern

9 Interpeduncular cistern

10 Cerebellar tonsil

11 Sup. cerebellar cistern

12 Quadrigeminal cistern

13 Sup. and inf. colliculi

14 Splenium of corpus callosum

15 Cerebellum

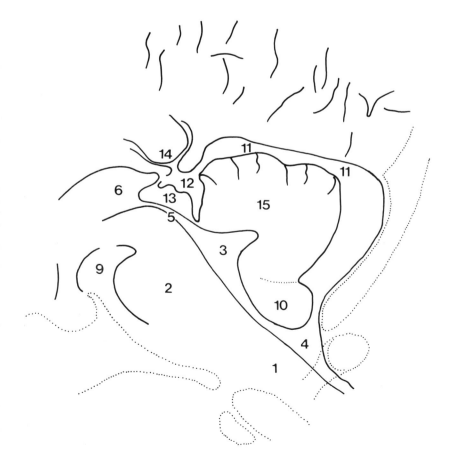

PNEUMOENCEPHALOGRAMS— THIRD VENTRICLE

The position of the third and fourth ventricles with reference to the aqueduct is particularly important when considering lesions of the brain stem and cerebellum. The third ventricle lies in the midline between the two thalami. The third ventricle has three openings: one inferiorly leading into the cerebral aqueduct and two on the anterolateral aspect, the interventricular foramina of Monro, which lead into the lateral ventricles. The quadrigeminal cistern lies above the superior and inferior colliculi and contains the large venous confluence of the inferior sagittal and straight sinuses, the vein of Galen and the basal vein of Rosenthal. These veins are demonstrated in the venous phases of cerebral angiograms shown later in this section.

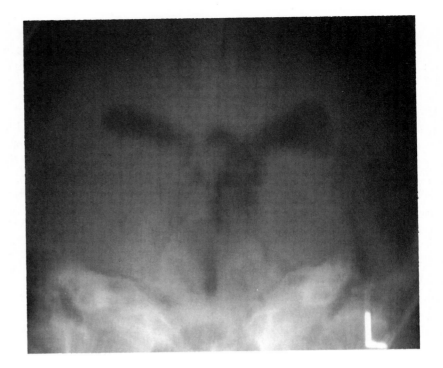

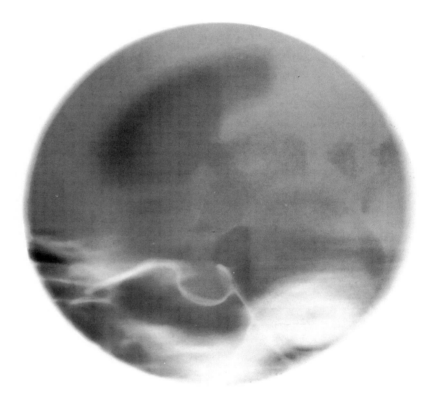

1   Lat. ventricle

2   Third ventricle

3   Position of falx cerebri

4   Fourth ventricle

5   Ambient cistern

6   Pontocerebellar cistern

7   Trigeminal n. (V)

8   Interpeduncular cistern

9   Chiasmatic cistern

10 Site of optic chiasma (II)

11 Interventricular foramen (Monro)

12 Interthalamic adhesion (massa intermedia, middle commissure)

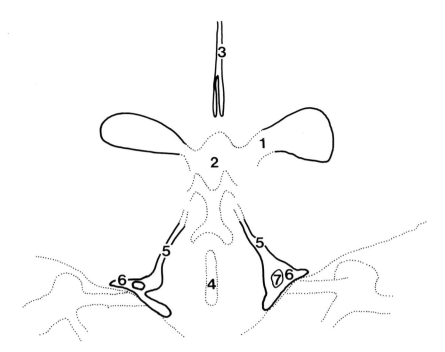

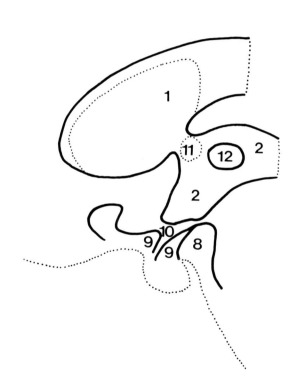

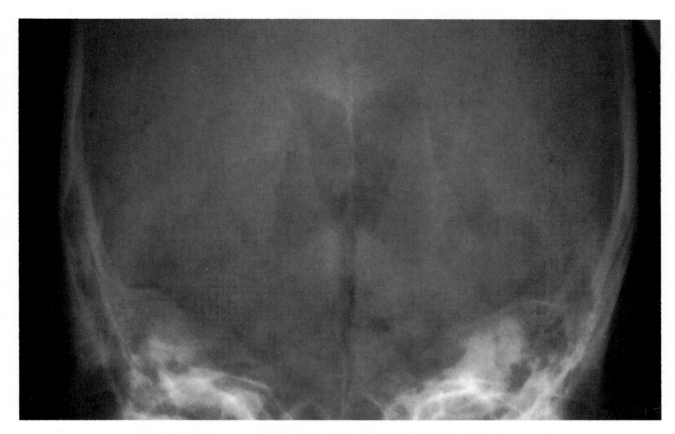

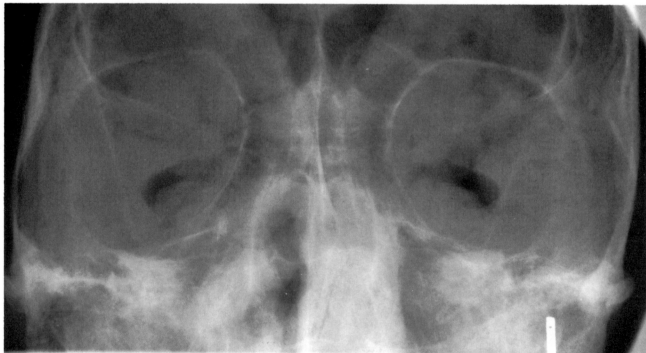

PNEUMOENCEPHALOGRAMS—LATERAL VENTRICLES

The two lateral ventricles are situated in the lower and medial parts of the cerebral hemispheres, and are almost completely separated by the septum pellucidum. Each lateral ventricle consists of a central part with three horns: frontal (anterior), occipital (posterior) and temporal (inferior). The trigone is at the junction of the body and the temporal and occipital horns. The lateral ventricles, the third ventricle and the fourth ventricle all contain choroid plexuses which secrete cerebrospinal fluid. Note the position of the temporal horns projecting through the orbits, and the indentation on their medial wall due to the pes hippocampi. The

third ventricle has a number of important recesses: the supraoptic recess above the optic chiasm; the infundibular recess lying above the pituitary stalk; the suprapineal recess above the pineal; and the pineal recess itself. There are three commissures which cause shadows in the third ventricle. These are: the anterior commissure, connecting the temporal lobes of the two hemispheres; the massa intermedia connecting the two thalami; and the posterior commissure which marks the posterior extent of the third ventricle.

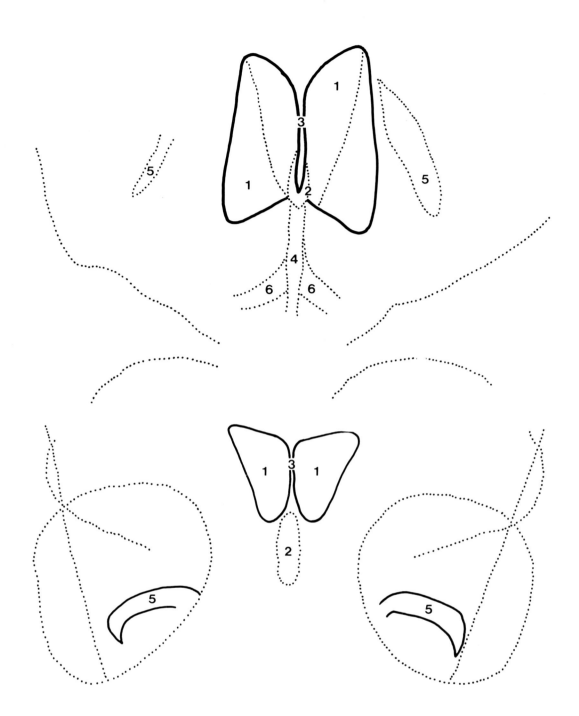

1   Lat. ventricle

2   Third ventricle

3   Septum pellucidum

4   Cerebral aqueduct (Sylvius)

5   Temporal horn of lat. ventricle

6   Ambient cistern

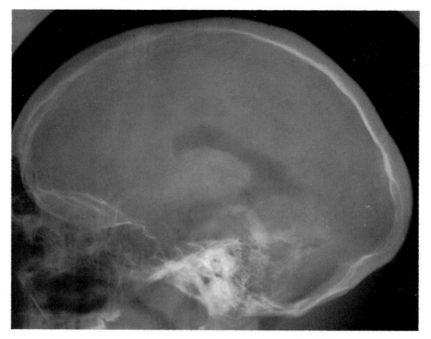

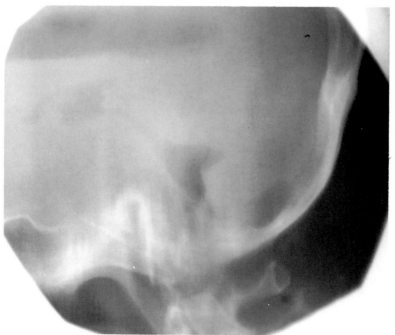

PNEUMOENCEPHALOGRAMS—THIRD AND LATERAL VENTRICLES

Pneumoencephalography is particularly valuable in the diagnosis of hydrocephalus (whether obstructive or non–obstructive), tumours in various intracranial sites and cerebral atrophy. Cerebral atrophy is characterized by dilatation of the ventricles and widening of the sulci. A major limitation of this technique is that it may fail to demonstrate small tumours such as multiple second-

ary deposits which do not cause any shift in the normal structures. It has very limited use in ischaemic and infective changes of the cerebral tissue. For detailed tumour localization, the reader is referred to specialized neuroradiological texts. Detailed neuro-anatomy is demonstrated in the 'Nuclear magnetic resonance' section.

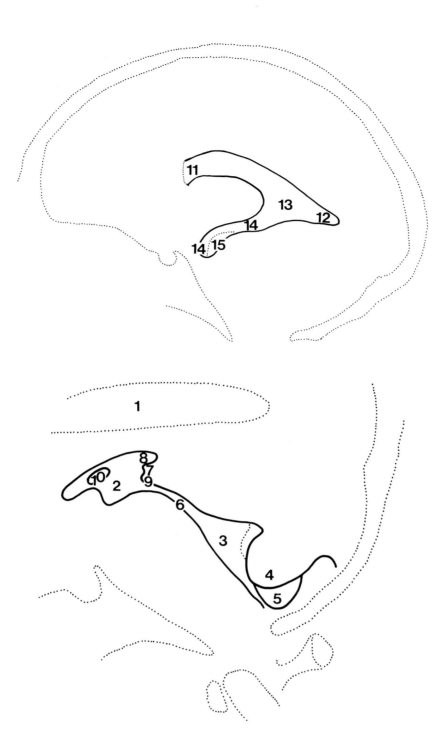

1   Lat. ventricle

2   Third ventricle

3   Fourth ventricle

4   Vermis of cerebellum

5   Cerebellar tonsil

6   Cerebral aqueduct (Sylvius)

7   Site of pineal body

8   Suprapineal recess of third ventricle

9   Site of post. commissure

10   Interthalamic adhesion (massa intermedia, middle commissure)

11   Frontal horn of lat. ventricle

12   Occipital horn of lat. ventricle

13   Trigone of lat. ventricle (isthmus)

14   Temporal horn of lat. ventricle

15   Site of pes hippocampi

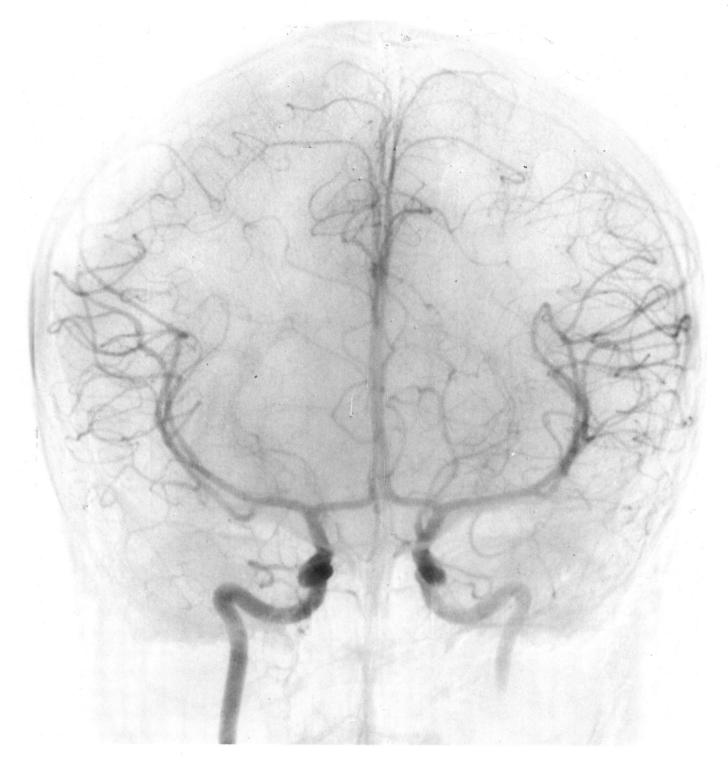

ANTEROPOSTERIOR VIEW OF INTERNAL CAROTID ARTERIOGRAM—ARTERIAL PHASE WITH SUBTRACTION

This and the following seven films demonstrate the anatomy of the brain circulation. Carotid angiography with arterial and venous phases is shown first, followed by similar studies of the vertebral circulation. Carotid and vertebral arteriography can be performed by direct puncture of the common carotid artery or vertebral artery respective. More recently there has been a tendency to perform both these procedures indirectly by selective catheterization via the femoral artery. Rapid serial films are obtained in the AP and lateral planes with axial and oblique views if necessary to demonstrate any pathology. The films shown on the next few pages are all subtraction views to allow clearer demonstration of the normal anatomy. The contrast used is water-soluble with an iodine content of approximately 280 mg/ml. As with all peripheral arteriography the amount of contrast used must be carefully controlled.

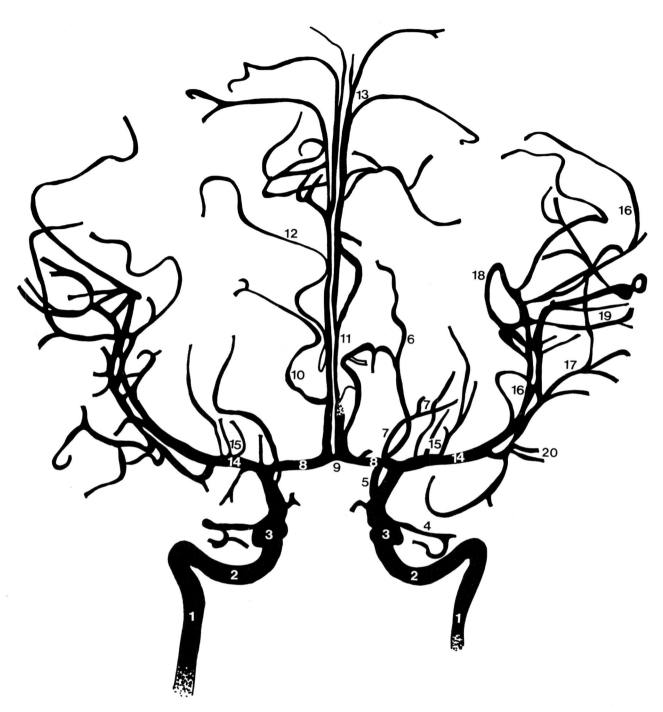

List of Arteries

1	Internal carotid, cervical part	8	Ant. cerebral	15	Lenticulostriate
2	Internal carotid, intrapetrous part	9	Ant. communicating	16	Post. parietal
3	Internal carotid, cavernous part	10	Frontopolar	17	Post. temporal
4	Ophthalmic	11	Pericallosal	18	Angular gyrus
5	Position of post. communicating	12	Callosomarginal	19	Parietal
6	Post. cerebral	13	Post. frontal	20	Frontoparietal
7	Ant. choroidal	14	Middle cerebral		

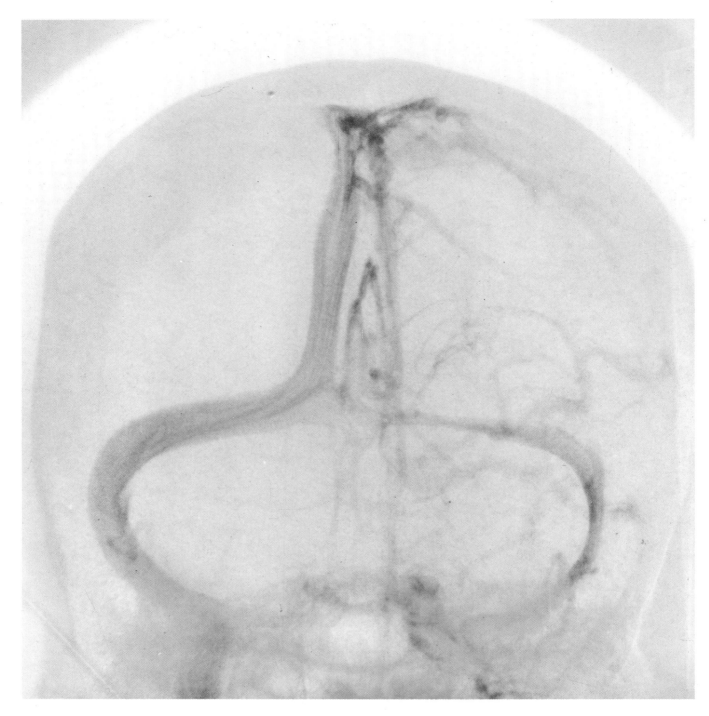

ANTEROPOSTERIOR VIEW OF INTERNAL CAROTID ARTERIOGRAM—VENOUS PHASE WITH SUBTRACTION

The carotid angiogram is divided into four phases. The first phase is the arterial phase lasting approximately 2 seconds; the second or capillary phase lasts about 1 second but is rarely seen clearly on the radiograph because of the length of time of contrast injection; the last two phases are the early and late venograms. The early venograms show the superficial cerebral veins which are variable in position and are less important than the deep cerebral veins which fill on the late venogram. These deep veins are more constant in position, and displacement may help localize a space-occupying lesion such as a tumour. The thalamostriate vein lies in the groove between the caudate nucleus and the thalamus, receiving tributaries from both these structures. It thus lies in the floor and lateral wall of the lateral ventricle and therefore is used to assess the size of the ventricle on this AP view.

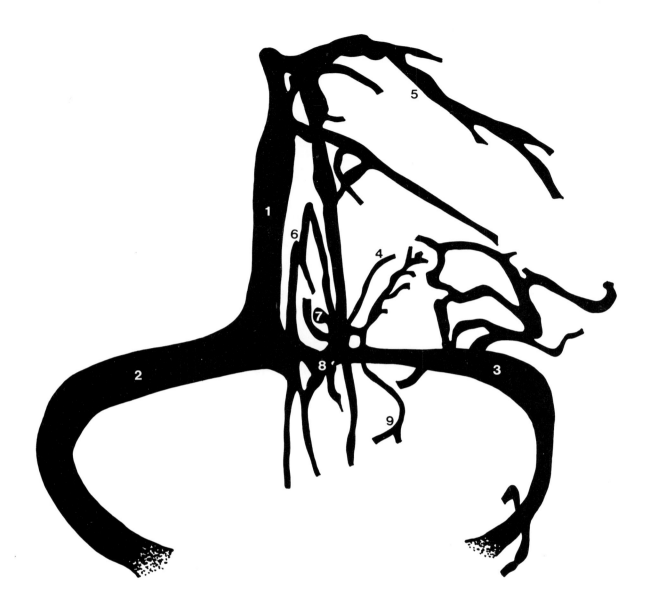

1	Sup. sagittal sinus	4	Thalamostriate v.	7	Great cerebral vein (Galen)
2	R. transverse sinus	5	Sup. cerebral vv.	8	Straight sinus
3	L. transverse sinus	6	Inf. sagittal sinus	9	Basal vein of cerebrum (Rosenthal)

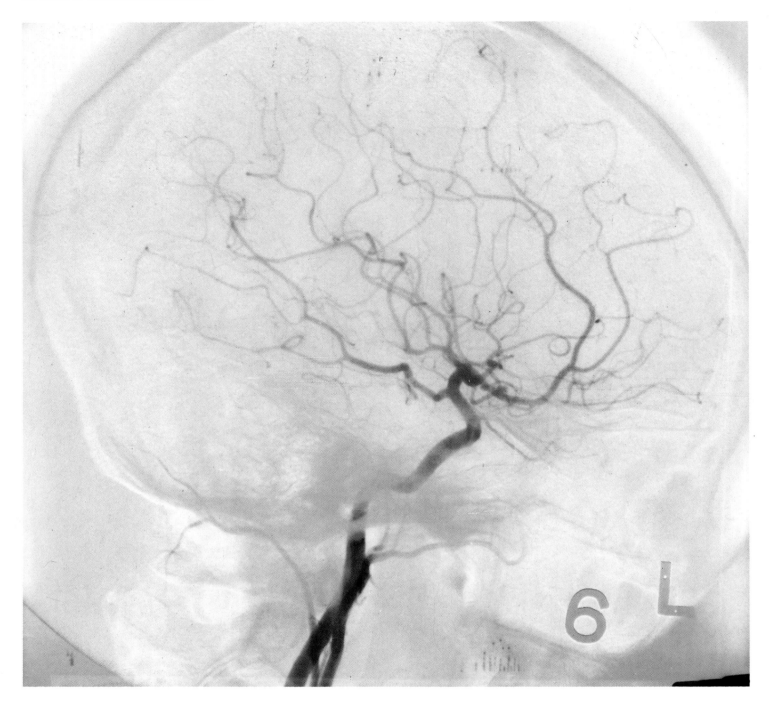

LATERAL VIEW OF INTERNAL CAROTID ARTERIOGRAM—ARTERIAL PHASE WITH SUBTRACTION

The carotid artery, which ascends from the neck, is divided into four portions: cervical, petrous, cavernous and intracranial. Note that the cervical portion has no branches. Five main branches come from the intracranial portion: the ophthalmic, anterior cerebral, middle cerebral, posterior communicating and anterior choroidal. The subdivisions of these branches can be seen labelled on the diagram. The posterior communicating artery fills in only about 30% of common carotid arteriograms but selective catheterization of the internal carotid artery demonstrates a much higher percentage. The anterior choroidal artery is small but constant;

arising near the posterior communicating artery, it passes backwards to cross the optic tract and lies in relation to the crura cerebri. It then turns lateral, again crossing the optic tract, and comes into relationship with the lateral aspect of the lateral geniculate body; it finally enters the inferior horn of the lateral ventricle through the choroidal fissure and terminates in the choroidal plexus. This artery is often of considerable importance when assessing cerebral tumours, and its particular displacement must be noted.

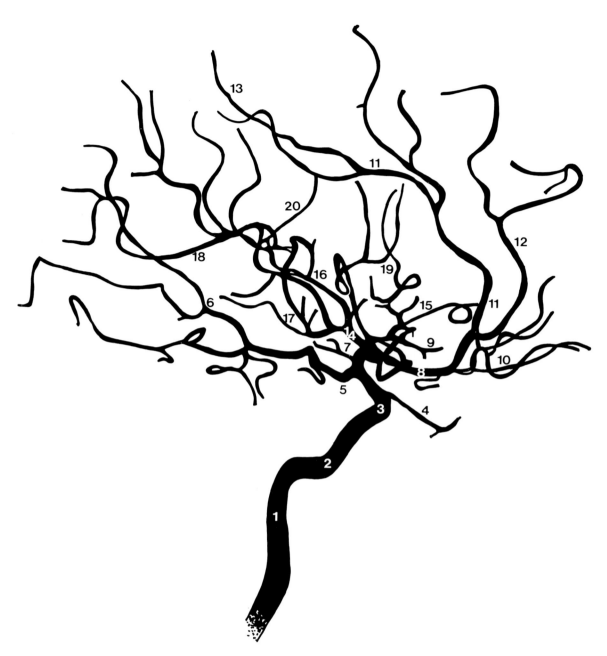

List of Arteries

1	Internal carotid, cervical part	8	Ant. cerebral	15	Precentral
2	Internal carotid, intrapetrous part	9	Orbitofrontal	16	Post. parietal
3	Internal carotid, cavernous part	10	Frontopolar	17	Post. temporal
4	Ophthalmic	11	Pericallosal	18	Angular gyrus
5	Post. communicating	12	Callosomarginal	19	Central
6	Post. cerebral	13	Post. frontal	20	Parietal opercular
7	Ant. choroidal	14	Middle cerebral		

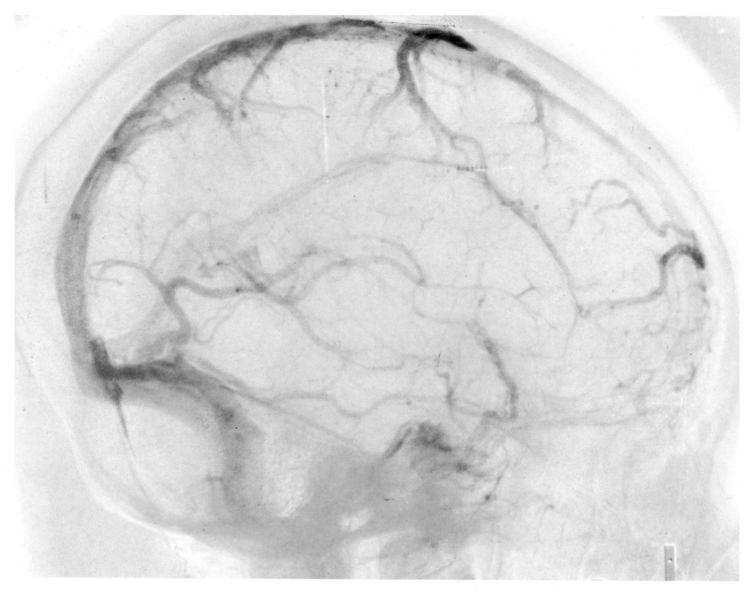

LATERAL VIEW OF INTERNAL CAROTID ARTERIOGRAM—VENOUS PHASE WITH SUBTRACTION

The veins of the brain are very thin due to the absence of muscle, and they possess no valves. They are divided into two sets: cerebral and cerebellar. Both drain into cranial dural venous sinuses. The cerebral veins are again divided into internal and external groups according to whether they drain the inner or outer surfaces of the hemispheres. The septal vein, the thalamostriate vein and the internal cerebral vein form the venous angle. This point usually marks the apex of the posterior and superior limits of the interventricular foramen of Monro. This angle appears in approximately 80% of all carotid angiographic studies but its anatomy is not constant and false venous angles may occur. The internal cerebral vein joins with the basal vein of Rosenthal to form the great cerebral vein of Galen. This in turn drains into the straight sinus, having joined the inferior sagittal sinus.

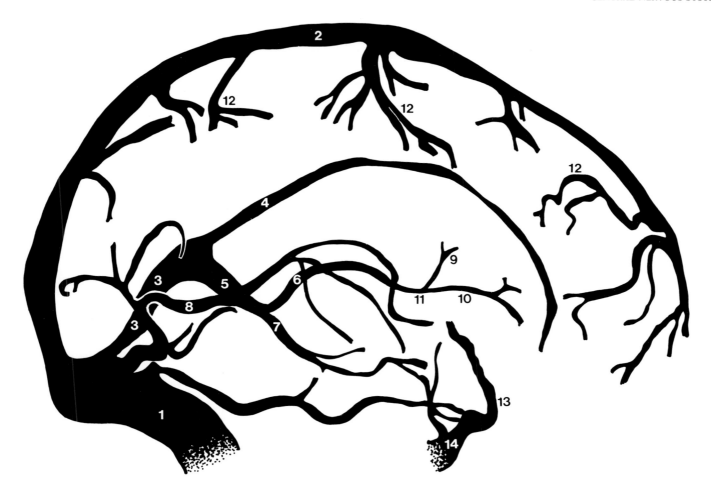

1	Transverse sinus	6	Internal cerebral v.	10	Septal v.	
2	Sup. sagittal sinus	7	Basal v. of cerebrum (Rosenthal)	11	Venous angle	
3	Straight sinus	8	Inf. anastomotic v. of cerebrum (Labbé)	12	Sup. cerebral vv.	
4	Inf. sagittal sinus			13	Sphenoparietal sinus	
5	Great cerebral v. (Galen)	9	Thalamostriate v.	14	Cavernous sinus	

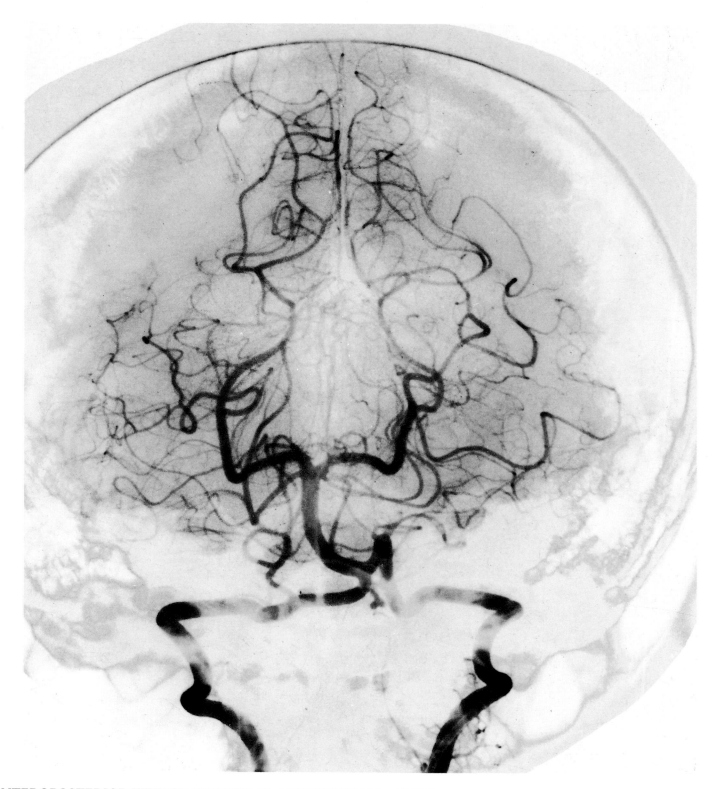

ANTEROPOSTERIOR VIEW OF VERTEBRAL ARTERIOGRAM—ARTERIAL PHASE WITH SUBTRACTION

The vertebral artery ascends through the foramina transversaria of the upper six cervical vertebrae, passes behind the lateral mass of the atlas and enters the cranial cavity through the foramen magnum where it joins the opposite vertebral artery to form the basilar artery, at the inferior border of the pons. Two spinal arteries arise from the vertebral artery in the region of the medulla oblongata. The anterior spinal artery descends in front of the medulla oblongata to unite with its fellow from the opposite side. This common trunk then passes inferiorly on the anterior aspect of the spinal cord and is very important in the cord's blood supply. The posterior inferior cerebellar artery (PICA) passes around the medulla oblongata posteriorly, and then ascends behind the origins of the glossopharyngeal and vagus nerves to the lower border of the pons, where it turns downwards to pass along the inferolateral border of the fourth ventricle. It then passes under the lower lateral edge of the cerebellar tonsil and divides into a medial and lateral branch. The PICA is of considerable importance in the diagnosis of posterior fossa lesions since it shows the anatomy of the brain stem, fourth ventricle and base of cerebellum.

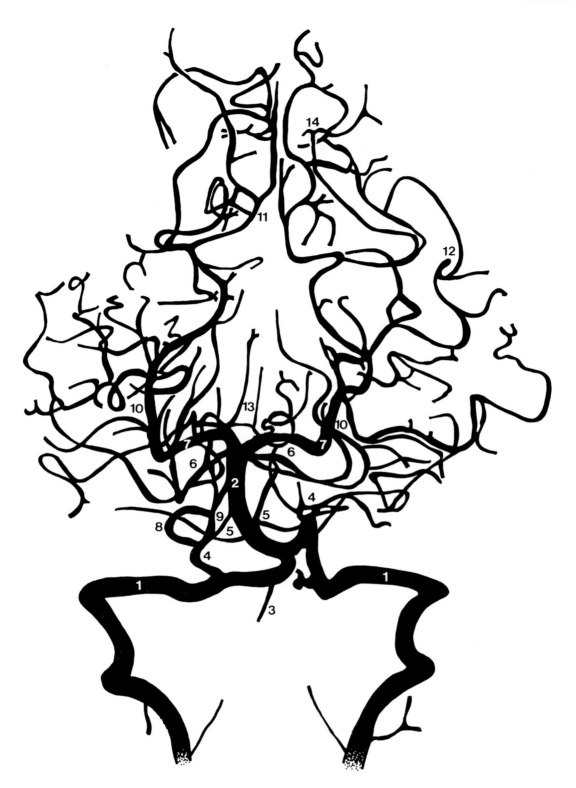

List of Arteries

1 Vertebral

2 Basilar

3 Ant. spinal

4 Post. inf. cerebellar (PICA)

5 Ant. inf. cerebellar

6 Sup. cerebellar

7 Post. cerebral (PCA)

8 Lat. medullary segment of PICA

9 Tonsillohemispheric branch of PICA

10 Internal occipital segment of PCA

11 Calcarine branch of PCA

12 Post. temporal branch of PCA

13 Thalamoperforate branch of PCA

14 Parieto-occipital branch of PCA

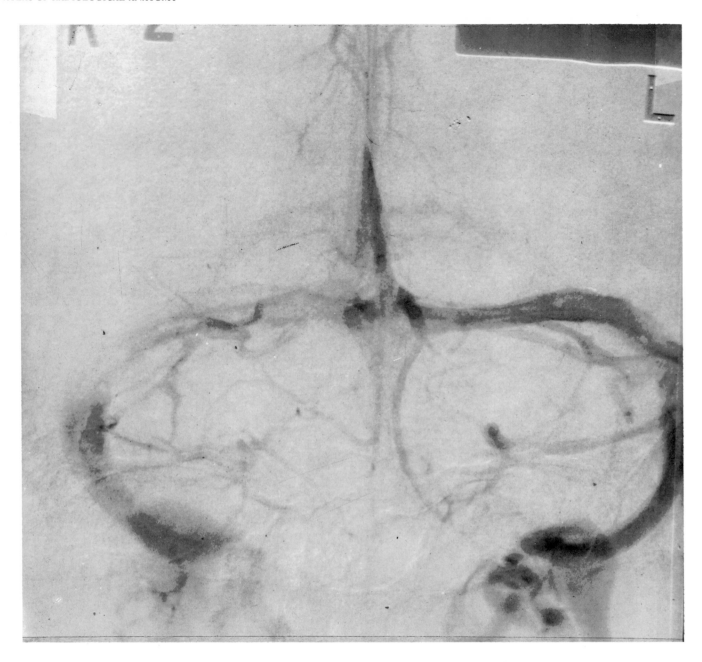

ANTEROPOSTERIOR VIEW OF VERTEBRAL ARTERIOGRAM—VENOUS PHASE WITH SUBTRACTION

The veins of the posterior fossa have played an increasingly important role in neuroradiology in the last few years, as their distinct anatomy has become more widely known. They are constant in position and their displacement is used in determining the size and shape of posterior fossa tumours. The veins are divided into three groups. The superior group consists of the precentral cerebellar vein, superior vermian veins, and posterior and lateral mesencephalic veins. These drain into the great cerebral vein. The anterior group consists of the petrosal cerebellar vein, the anterior pontomesencephalic vein, the transverse pontine veins and several superior and inferior hemispheric veins. This group drains to the superior or inferior petrosal sinuses. The last collection of veins is the posterior group which include some superior and inferior hemispheric veins, inferior veins of the vermis and the medial superior cerebellar veins. This group drains into the transverse sinus.

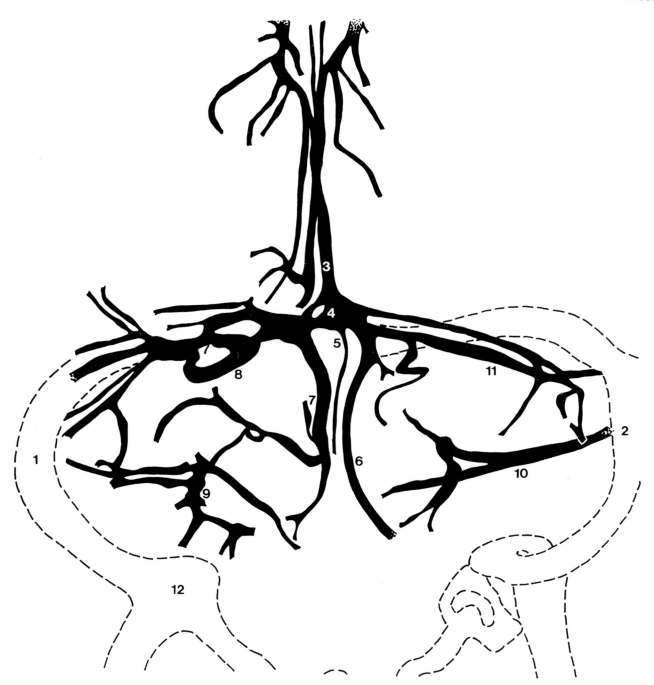

1 Position of r. transverse sinus

2 Position of l. transverse sinus

3 Straight sinus

4 Great cerebral v. (Galen)

5 Precentral cerebellar v.

6 Inf. hemispheric v.

7 Inf. vermian v.

8 Post. mesencephalic v.

9 Petrosal v.

10 Sup. petrosal sinus

11 Sup. hemispheric v.

12 Position of jugular bulb

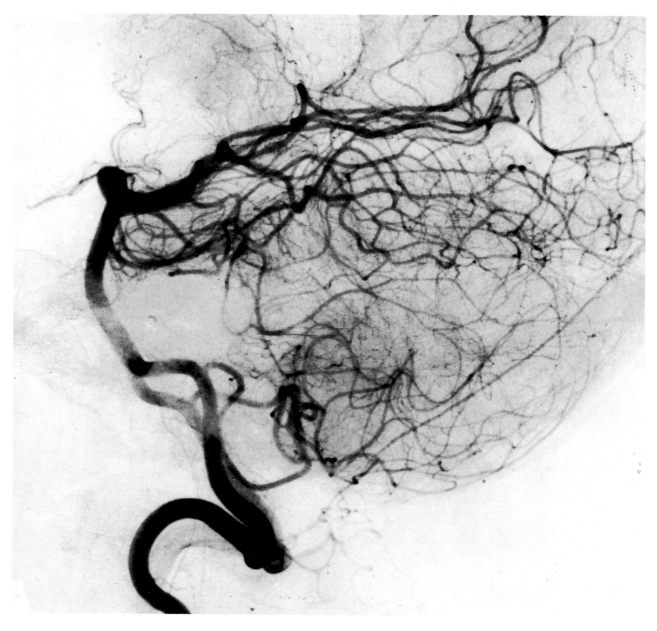

LATERAL VIEW OF VERTEBRAL ARTERIOGRAM— ARTERIAL PHASE WITH SUBTRACTION

The posterior inferior cerebellar artery is again seen on this view with its characteristic contour visualized. There is wide variation in the course and distribution of this artery and occasionally it may be absent. The superior cerebellar artery arises near the termination of the basilar artery and passes laterally below the oculomotor nerve. It then passes round the cerebral peduncle to reach the superior surface of the cerebellum. It anastomoses with branches from the inferior cerebellar arteries and also gives branches to the pons, the pineal, the superior medullary velum and the tela choroidea of the third ventricle. The posterior cerebral arteries are the terminal branches of the basilar artery. They curve round the cerebral peduncles to pass through the tentorium and reach the inferior surface of the temporal lobe. Two major divisions of these arteries are the posterior temporal and internal occipital, the latter dividing again into the calcarine and parieto-occipital arteries. Note that the posterior cerebral arteries supply the visual area of the cerebral cortex.

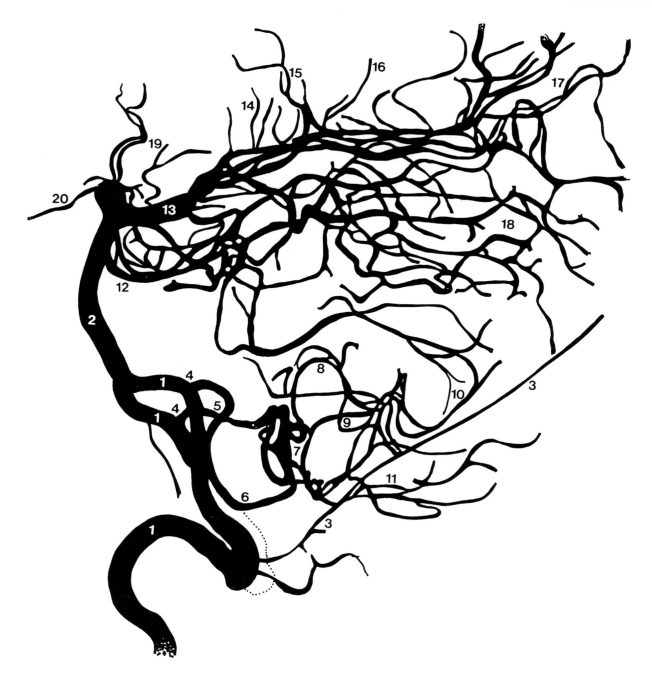

List of Arteries

1	Vertebral	8	Supratonsillar segment of PICA	15	Lat. post. choroidal branch of PCA
2	Basilar	9	Retrotonsillar segment of PICA	16	Splenial branch of PCA
3	Meningeal branch	10	Inf. vermian segment of PICA	17	Parieto-occipital branch of PCA
4	Post. inf. cerebellar (PICA)	11	Hemispheric branches of PICA	18	Post. temporal branch of PCA
5	Ant. medullary segment of PICA	12	Sup. cerebellar	19	Thalamoperforate branch of PCA
6	Lat. medullary segment of PICA	13	Post. cerebral (PCA)	20	Post. communicating
7	Post. medullary segment of PICA	14	Med. post. choroidal branch of PCA		

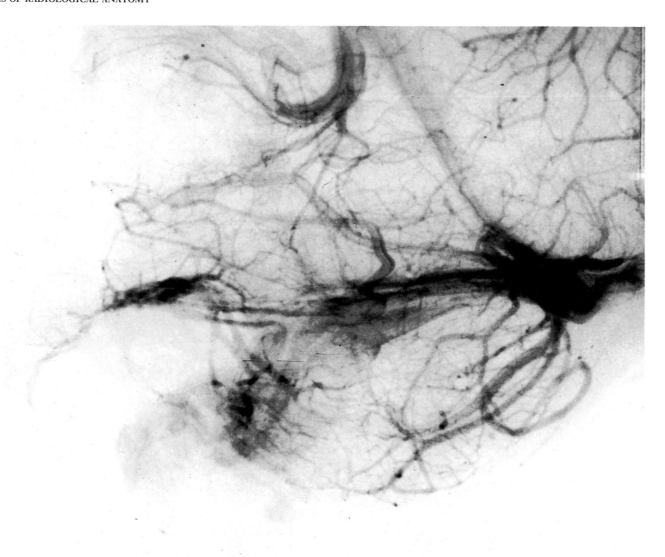

LATERAL VIEW OF VERTEBRAL ARTERIOGRAM— VENOUS PHASE WITH SUBTRACTION

The precentral cerebellar vein is small and is easily recognized on this lateral projection. It passes upwards between the superior vermis of the cerebellum and the tectum of the mid brain, across the quadrigeminal cistern, to lie dorsal to the mid brain. This is therefore an important structure, as tumours in the region of the pineal, upper vermis, aqueduct and fourth ventricle will cause characteristic displacements of its position. The vein drains into the great cerebral vein. The petrosal vein is also of considerable importance as it runs within the cerebellopontine angle and can help in the evaluation of tumours in this region.

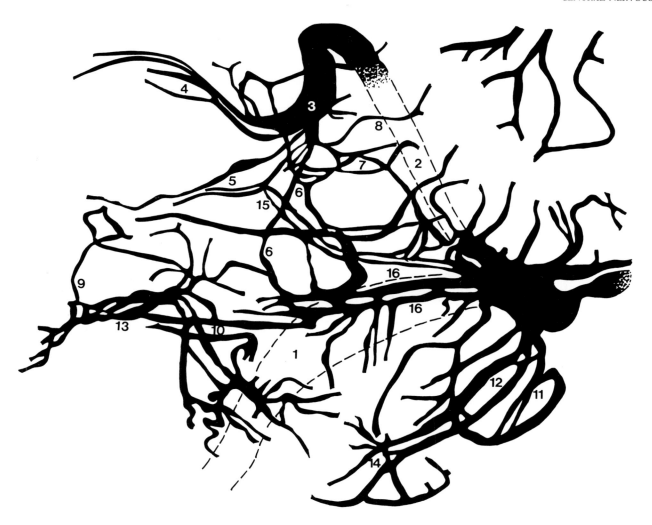

1	Position of transverse sinus	7	Sup. hemispheric v.	13	Sup. petrosal sinus
2	Position of straight sinus	8	Inf. occipital v.	14	Tonsillar vv.
3	Great cerebral v. (Galen)	9	Ant. pontomesencephalic v.	15	Lat. mesencephalic v.
4	Sup. choroidal v.	10	Petrosal v.	16	V. of the great horizontal fissure
5	Post. mesencephalic v.	11	Inf. hemispheric v.		
6	Precentral cerebellar v.	12	Inf. vermian v.		

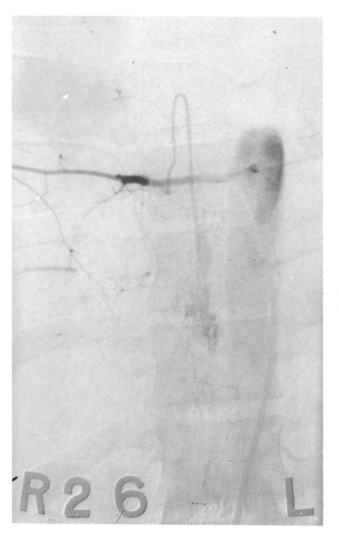
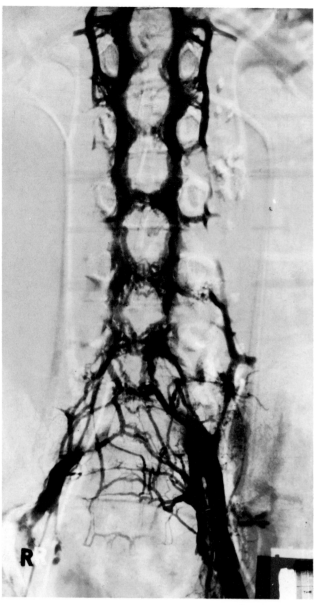

SELECTIVE SPINAL CORD ARTERIOGRAM AND LUMBAR VERTEBRAL VENOGRAM

Both these specialized techniques are used for locating spinal, intradural and extradural tumours, especially vascular malformations. Note the arteria radicularis magna or artery of Adamkiewicz supplying the dorsolumbar cord. It usually arises from a left dorsal branch of the posterior intercostal arteries of T9–12. Here, it arises at the level of T9 on the right. Therefore, beware the level of around T10 for performing aortography with pressure injection, as spinal cord damage may result. Venous drainage of the spinal cord is via six longitudinally arranged plexi, which anastomose freely with the internal and external vertebral venous plexi. A segmental arrangement offers direct communication with intercostal, lumbar and sacral veins, especially those of the pelvis, thus explaining this common site for metastases.

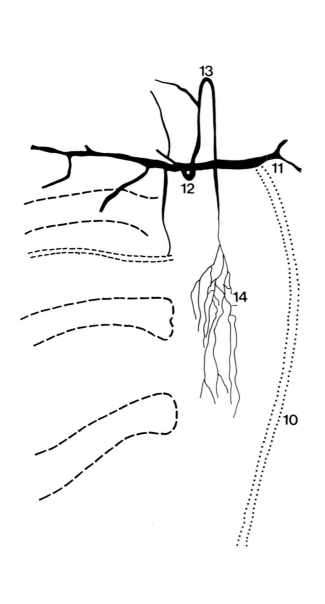
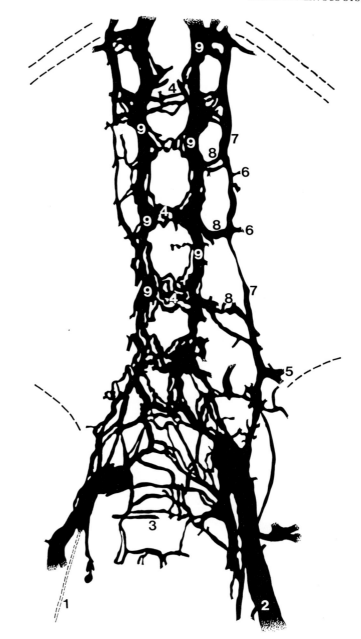

1 Catheter in common iliac v.	6 Segmental lumbar vv.	11 Catheter tip in post. intercostal a. of T9
2 External iliac v.	7 Ascending lumbar v.	12 Origin of arteria radicularis magna
3 Sacral venous plexus	8 Intervertebral vv.	
4 Basivertebral vv.	9 Longitudinal vertebral venous plexi	13 'Hairpin' of normal a. of Adamkiewicz
5 Iliolumbar v.	10 Catheter in thoracic aorta	14 Sinuous termination of a.

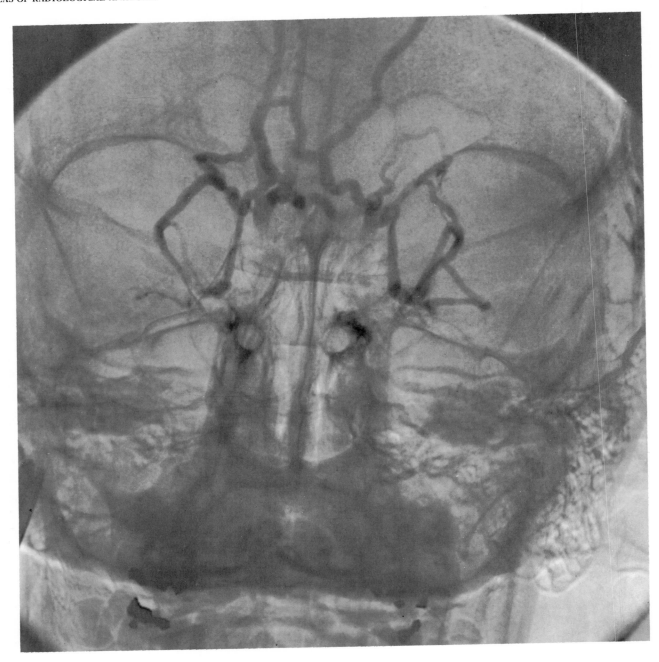

ORBITAL VENOGRAM WITH SUBTRACTION

This technique is performed by injection of soluble contrast medium into the frontal vein, usually under local anaesthetic. A compression band is placed around the hairline to prevent reflux of contrast into the superficial skull veins. The facial veins are also occluded by pressure. In this manner the venous system of the orbits is demonstrated. Both superior ophthalmic veins fill from this single frontal vein injection, so it is possible to compare the two sides. The radiological diagnosis of orbital tumours depends on three main features: first, displacement of veins; secondly, a pathological circulation; and, thirdly, non-filling of the superior ophthalmic vein due to compression or thrombosis

The superior ophthalmic vein is the largest of the two draining veins and is divided into three parts: the first part along the inner wall of the orbit, the second part passing posteriorly and laterally under the superior rectus muscle and above the optic nerve. The third part runs posteriorly and slightly medially to pass through the superior orbital fissure. The other draining vein of the orbit is the inferior ophthalmic vein, which begins at the venous plexus in the floor of the orbit; it drains to the cavernous sinus either separately or having previously joined the superior ophthalmic vein.

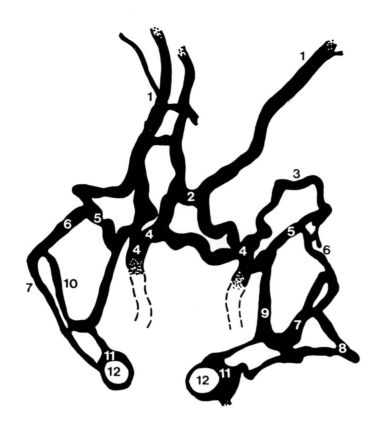

1	Frontal vv.	5	Sup. ophthalmic v. (first part)	9	Ant. collateral v.
2	Superficial connecting v.	6	Sup. ophthalmic v. (second part)	10	Med. collateral v.
3	Supraorbital v.	7	Sup. ophthalmic v. (third part)	11	Cavernous sinus
4	Angular vv.	8	Inf. ophthalmic v.	12	Internal carotid a.

RESPIRATORY SYSTEM

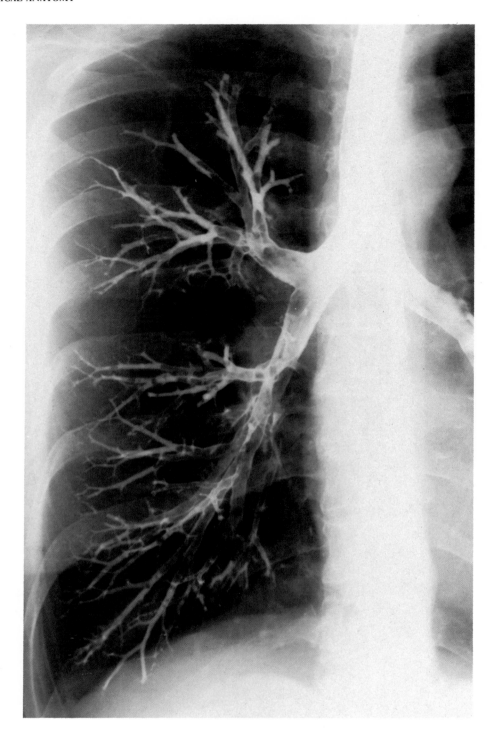

POSTEROANTERIOR BRONCHOGRAM OF RIGHT LUNG

This and the following five films are devoted to demonstration of the bronchopulmonary segments. The contrast which has been used is propyliodone in arachis oil 60% (Dionosil Oily). This contrast medium leaves the lungs within four days and has few side effects, though mild pyrexia may follow the examination and granulomas have been reported. The right lung consists of three lobes: upper, middle and lower. These lobes are further sub-divided into bronchopulmonary segments. It is vital that the distribution and position of these bronchopulmonary segments be appreciated on all chest radiograms. The segmental anatomy is of considerable importance when conditions such as pneumonia, bronchiectasis, neoplasia and tuberculosis are suspected. It is also important in dealing with patients with pulmonary infarction as the arteries of the lung closely parallel the bronchi.

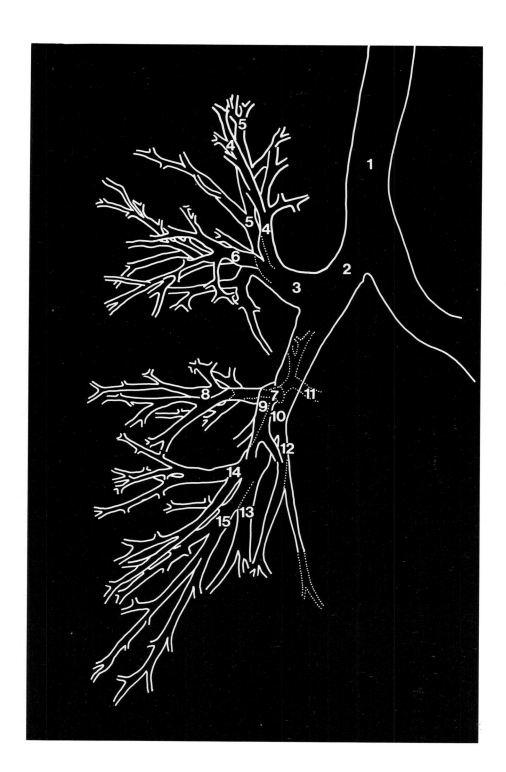

1   Trachea

2   R. main bronchus

3   R. upper lobe bronchus

4   Apical segmental bronchus

5   Post. segmental bronchus

6   Ant. segmental bronchus

7   Middle lobe bronchus

8   Lat. segmental bronchus

9   Med. segmental bronchus

10   R. lower lobe bronchus

11   Sup. segmental bronchus (apical basal)

12   Med. basal segmental bronchus

13   Ant. basal segmental bronchus

14   Lat. basal segmental bronchus

15   Post. basal segmental bronchus

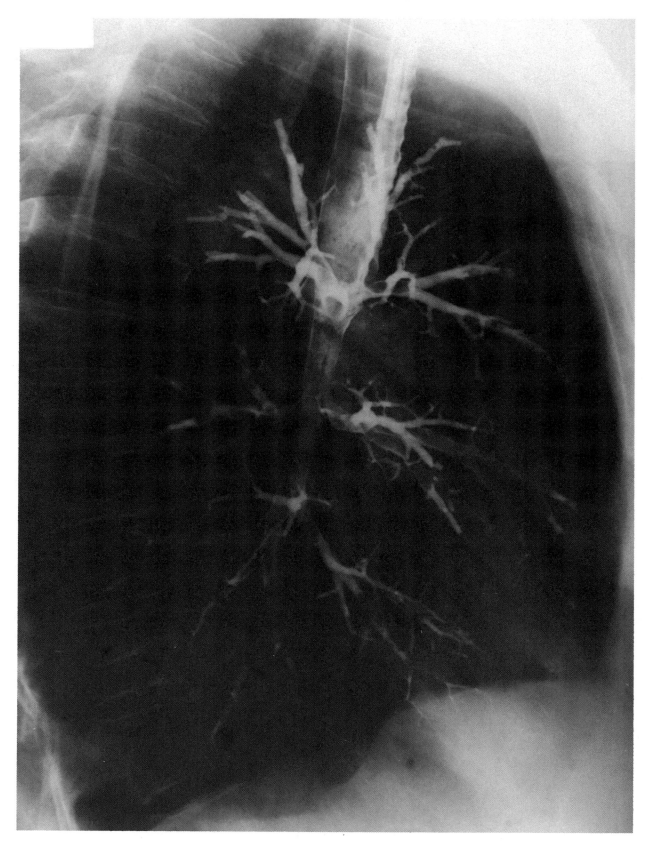

RIGHT LATERAL BRONCHOGRAM OF RIGHT LUNG

The trachea bifurcates into the right and left main bronchi at the level of the sternal angle or the vertebral level of T4/5. The right main bronchus descends at a sharper angle than the left due to the left atrium, and gives off the right upper lobe bronchus after about 2.5 cm. This bronchus then divides into the three segments of the upper lobe: apical, posterior and anterior. Note that this right upper lobe bronchus is the only bronchus to arise above its accompanying pulmonary artery. The right bronchus then contin-

ues and gives off the middle lobe bronchus which divides into two segments: lateral and medial. The apical bronchus of the lower lobe originates at the same level as the middle lobe bronchus. The right bronchus continues, forming the four basal segments: medial, anterior, lateral and posterior, of which the posterior is the largest. Note that the right main bronchus is larger than the left due to the fact that the right lung is larger than the left (60%:40%).

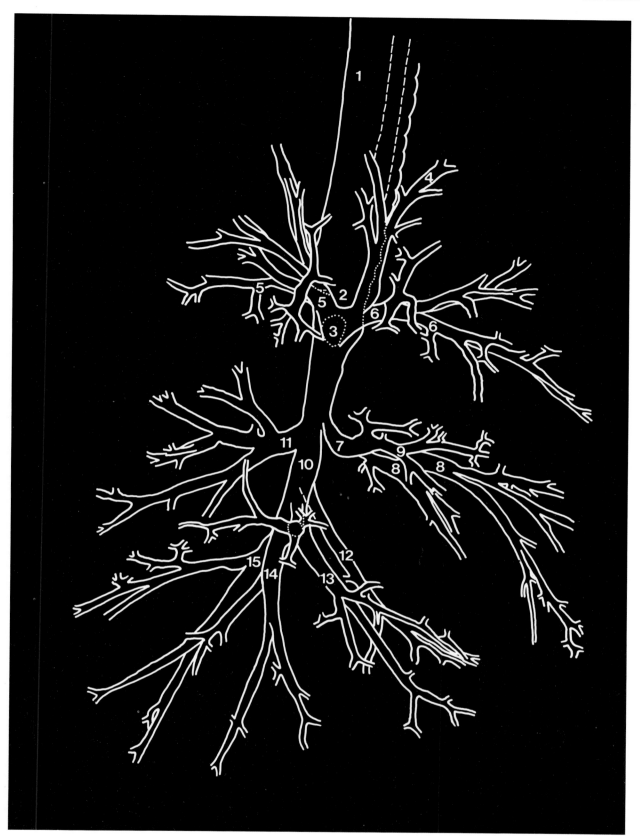

1	Trachea	6	Ant. segmental bronchus	11	Sup. segmental bronchus (apical basal)
2	R. main bronchus	7	Middle lobe bronchus	12	Med. basal segmental bronchus
3	R. upper lobe bronchus	8	Lat. segmental bronchus	13	Ant. basal segmental bronchus
4	Apical segmental bronchus	9	Med. segmental bronchus	14	Lat. basal segmental bronchus
5	Post. segmental bronchus	10	R. lower lobe bronchus	15	Post. basal segmental bronchus

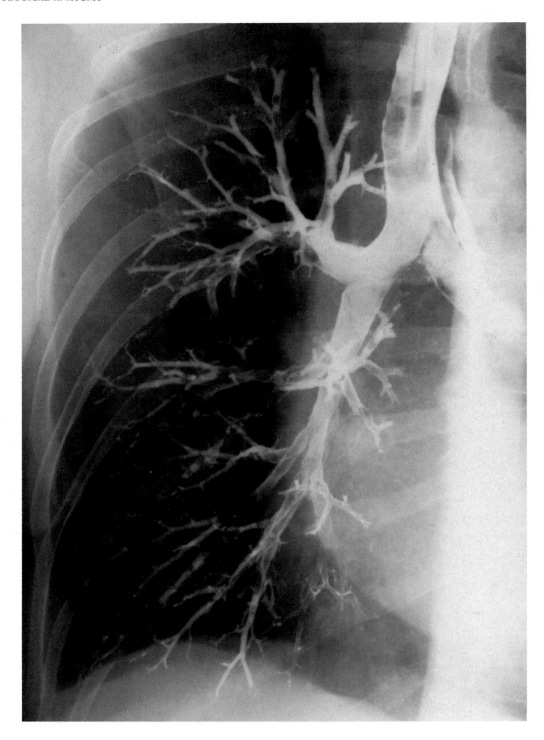

LEFT ANTERIOR OBLIQUE BRONCHOGRAM OF RIGHT LUNG

There are three main techniques for performing bronchography. The first method is to protrude the tongue anteriorly and to lean the patient forward so that contrast medium can be poured over the back of the tongue, through the larynx and into the trachea and major bronchi. The second method is to pass a soft tube, either via the nose or less commonly via the mouth, into the trachea and to inject contrast medium directly into the major bronchi. Both these methods require local anaesthesia of the pharynx and larynx, administered by spray. The amount of local anaesthetic should not exceed 20 ml of 1%, or side effects due to mucosal uptake may develop. The third method is to puncture the trachea either through the cricothyroid membrane or just below the cricoid. Contrast is then injected directly into the trachea. Although this method is quick there are two main disadvantages: first, the leakage of air into the surrounding subcutaneous tissue, which may cause compression and lead to infection; and secondly, accidental injection of contrast medium into the paratracheal tissues may cause subsequent damage.

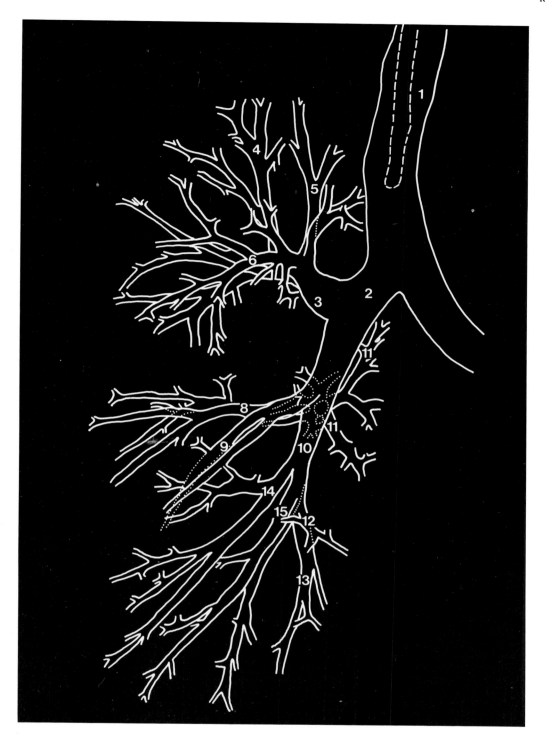

1   Trachea

2   R. main bronchus

3   R. upper lobe bronchus

4   Apical segmental bronchus

5   Post. segmental bronchus

6   Ant. segmental bronchus

7   Middle lobe bronchus

8   Lat. segmental bronchus

9   Med. segmental bronchus

10 R. lower lobe bronchus

11 Sup. segmental bronchus (apical basal)

12 Med. basal segmental bronchus

13 Ant. basal segmental bronchus

14 Lat. basal segmental bronchus

15 Post. basal segmental bronchus

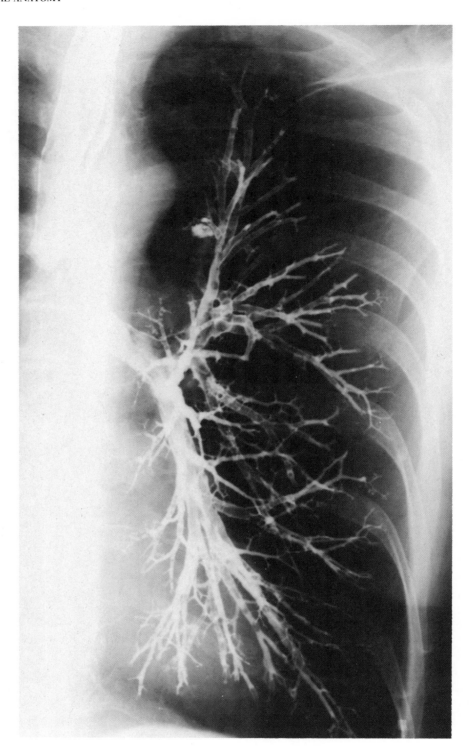

POSTEROANTERIOR BRONCHOGRAM OF LEFT LUNG

The anatomy of the bronchopulmonary segments in the left lung are shown on this and the next two films. Note that there are several differences between the left and the right lung. On the left side there are two lobes divided by the oblique fissure. The left main bronchus is 3.5 cm in length and divides into the left upper lobe and left lower lobe bronchi. The left upper lobe bronchus bifurcates into an upper lobe proper and a lingular segment in about 80% of cases. In 20% there is a trifurcation with the anterior segmental bronchus coming between the upper lobe proper and the lingula below. The left upper lobe has four main bronchopulmonary segments: apicoposterior, anterior, superior lingular and inferior lingular. Notice that the apicoposterior bronchus quickly divides into the apical and posterior subsegments. The lingula on the left is the equivalent of the middle lobe on the right.

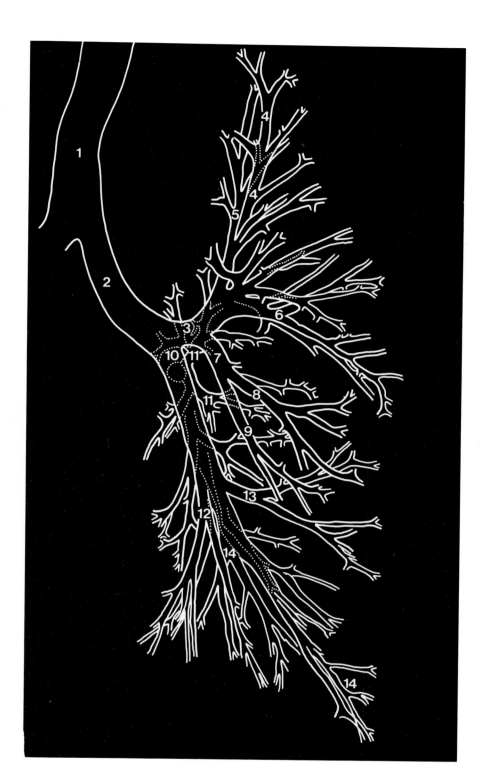

1	Trachea	6	Ant. segmental bronchus	11	Sup. segmental bronchus (apical basal)
2	L. main bronchus	7	Lingular lobe bronchus	12	Anteromedial basal segmental bronchus
3	L. upper lobe bronchus	8	Sup. lingular segmental bronchus		
4	Apical segmental bronchus	9	Inf. lingular segmental bronchus	13	Lat. basal segmental bronchus
5	Post. segmental bronchus	10	L. lower lobe bronchus	14	Post. basal segmental bronchus

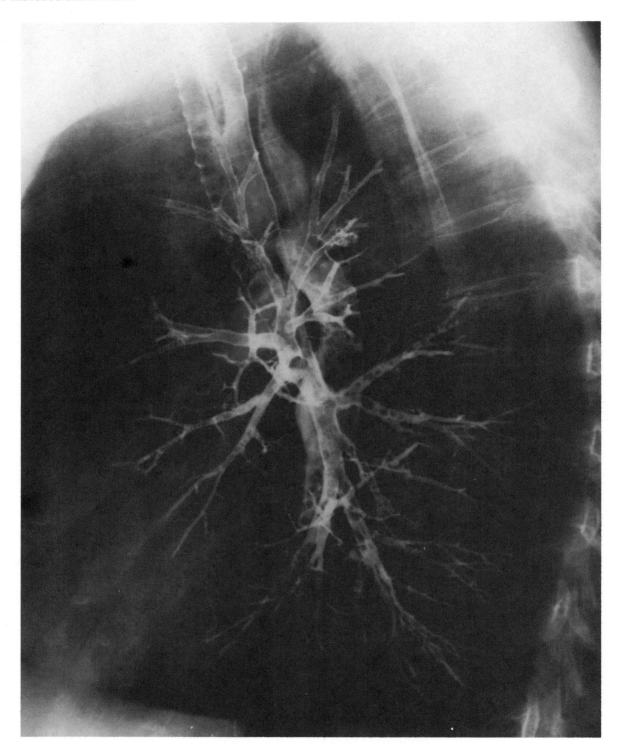

LEFT LATERAL BRONCHOGRAM OF LEFT LUNG

The left lower lobe bronchus divides into four segments: apical, anteromedial basal, lateral basal and posterior basal. Once again, the posterior basal segment is the largest segmental bronchus in the left lung. Note the common origin of the anteromedial basal segment, which is normal. There is considerable variation in bronchopulmonary segmentation, therefore bronchography is a less reliable method of correct labelling than anatomical sections.

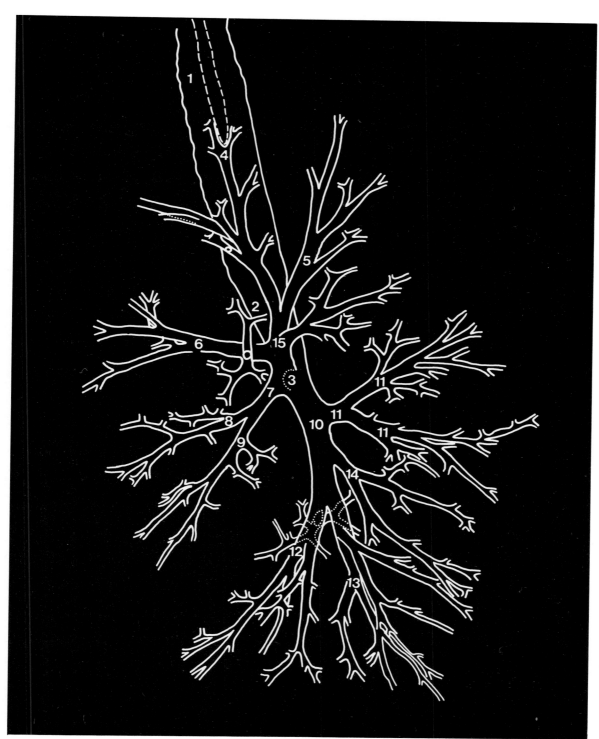

1 Trachea

2 L. main bronchus

3 L. upper lobe bronchus

4 Apical segmental bronchus

5 Post. segmental bronchus

6 Ant. segmental bronchus

7 Lingular lobe bronchus

8 Sup. lingular segmental bronchus

9 Inf. lingular segmental bronchus

10 L. lower lobe bronchus

11 Sup. segmental bronchus (apical basal)

12 Anteromedial basal segmental bronchus

13 Lat. basal segmental bronchus

14 Post. basal segmental bronchus

15 Apicoposterior segmental bronchus

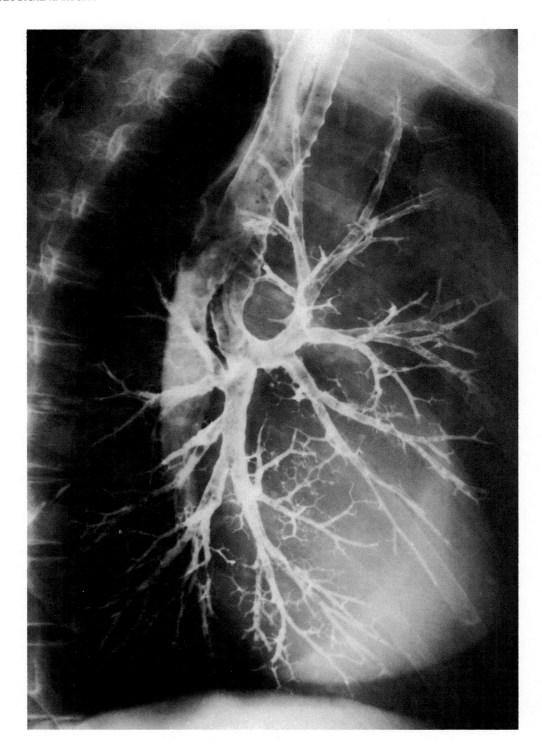

RIGHT ANTERIOR OBLIQUE BRONCHOGRAM OF LEFT LUNG

Bronchography is of particular use in bronchiectasis where a knowledge of the degree of disease is required prior to surgery. The technique is also of use when trying to distinguish between an adenoma and a carcinoma, as the appearances are different.

Recently superselective bronchography using a guided catheter has been introduced so that individual bronchopulmonary segments can be visualized. Further methods include barium and tantalum inhalation.

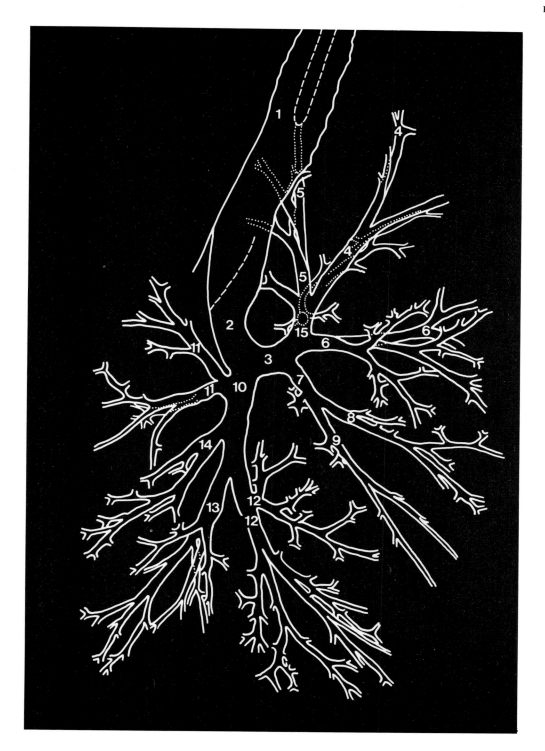

1   Trachea

2   L. main bronchus

3   L. upper lobe bronchus

4   Apical segmental bronchus

5   Post. segmental bronchus

6   Ant. segmental bronchus

7   Lingular lobe bronchus

8   Sup. lingular segmental bronchus

9   Inf. lingular segmental bronchus

10 L. lower lobe bronchus

11 Sup. segmental bronchus (apical basal)

12 Anteromedial basal segmental bronchus

13 Lat. basal segmental bronchus

14 Post. basal segmental bronchus

15 Apicoposterior segmental bronchus

ARTERIAL SYSTEM

RIGHT SELECTIVE CORONARY ARTERIOGRAMS

The right main coronary artery arises from the anterior aortic sinus. It passes forwards and to the right, to emerge between the pulmonary trunk and the right atrium. It then runs inferiorly and to the right in the atrioventricular groove to reach the crux. It then runs on the back of the heart as far as the posterior interventricular groove, where it anastomoses with the left coronary artery. In approximately 70% of patients the right coronary is dominant, i.e. it crosses the crux of the heart and supplies part of the left ventricular wall and interventricular septum. The selective catheter in the right coronary artery has been introduced by Judkins' technique via the femoral artery. There are three different systems of naming the aortic cusps. The official names are posterior, right and left (*Nomina Anatomica*, 1977). *Gray's Anatomy* (Warwick & Williams, 1980, p. 651) names the cusps anterior, left posterior and right posterior. In clinical practice, the cusps are named by reference to their coronary arteries; hence the anterior is the right coronary, the left posterior the left coronary and the right posterior the non-coronary.

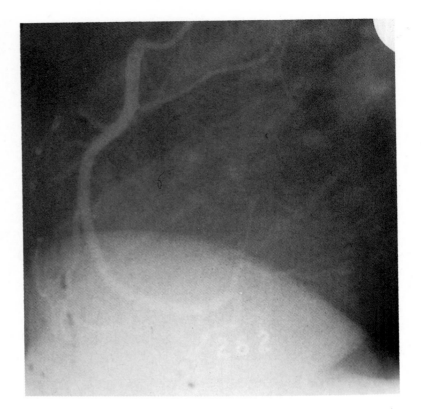

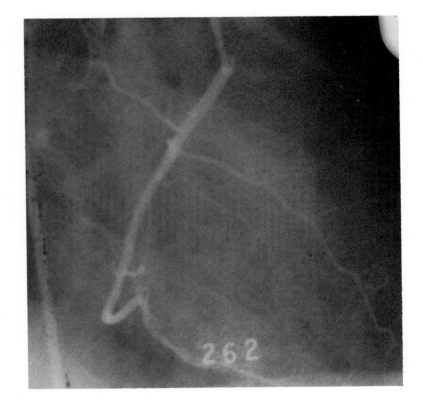

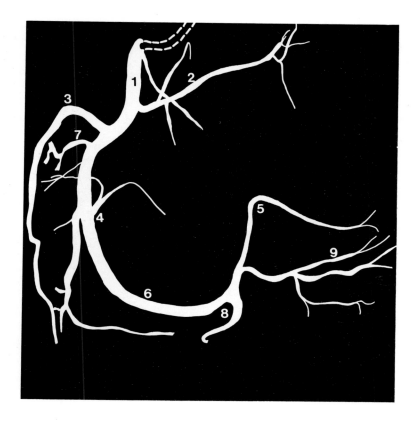

A   Lateral

1   R. main coronary a.

2   Branch to sinuatrial node

3   R. ventricular a.

4   Branch to atrioventricular node

5   Post. interventricular branch

6   Marginal a.

7   Acute marginal branch

8   Post. descending branch

9   Posterolateral branch

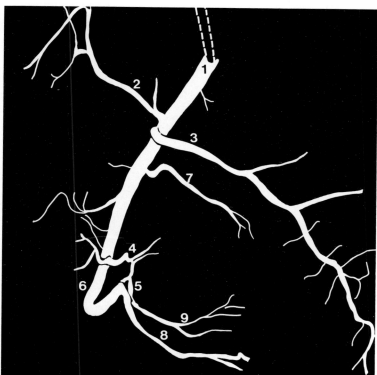

B   Right anterior oblique

LEFT SELECTIVE CORONARY ARTERIOGRAMS

The left main coronary artery arises from the left posterior aortic sinus and runs between the pulmonary trunk and the left atrial appendage. It then turns into the coronary sulcus after dividing into its two major branches—the anterior descending branch which runs in the anterior interventricular groove to the apex of the heart, and the circumflex branch which runs in the left atrioventricular sulcus giving off branches to the upper lateral left ventricular wall and left atrium. This selective coronary arteriogram was again performed using Judkins' technique. Coronary arteriography has become increasingly important with the investigation and surgery of ischaemic heart disease, and the number of examinations performed each year is ever increasing. It is important to note the variations of the normal anatomy and to know the branches so that they can be recognized in any plane.

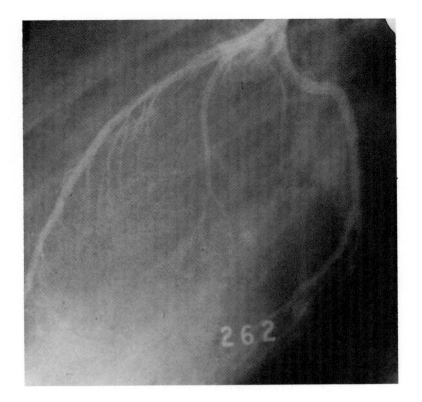

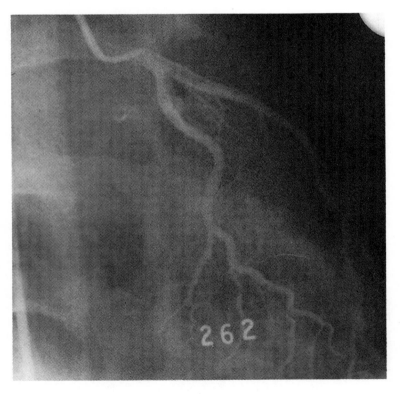

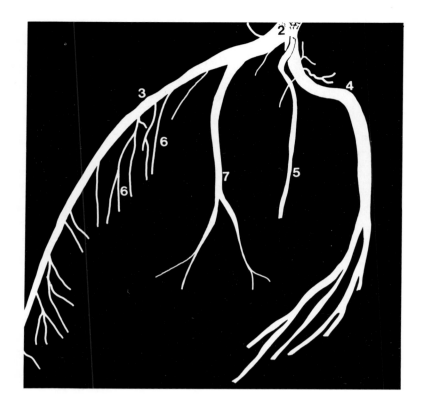

1   Catheter tip in l. coronary a.

2   Main trunk of l. coronary a.

3   Ant. descending interventricular
     branch

4   Circumflex a.

5   Obtuse marginal branch

6   Septal branches

7   Diagonal branch

8   Med. circumflex a.

9   Lat. circumflex a.

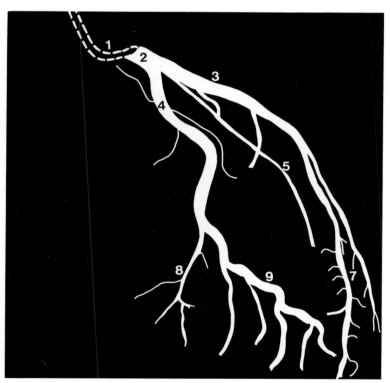

B   Posteroanterior

143

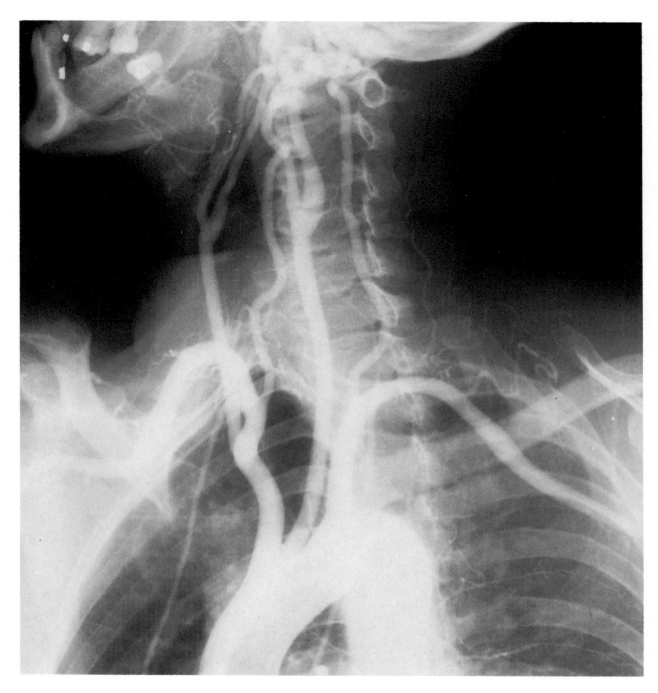

AORTIC ARCH ARTERIOGRAM—LEFT ANTERIOR OBLIQUE VIEW

The aorta gives off three branches from the upper aspect of its arch: the brachiocephalic, the left common carotid and the left subclavian. The left anterior oblique projection is used so that the arch and vessel origins are demonstrated more clearly. There are several congenital variations of the distribution of the major vessels, the commonest being a common brachiocephalic trunk giving rise to both common carotid arteries. The brachiocephalic artery is the largest branch of the aorta and its course takes it to lie on the right side of the trachea. In old people, this artery commonly elongates and becomes tortuous, giving rise to a soft tissue impression on the right side of the upper mediastinum on a PA

chest radiograph. It divides into the right common carotid and right subclavian arteries at the upper border of the right sterno-clavicular joint. The subclavian artery supplying the arm extends from its origin to the outer border of the first rib, where it becomes the axillary artery. The catheter has been introduced into the aortic arch via the femoral route and the contrast medium (water-soluble with an iodine content of around 400 mg/ml) injected under pressure. A lower concentration of iodine of about 280 mg/ml is used for all the following peripheral angiography demonstrated and for the cerebral angiography.

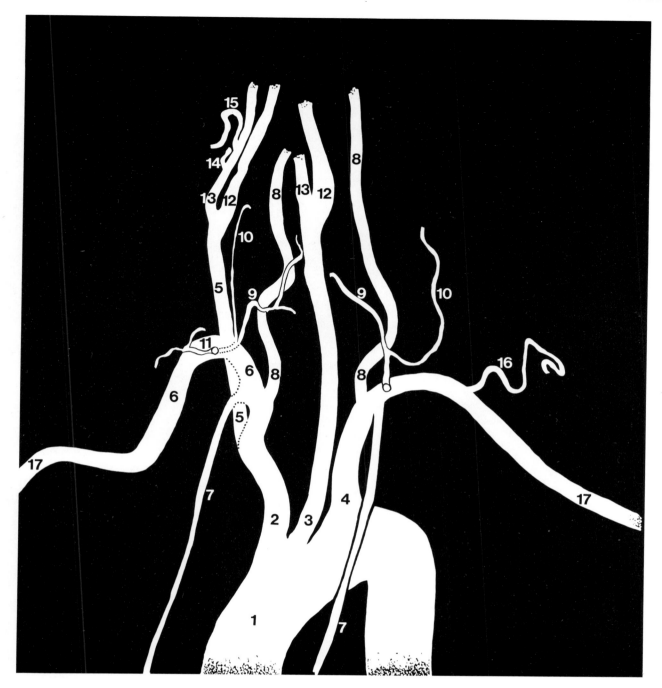

1	Ascending aorta	7	Internal thoracic (mammary) a.	13	External carotid a.
2	Brachiocephalic (innominate) a.	8	Vertebral a.	14	Lingual a.
3	L. common carotid a.	9	Inf. thyroid a.	15	Facial a.
4	L. subclavian a.	10	Ascending cervical a.	16	Suprascapular a.
5	R. common carotid a.	11	Costocervical trunk	17	Axillary a.
6	R. subclavian art.	12	Internal carotid a.		

EXTERNAL CAROTID ARTERIOGRAMS

The branches of the external carotid artery from its origin are superior thyroid, ascending pharyngeal, lingual, facial, occipital, posterior auricular, superficial temporal and maxillary. The external carotid artery begins at the level of the C3/4 disc and ascends to the angle of the jaw where it enters the parotid gland, to divide into the terminal branches of the superficial temporal and maxillary arteries. One reason for performing selective catheterization of the external carotid is to assess the blood supply to tumours. Two examples of this are the vault meningioma, which often has a dual blood supply from the common carotid as well as the external carotid, and the rare juvenile nasopharyngeal fibroma (fibrohaemangioma). It is possible to inject directly the superficial temporal artery in patients with temporal arteritis to show the position of lesions, which can then be biopsied.

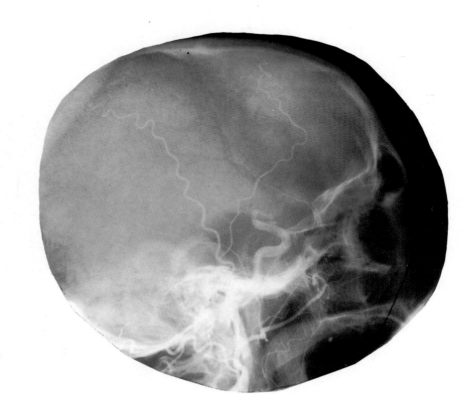

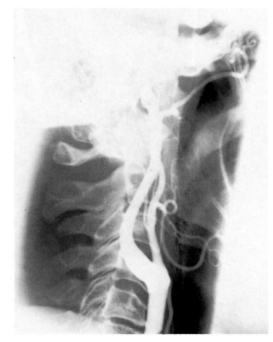

146

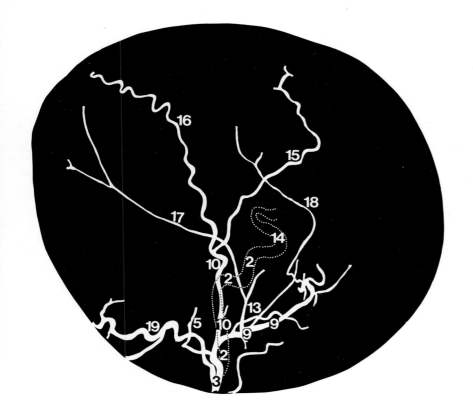

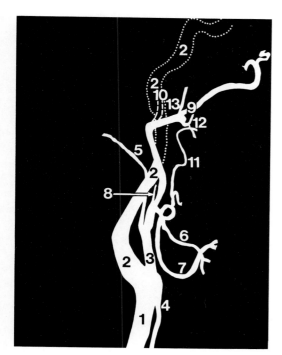

1 Common carotid a.

2 Internal carotid a.

3 External carotid a.

4 Sup. thyroid a.

5 Post. auricular a.

6 Lingual a.

7 Facial a.

8 Ascending pharyngeal a.

9 Maxillary (internal maxillary) a.

10 Superficial temporal a.

11 Ascending palatine a.

12 Inf. alveolar (dental) a.

13 Middle meningeal a.

14 Internal carotid siphon (cavernous part)

15 Frontal branch, superficial temporal a.

16 Parietal branch, superficial temporal a.

17 Parietal branch, middle meningeal a.

18 Frontal branch, middle meningeal a.

19 Occipital a.

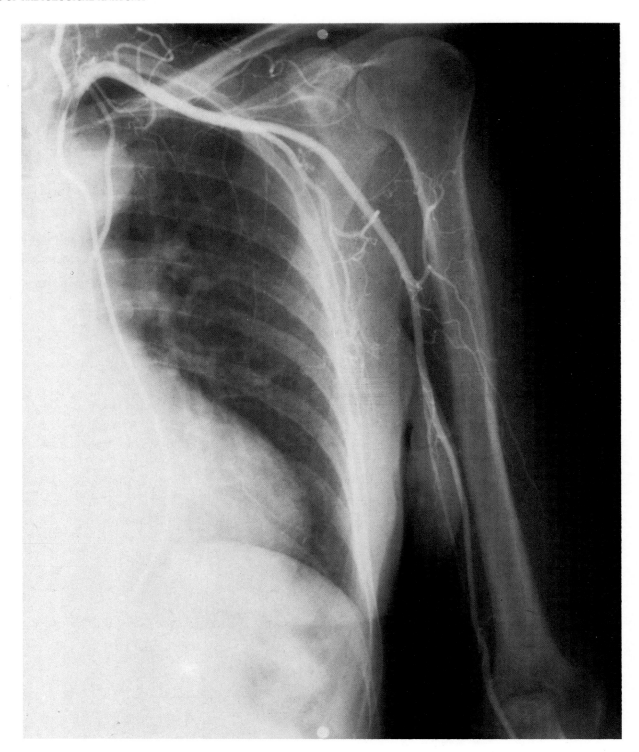

SUBCLAVIAN-AXILLARY ARTERIOGRAM

The axillary artery runs from the outer border of the first rib to the lower border of the teres major muscle whence it becomes the brachial artery. The branches of the subclavian artery are the vertebral, internal thoracic, thyrocervical trunk and costocervical trunk. On the left side of the neck the four branches arise from the first part of the subclavian artery whereas on the right side the costocervical trunk often springs from the second part. The subclavian artery is divided into its three parts by the scalenus anterior muscle. Note the anastomosis between the suprascapular and acromial arteries. Note also the anastomosis of the circumflex humeral arteries which give branches to the shoulder joint. One of the common reasons for performing this selective arteriogram is to demonstrate compression of the subclavian artery by a cervical rib or fibrous band. Careful positioning of the patient's arm may be needed to show this vascular abnormality.

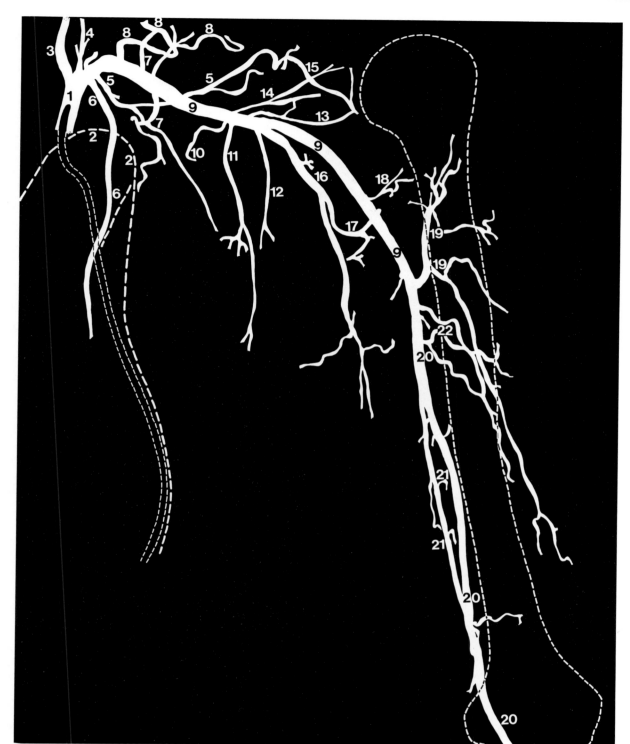

1	Catheter in l. subclavian a.	9	Axillary a.	15	Anastomoses between suprascapular and acromial aa.
2	Aortic knuckle or knob	10	Sup. thoracic a.	16	Subscapular a.
3	Vertebral a.	11	Lat. thoracic a.	17	Circumflex scapular a.
4	Inf. thyroid a.	12	Pectoral branch, thoracoacromial a.	18	Ant. circumflex humeral a.
5	Suprascapular a.	13	Acromial branch, thoracoacromial a.	19	Post. circumflex humeral a.
6	Internal thoracic (mammary) a.	14	Deltoid branch, thoracoacromial a.	20	Brachial a.
7	Dorsal scapular a.			21	Profunda brachii a.
8	Transverse cervical (superficial cervical) a.			22	Deltoid branch, profunda brachii a.

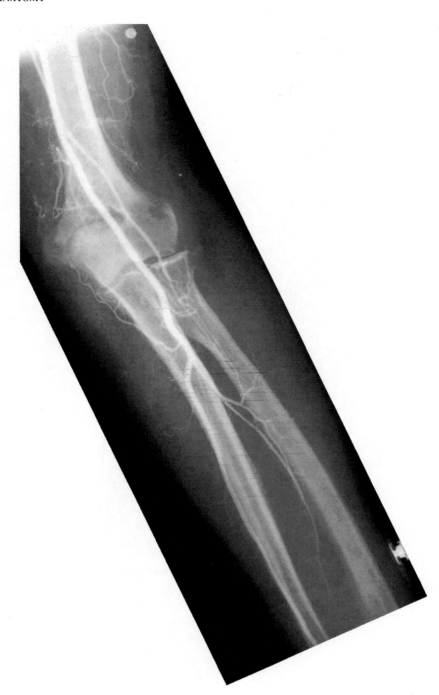

BRACHIAL ARTERIOGRAM

The brachial artery is a continuation of the axillary artery; it begins at the lower border of teres major and ends about 1 cm below the elbow joint by dividing into the radial and ulnar arteries. The distal division is often variable with a high take-off point, particularly of the radial artery. The profunda brachii artery is a large vessel which arises from the brachial artery below the teres major muscle. It closely follows the radial nerve, running in the groove covered by the lateral head of the triceps muscle. The ulnar artery is the larger of the two terminal branches of the brachial artery and passes to the medial side of the forearm to cross the flexor retinaculum on the lateral side of the ulnar nerve. The anterior and posterior interosseous arteries arise from the ulnar artery via the common interosseous artery. They descend on the surfaces of the interosseous membrane itself. Note the congenital variation present with no radial artery shown.

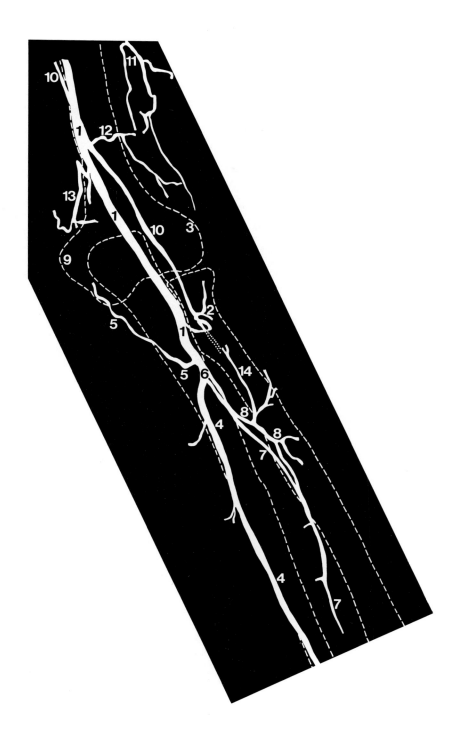

1	Brachial a.	6	Common interosseous a.	11	Descending branch of post. humeral circumflex a.
2	Radial recurrent a.	7	Ant. interosseous a.	12	Ascending branch of profunda brachii a.
3	Lat. epicondyle	8	Post. interosseous a.	13	Inf. ulnar collateral a.
4	Ulnar a.	9	Med. epicondyle	14	Interosseous recurrent a.
5	Ulnar recurrent a.	10	Profunda brachii a.		

ANTEROPOSTERIOR VIEW OF HAND ARTERIOGRAM

The median artery arises from the anterior interosseus artery and accompanies the median nerve. It is of variable size and, when large, may join the superficial palmar arch. The superficial palmar arch is formed mainly by the ulnar artery which crosses on the medial side of the hook of the hamate to spread across the palm and become the arch. The anatomy of the superificial and deep arches is shown. Two pathological conditions which can be visualized on hand arteriography are the digital vessel occlusion seen in Raynaud's disease and the small microaneurysms seen in the collagen disease, polyarteritis nodosa.

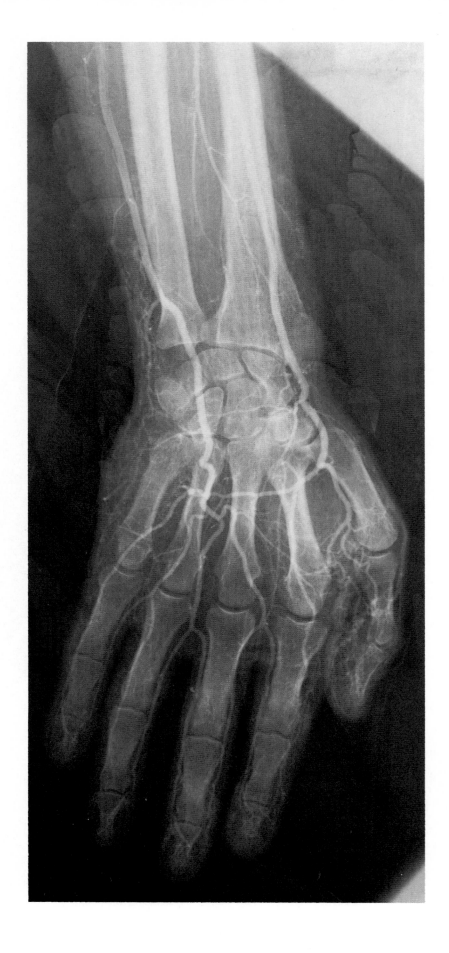

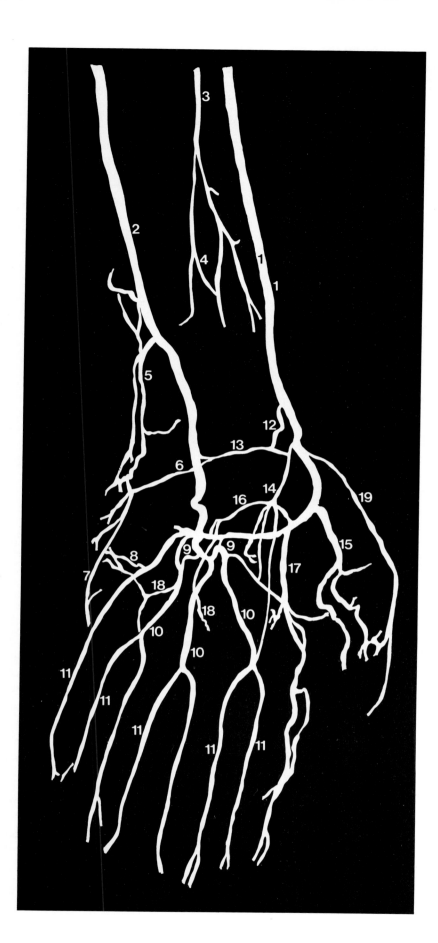

1   Radial a.

2   Ulnar a.

3   Ant. interosseus a.

4   Median a.

5   Deep palmar branch of ulnar a.

6   Palmar carpal branch of ulnar a.

7   Dorsal carpal branch of ulnar a.

8   Deep palmar branch of ulnar a.

9   Superficial palmar arch

10 Common palmar digital aa.

11 Proper palmar digital aa.

12 Palmar carpal branch of radial a.

13 Palmar carpal arch

14 Superficial palmar branch of
    radial a.

15 Princeps pollicis a.

16 Deep palmar arch

17 Radialis indicis a.

18 Palmar metacarpal a.

19 A. to radial aspect of thumb

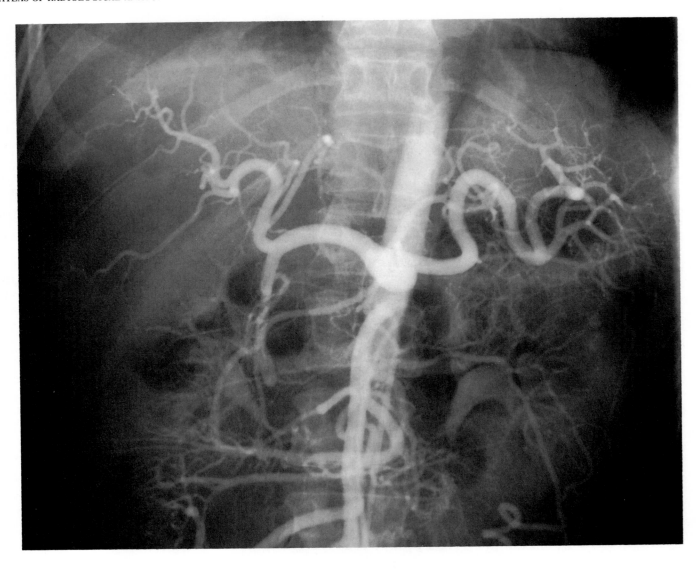

COELIAC ARTERIOGRAM

The coeliac artery comes off the ventral aspect of the abdominal aorta at the level of the T12/L1 disc. The three major branches are the left gastric, common hepatic and splenic. The common hepatic artery gives off the gastroduodenal artery and continues as the hepatic proper which ascends via the porta hepatis to divide into left and right branches supplying the corresponding lobes of the liver. In the lesser omentum, the hepatic artery lies in front of the portal vein and on the left side of the common bile duct, with its right branch usually crossing behind the common hepatic duct. With recent techniques of catheterization, superselective arteriograms can be performed with subtraction. These are of particular value when looking for pancreatic lesions.

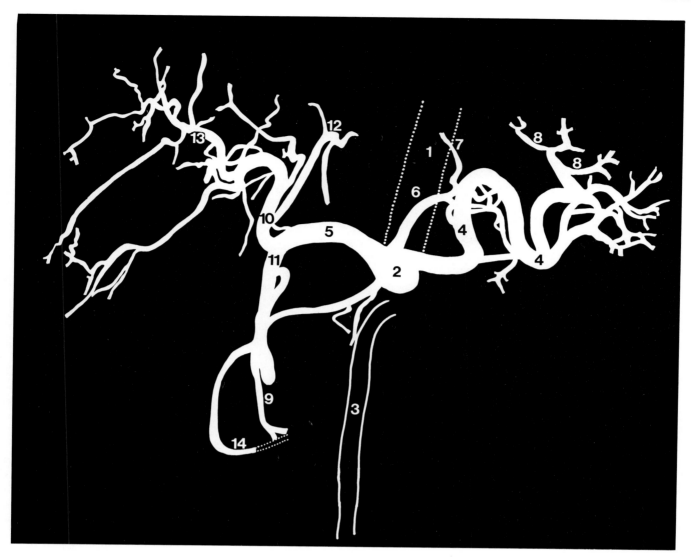

1	Abdominal aorta	6	L. gastric a.	10	Hepatic a. proper
2	Coeliac trunk	7	Oesophageal branches of l. gastric a.	11	Gastroduodenal a.
3	Sup. mesenteric a.			12	L. hepatic a.
4	Splenic a.	8	Splenic a. branches	13	R. hepatic a.
5	Common hepatic a.	9	Sup. pancreaticoduodenal a.	14	R. gastroepiploic a.

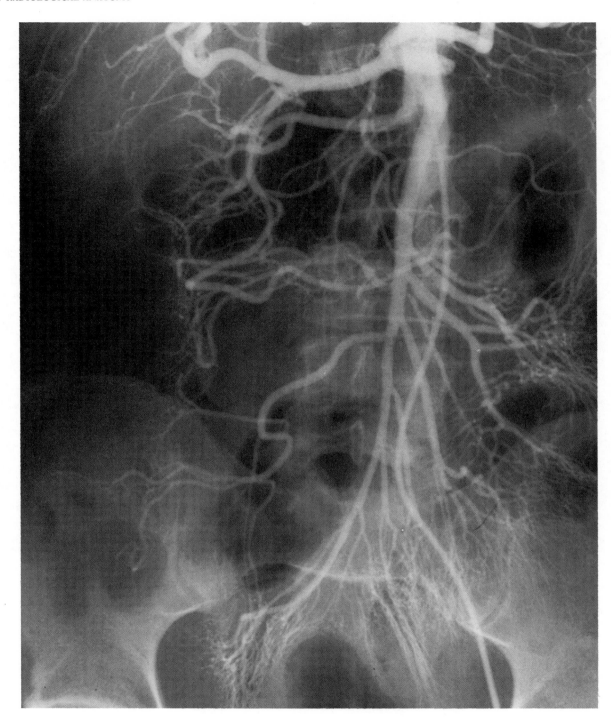

SUPERIOR MESENTERIC ARTERIOGRAM

The superior mesenteric artery supplies the whole of the small intestine, except the upper part of the duodenum. It also supplies the caecum, ascending colon and most of the transverse colon. It originates about 1 cm below the coeliac artery, is crossed anteriorly by the splenic vein and body of the pancreas and then passes downwards and forwards, anterior to the head of the pancreas to reach the mesentery. Note the congenital variation of an accessory right hepatic artery coming from the superior mesenteric artery. The coeliac and superior mesenteric artery systems have numerous congenital variations, particularly concerning the vascular supply of the pancreas. If a patient is suspected of having mesenteric ischaemia, then a lateral film of the abdominal aorta should be performed so that the origins of both the coeliac and superior mesenteric arteries may be seen and checked for narrowing. Occasionally, the superior mesenteric artery is seen to cause an impression on the third part of the duodenum on a barium meal as it crosses anteriorly, and this can very rarely cause a degree of duodenal obstruction.

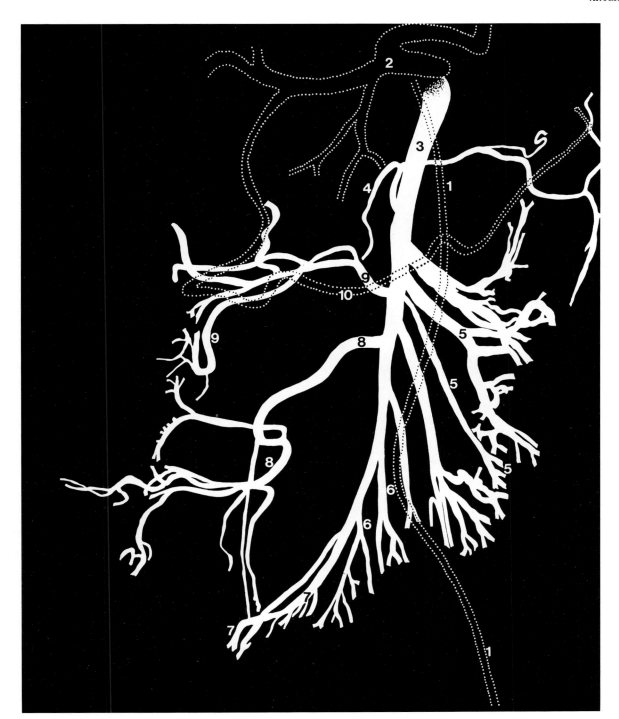

1	Catheter via femoral route	4	Inf. pancreaticoduodenal a.	8	R. colic a.
2	Coeliac trunk and branches (dotted)	5	Jejunal branches	9	Middle colic a.
3	Sup. mesenteric a.	6	Ileal branches	10	L. gastroepiploic a. (branch of coeliac trunk)
		7	Ileocolic a.		

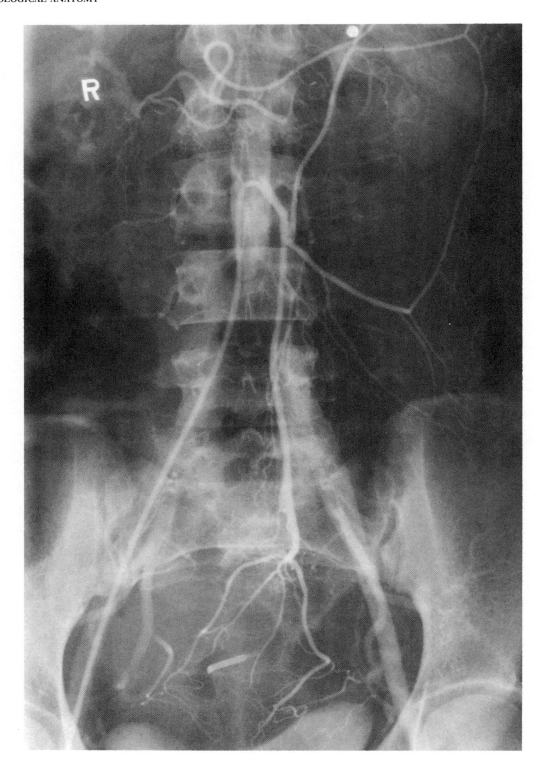

INFERIOR MESENTERIC ARTERIOGRAM

The inferior mesenteric artery supplies blood to the distal transverse colon, descending colon, sigmoid colon and rectum. It originates about 3–4 cm above the aortic bifurcation at the level of L3 or just above the lower border of the third part of the duodenum. It crosses the left common iliac artery on the medial side of the left ureter and continues into the sigmoid mesocolon to become the superior rectal artery. Note the anastomosis of the marginal artery of Drummond. The anastomoses in the region of the splenic flexure of the colon constitute the most vulnerable part of the intestine's blood supply and are therefore most prone to ischaemia. The grades of ischaemia can be diagnosed on a barium enema and divided into acute, subacute and chronic changes. The inferior mesenteric artery may considerably enlarge when there is disease of the common iliac vessels and be an important collateral route for the blood supply of the pelvis and lower limbs.

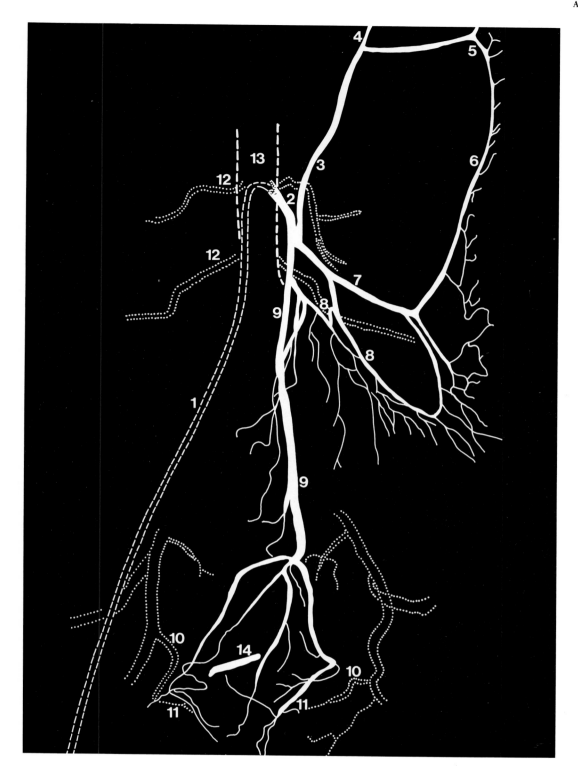

1 Percutaneous catheter into inf. mesenteric a.

2 Inf. mesenteric a.

3 L. colic a.

4 Ascending branch of l. colic a.

5 Descending branch of l. colic a.

6 Marginal a. (Drummond)

7 Sigmoid a (inf. l. colic)

8 Anastomosis between sigmoid and sup. rectal aa.

9 Sup. rectal a.

10 Middle rectal a.—branch of internal iliac a.

11 Anastomosis of sup. and middle rectal aa.

12 Reflux in lumbar aa.

13 Reflux in aorta

14 Intrauterine contraceptive device (IUCD)

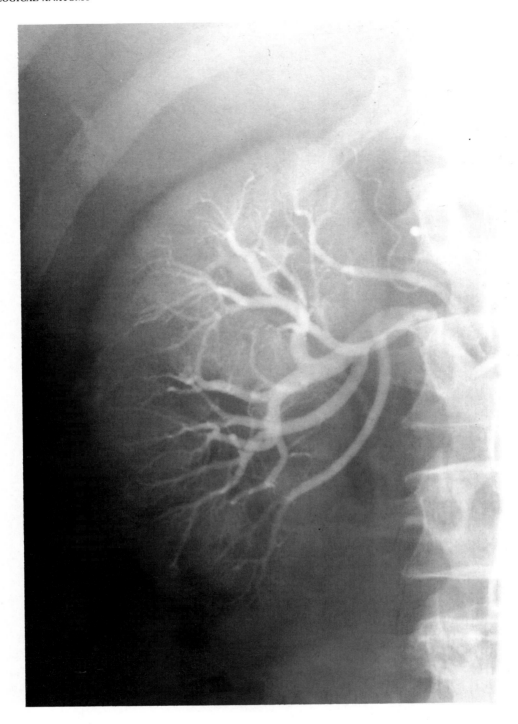

SELECTIVE RENAL ARTERIOGRAM

For most selective catheterizations, preshaped catheters are used so that injection into the vessel of choice is possible. The renal arteries arise from the lateral walls of the aorta at the level of the L1/2 disc. The right renal artery is longer than the left due to the position of the aorta, and it passes behind the inferior vena cava to reach the hilum of the kidney. The left renal artery is slightly higher than the right and lies behind the left renal vein. Accessory renal arteries are often found; they most commonly arise from the aorta either above or below the main artery and usually enter either the upper or lower parts of the kidneys away from the hilum. These accessory arteries may very occasionally arise from the iliac vessels. Renal arteriography is performed for two major reasons: first, to demonstrate the main renal artery to look for narrowing in cases of hypertension and, secondly, for the differential diagnosis of renal masses. It is important when diagnosing renal artery narrowing that the whole of the main artery, including its origin, is seen. It is often necessary to perform a non-selective lower abdominal aortogram to show these details.

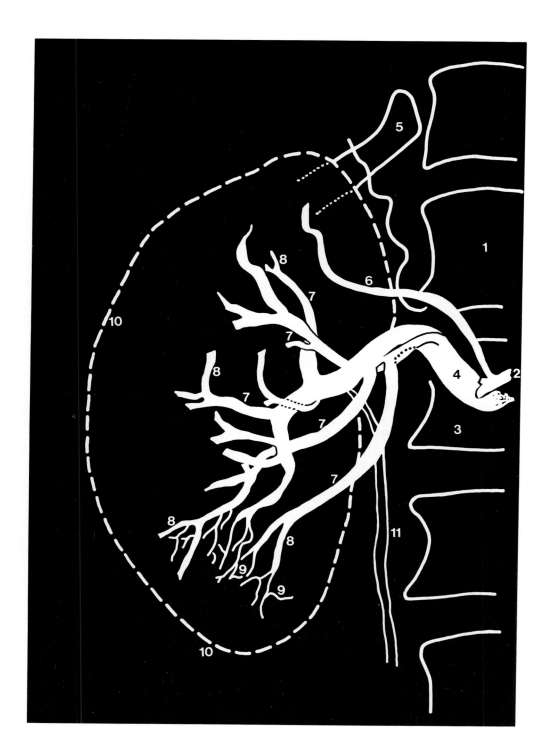

1	Body of L1 vertebra	5	Twelfth rib	9	Arcuate aa.
2	Catheter tip in r. renal a.	6	Inf. suprarenal a.	10	Renal outline
3	Body of L2 vertebra	7	Lobar aa.	11	Ureter overlying transverse process of L3
4	Principal renal a.	8	Interlobular aa.		

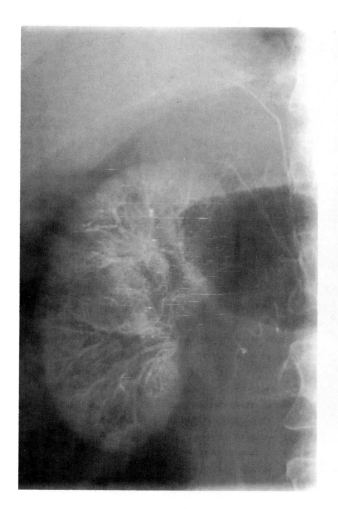
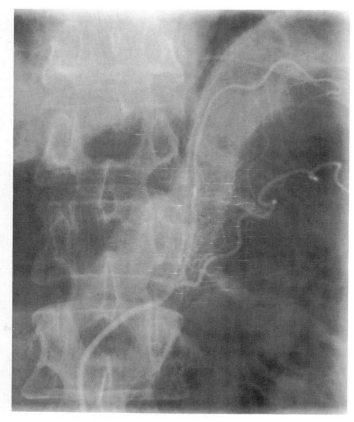

RIGHT AND LEFT SUPRARENAL ARTERIOGRAMS

The blood supply to the suprarenal glands is from three main sources: an inferior suprarenal artery arising from the renal artery, a middle suprarenal artery arising from the aorta and a superior suprarenal artery arising from the inferior phrenic artery. However, this supply is subject to a lot of variation and the glands may be supplied by a variety of other small vessels. A non-selective abdominal aortogram may be sufficient to show large supra-renal tumours, but selective catheterization of the three main blood vessels may be needed to show small tumours. The cortex of the suprarenal gland usually shows as a dense blush about 2 mm wide on angiography with a less opaque medulla. The three main tumours diagnosed by arteriography are carcinomas, neuroblastomas and phaeochromocytomas.

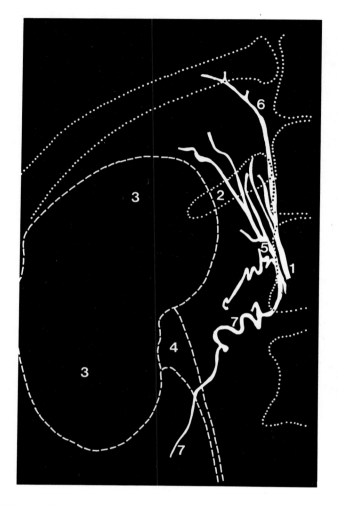
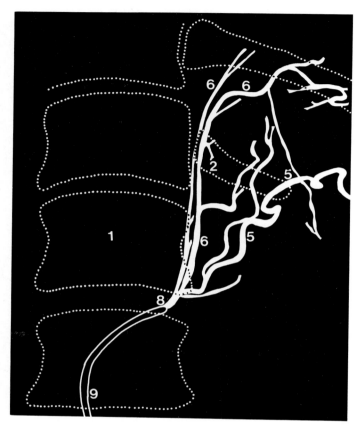

1	Body of L1 vertebra	4	Pelvis of kidney
2	Twelfth rib	5	Inf. suprarenal (adrenal) a.
3	Renal pattern	6	Inf. phrenic a.

7 Ureteric a.

8 Catheter tip in suprarenal (adrenal) a.

9 Catheter in abdominal aorta

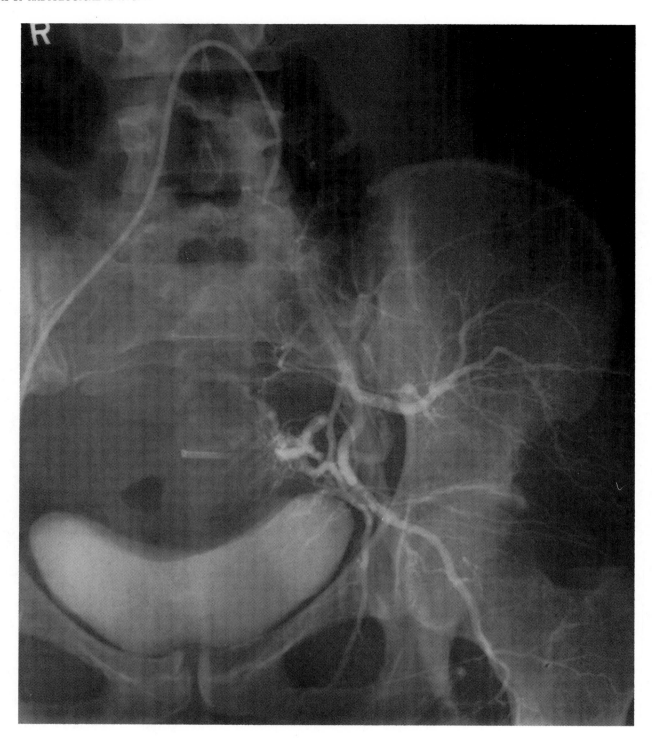

SELECTIVE INTERNAL ILIAC ARTERIOGRAM

The catheter has been introduced into the contralateral femoral artery, negotiated through the aortic bifurcation and down into the opposite internal iliac artery. This is often the easiest method of cannulation because of the acute angle of the origin of this artery. The internal iliac artery arises at about the level of the lumbrosacral disc, in front of the sacroiliac joint. It descends to the margin of the greater sciatic foramen where it divides into anterior and posterior trunks. The anterior trunk is the direct continuation of the internal iliac artery and proceeds towards the ischial spine. The posterior trunk runs backwards towards the foramen. Notice that this patient is female with an intrauterine contraceptive device showing clearly the position of the uterus in relation to the bladder. Note the normal early filling of the uterine venous plexus. In approximately 25% of patients, the obturator artery is replaced by a large pubic branch of the inferior epigastric artery. Rarely, this artery runs along the free margin of the lacunar ligament and may be cut accidentally when a femoral hernia is repaired.

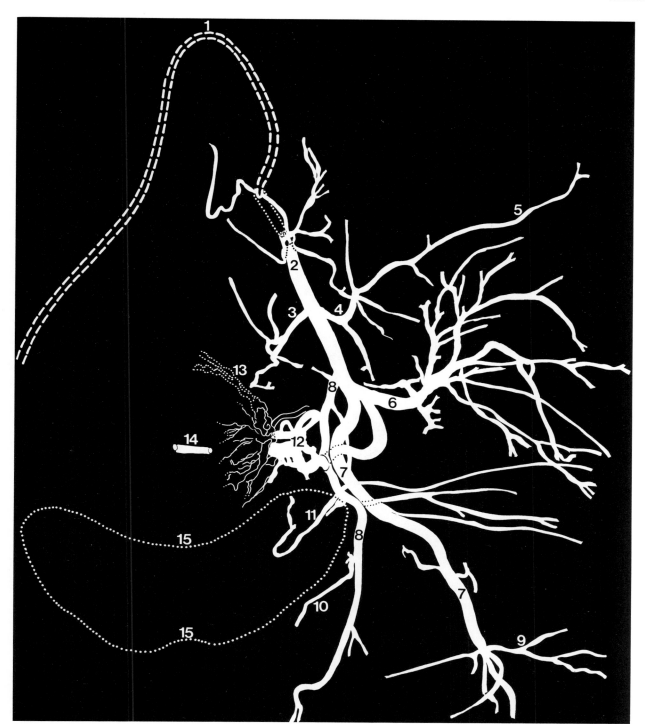

1	Catheter via contralateral femoral route	6	Sup. gluteal a.	11	Sup. vesical aa.
2	Internal iliac a.	7	Inf. gluteal a.	12	Uterine a.
3	Lat. sacral a.	8	Obturator a.	13	Uterine venous plexus
4	Iliolumbar a.	9	Anastomosis with medial circumflex femoral a.	14	Intrauterine contraceptive device (IUCD)
5	Iliac branch of iliolumbar a.	10	Pubic branch of obturator a.	15	Bladder outlined by contrast medium

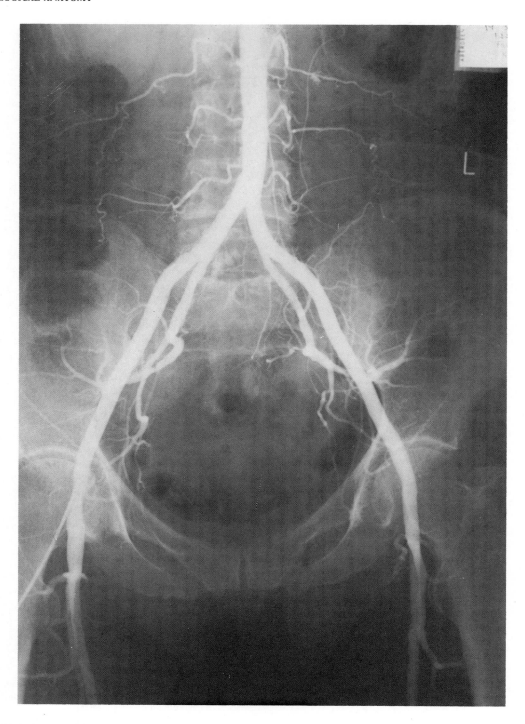

AORTIC AND ILIAC ARTERIOGRAM

The lower abdominal aorta and arterial branches to the mid thigh are demonstrated in this projection. There are two main methods of performing this arteriogram: the one shown is by retrograde catheterization via the femoral artery, the other is by performing a translumbar injection. This latter procedure is performed, usually under general anaesthetic, by introducing a needle into the abdominal aorta via the left flank. Two main approaches are used: high and low, the high injection being approximately at the level of T12, above the renal arteries, and the low injection at approximately L2, below the renal arteries. The site is determined by clinical conditions relating to that particular patient's investigation. To see the origin of the profunda femoris artery, it is necessary to take an oblique projection so that atheromatous disease will not be missed. The femoral artery is the continuation of the external iliac artery and originates deep to the inguinal ligament. It terminates by passing through a hiatus in the adductor magnus muscle to become the popliteal artery. The first 3–4 cm of the femoral artery and vein are enclosed within the femoral sheath. The femoral artery lies lateral to the femoral vein and the femoral nerve lies lateral to the sheath.

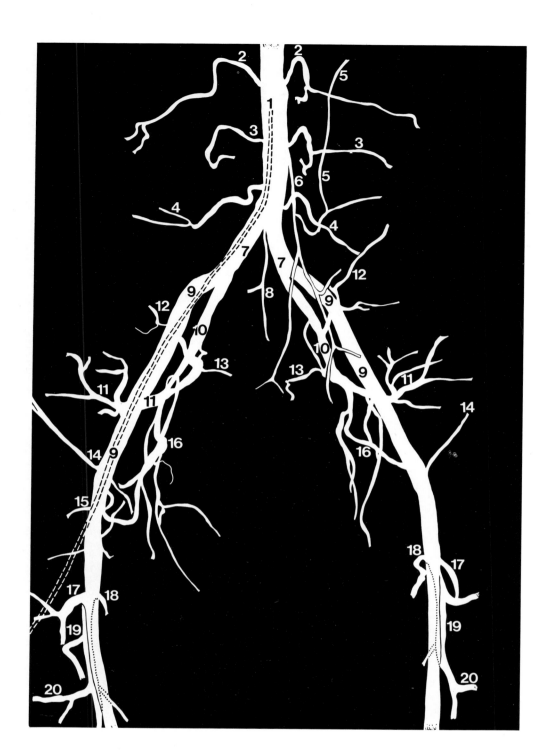

1	Catheter tip in aorta via retrograde femoral route	7	Common iliac a.	14	Deep circumflex iliac a.
2	Third lumbar a.	8	Median sacral a.	15	Superficial circumflex iliac a.
3	Fourth lumbar a.	9	External iliac a.	16	Inf. gluteal a.
4	Fifth lumbar a.	10	Internal iliac a.	17	Lat. circumflex femoral a.
5	L. colic a.	11	Sup. gluteal a.	18	Med. circumflex femoral a.
6	Inf. mesenteric a.	12	Iliolumbar a.	19	Profunda femoris a.
		13	Lat. sacral a.	20	Perforating a.

POPLITEAL ARTERIOGRAM

Femoral and popliteal arteriography can be performed by the techniques described on the previous page or by direct needle puncture and injection of the femoral artery. The popliteal artery begins at the adductor hiatus and runs deep through the popliteal fossa to reach the lower border of the popliteus muscle, where it divides into the anterior and posterior tibial arteries. The anterior tibial artery passes forwards between the heads of the tibialis posterior muscle and through the interosseous membrane to the front of the leg, where it descends on the anterior surface of the membrane and becomes, in the foot, the dorsalis pedis artery. The posterior tibial artery descends medially on the posterior aspect of the leg and terminates as the medial and lateral plantar arteries. The peroneal artery originates from the posterior tibial artery to run in the tibiofibular syndesmosis, to reach the calcaneus.

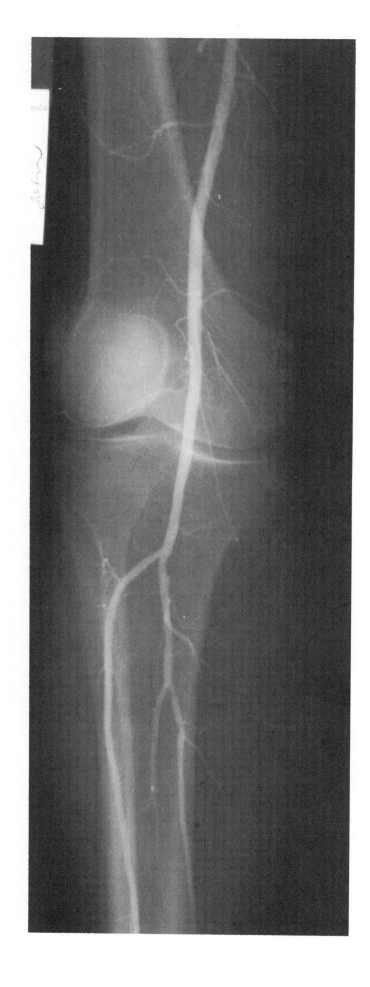

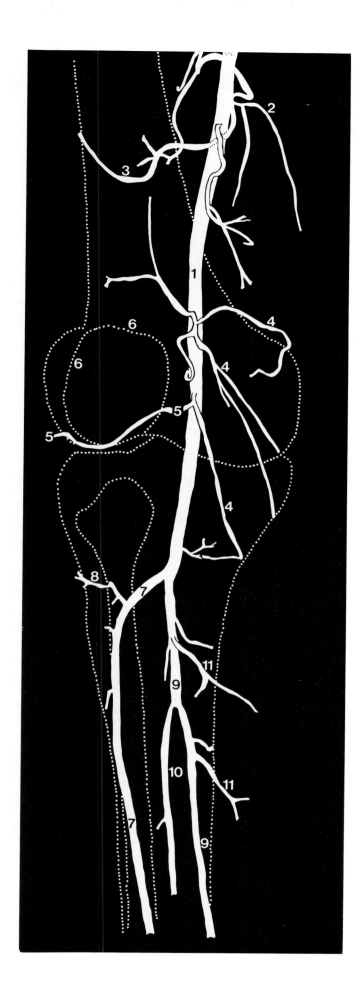

1 Popliteal a.

2 Sup. med. genicular a.

3 Sup. lat. genicular a.

4 Inf. med. genicular aa.

5 Inf. lat. genicular a.

6 Patella

7 Ant. tibial a.

8 Recurrent tibial a.

9 Post. tibial a.

10 Peroneal a.

11 Muscular branches of posterior tibial a.

LOWER LEG ARTERIOGRAM

The anterior tibial artery becomes the dorsalis pedis artery at the level of the ankle joint. At the proximal end of the first intermetatarsal space a branch enters the sole of the foot and the dorsalis pedis becomes the first dorsal metatarsal artery. Occasionally the anterior tibial artery runs a short way down the leg, and the dorsalis pedis artery then arises from the peroneal artery.

The peroneal artery descends on the tibialis posterior muscle and lies deep to the flexor hallucis longus. It ends on the lateral surface of the calcaneum.

The posterior tibial artery begins at the upper border of the soleus and finishes deep to the flexor retinaculum by dividing into the medial and lateral plantar arteries.

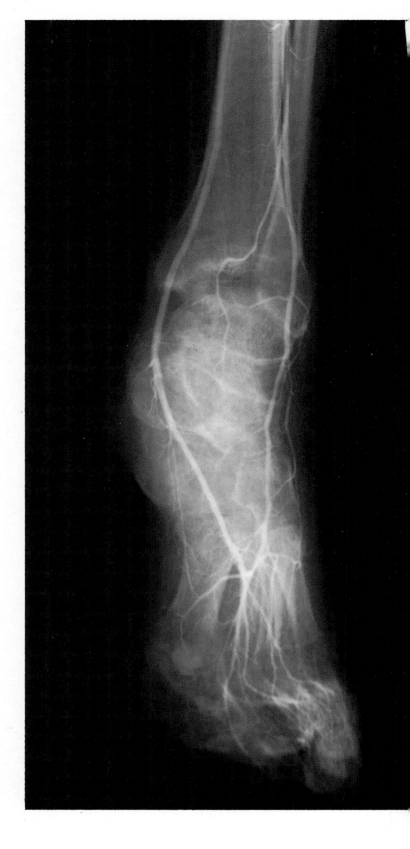

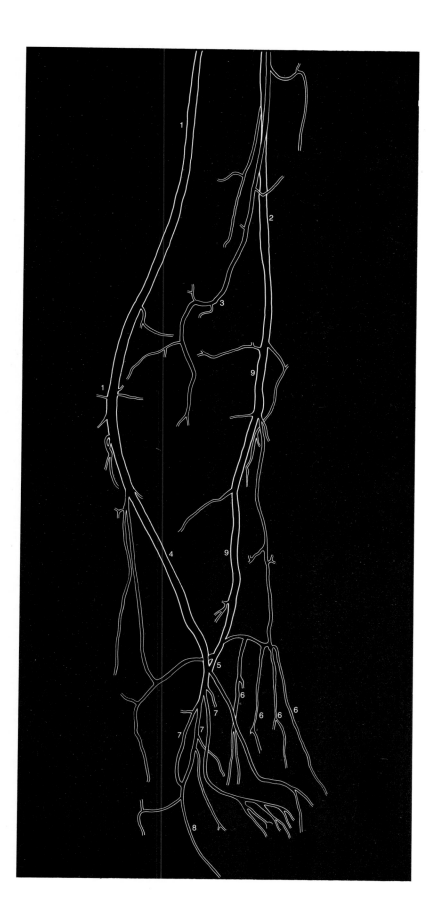

1   Post. tibial a.

2   Ant. tibial a.

3   Peroneal a.

4   Lat. plantar a.

5   Plantar arch

6   Dorsal metatarsal a.

7   Plantar metatarsal a.

8   Med. plantar a.

9   Dorsalis pedis a.

VENOUS AND PULMONARY SYSTEM

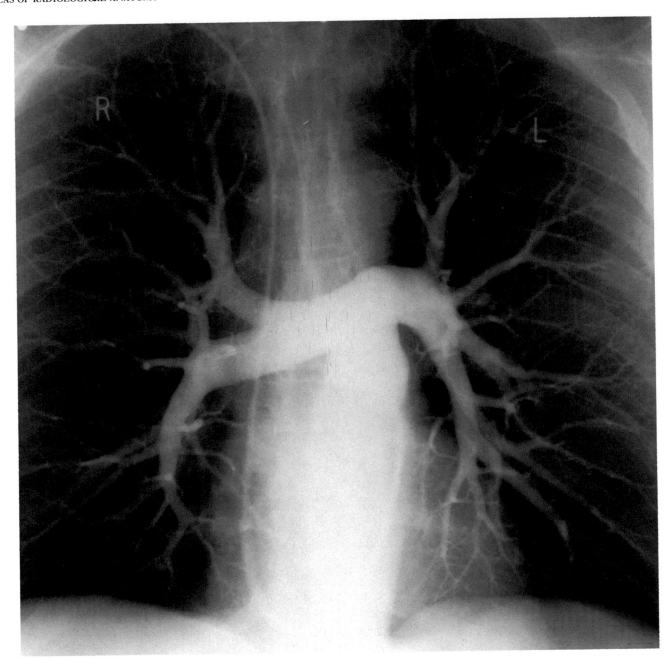

PULMONARY ARTERIOGRAM

Pulmonary arteriography is usually performed by cannulating the median cubital vein at the elbow and passing the catheter through the right atrium and right ventricle into the pulmonary artery. The whole of the pulmonary trunk is contained within the pericardium. The trunk arises from the base of the right ventricle to run upwards and posteriorly in front and then to the left of the ascending aorta. It divides into the right and left pulmonary arteries beneath the aortic arch. The right pulmonary artery is slightly longer and larger than the left and runs horizontally behind the ascending aorta, the superior vena cava and the upper right pulmonary vein. It runs in front of the oesophagus and the right main bronchus, to the root of the right lung, where it divides into two branches. The left pulmonary artery runs horizontally in front of the descending thoracic aorta and the left main bronchus to the root of the left lung where again it divides into two branches. On the upper surface of the left pulmonary artery there is a connection to the aortic arch by the ligamentum arteriosum, which bears a close relationship to the left recurrent laryngeal nerve.

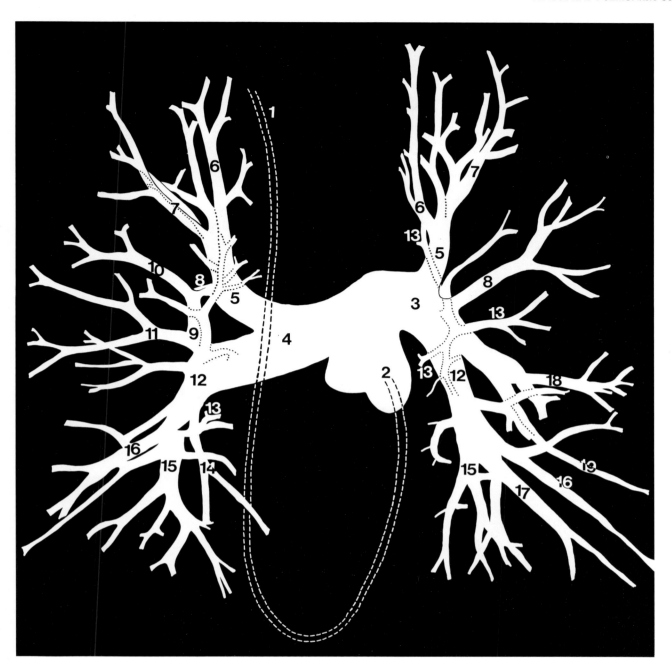

1	Catheter in sup. vena cava	7	Post. a. (upper lobe)
2	Catheter tip in pulmonary trunk	8	Ant. a. (upper lobe)
3	L. pulmonary a.	9	Middle lobe a.
4	R. pulmonary a.	10	Lat. a. (middle lobe)
5	Upper lobe a.	11	Medial a. (middle lobe)
6	Apical a. (upper lobe)	12	Lower lobe a.

13	Sup. (apical basal) a.
14	Med. basal a.
15	Post. basal a.
16	Lat. basal a.
17	Ant. basal a.
18	Sup. lingular a.
19	Inf. lingular a.

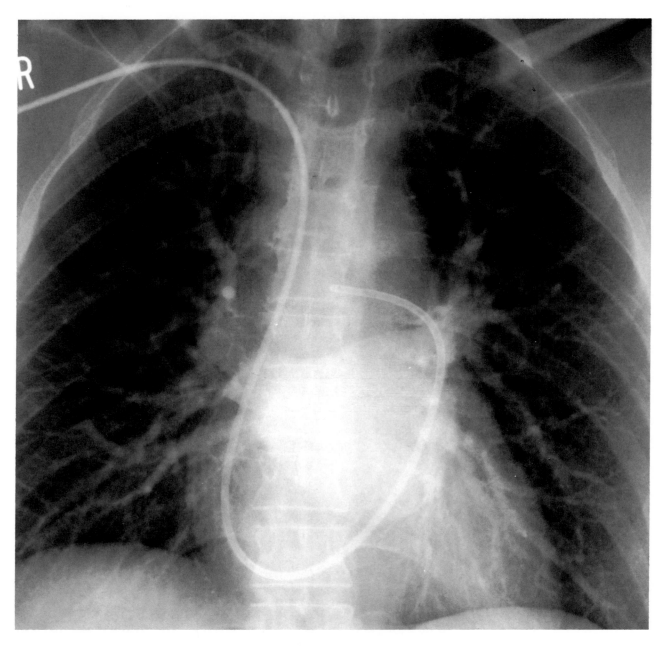

PULMONARY ARTERIOGRAM—VENOUS PHASE

The pulmonary veins, unlike the pulmonary arteries, do not accompany the corresponding bronchi and consequently a bronchopulmonary segment is not a complete vascular unit as veins cross from one segment to another. The veins drain into the left atrium which lies high and posterior. Note that the pulmonary arteries and veins are not the only vascular system present in the lungs as there is a systemic bronchial circulation, consisting of bronchial arteries arising from the descending thoracic aorta. The bronchial veins have two systems: a deep and a superficial; the deep veins join the main pulmonary veins at the left atrium, and the superficial veins drain on the right side into the azygos vein and on the left side into the accessory hemiazygos vein or one of the superior intercostal veins.

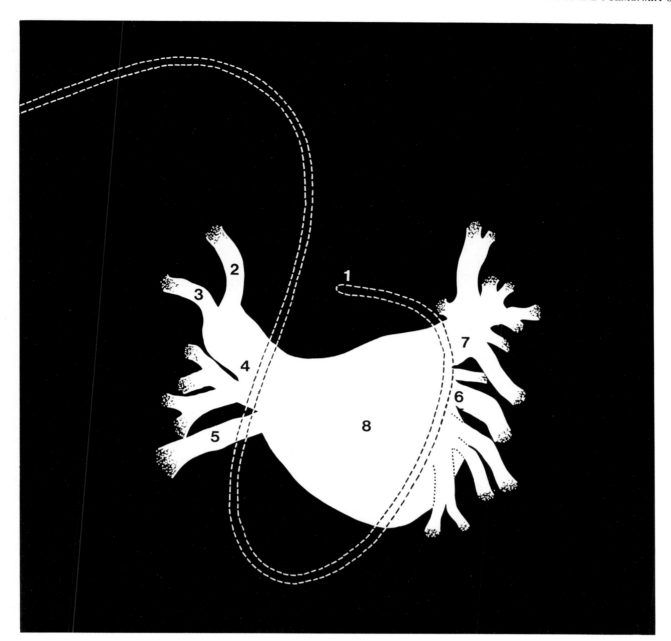

1 Catheter tip in pulmonary a.

2 Pulmonary v.—r. apical upper lobe

3 Pulmonary v.—r. post. upper lobe

4 R. sup. pulmonary v.

5 R. inf. pulmonary v.

6 L. inf. pulmonary v.

7 L. sup. pulmonary v.

8 L. atrium overlying vertebral column

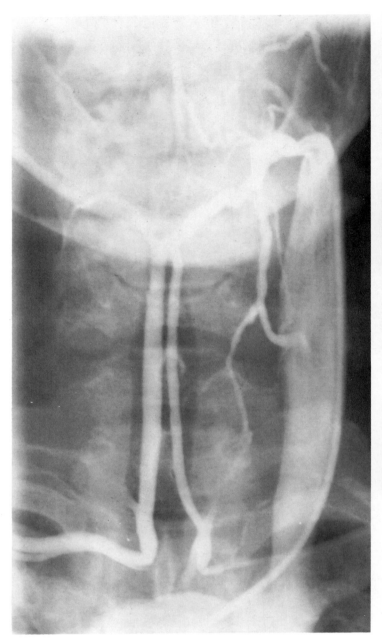
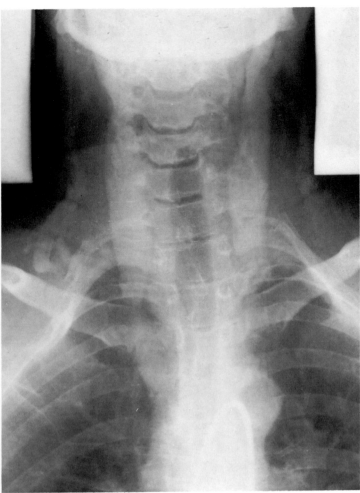

VEINS OF THE NECK

The catheter has been introduced into the left brachiocephalic vein from the femoral vein. The catheter is advanced from the femoral vein into the inferior vena cava, through the right atrium into the superior vena cava and then into the left brachiocephalic. The veins of the neck are divided into two sets, one lying superficial to the deep fascia and the other lying deep to it. The external jugular vein is formed by the union of the posterior division of the retromandibular vein and the posterior auricular vein, and originates at the angle of the mandible. It terminates by draining into the subclavian vein about 4 cm above the clavicle. The internal jugular vein begins in the base of the skull and is continuous with the sigmoid sinus. The vein passes inferiorly through the neck within the carotid sheath to unite with the subclavian vein, thus forming the brachiocephalic vein. Note the position of the thyroid veins, the superior and middle being shown. The inferior thyroid veins arise in the thyroid gland, after a free anastomosis with the middle and superior veins, to drain into the brachiocephalic veins. This technique of superselective catheterization of thyroid veins is of particular use when assaying blood for increased parathyroid hormone levels due to a parathyroid tumour (parathyroid venous sampling).

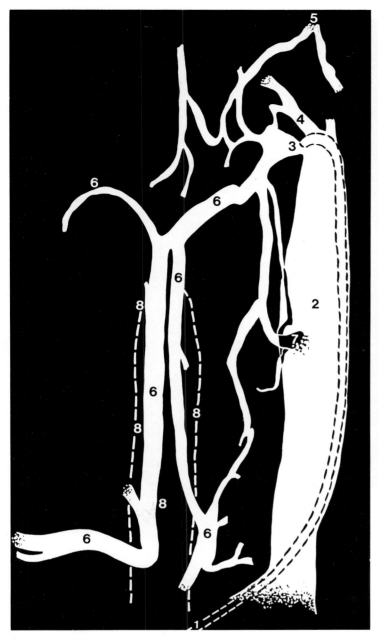
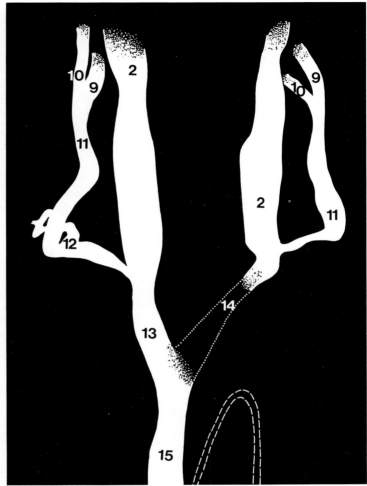

1	Catheter in l. brachiocephalic v.	6	Ant. jugular vv.	11	External jugular v.
2	Internal jugular v.	7	Middle thyroid v.	12	Transverse cervical v.
3	Sup. thyroid v.	8	Air within trachea	13	R. brachiocephalic v.
4	Lingual v.	9	Post. division of retromandibular v.	14	Position of l. brachiocephalic v.
5	Facial v.	10	Post. auricular v.	15	Sup. vena cava

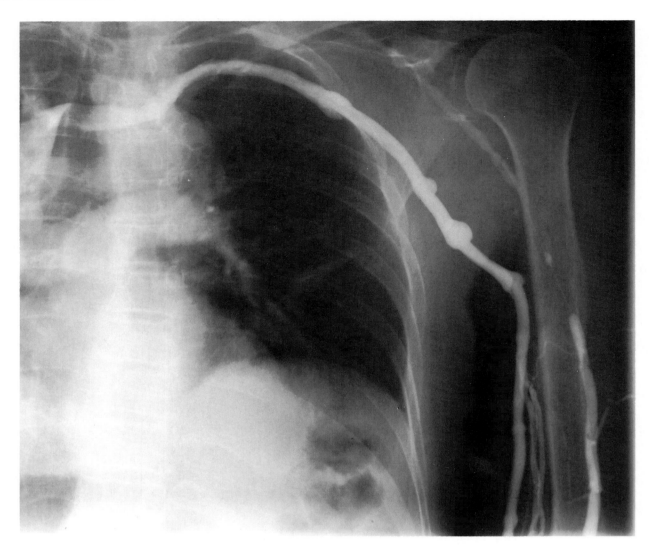

AXILLARY AND SUBCLAVIAN VENOGRAM

The cephalic vein runs upwards along the lateral border of the biceps muscle and lies in the deltopectoral groove before entering the infraclavicular fossa. It pierces the clavipectoral fascia, crosses the axillary artery and joins the axillary vein below the clavicle. The basilic vein runs upwards from the elbow along the medial border of the biceps muscle, to perforate the deep fascia in the middle of the arm, and ascends beside the brachial artery to the lower border of teres major where it becomes the axillary vein. The axillary vein extends from this point to become the subclavian vein at the outer border of the first rib.

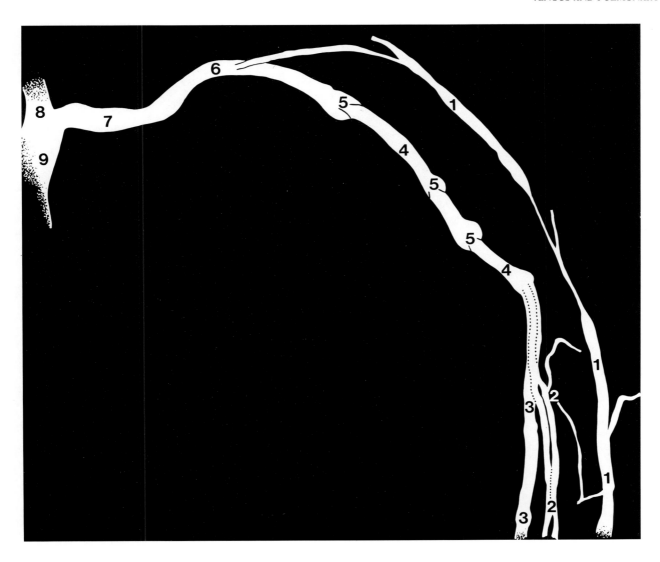

1	Cephalic v.	4	Axillary v.
2	Brachial vv. (venae comitantes of brachial a.)	5	Site of valves (three in axillary v.)
		6	L. subclavian v.
3	Basilic v.		

7	L. brachiocephalic (innominate) v.
8	R. brachiocephalic (innominate) v.
9	Sup. vena cava

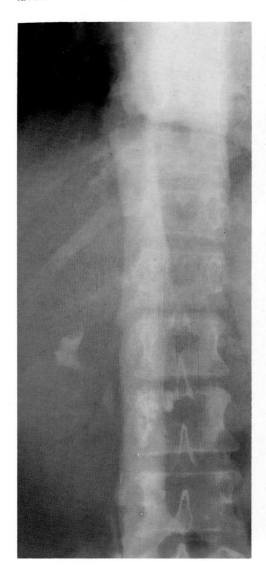 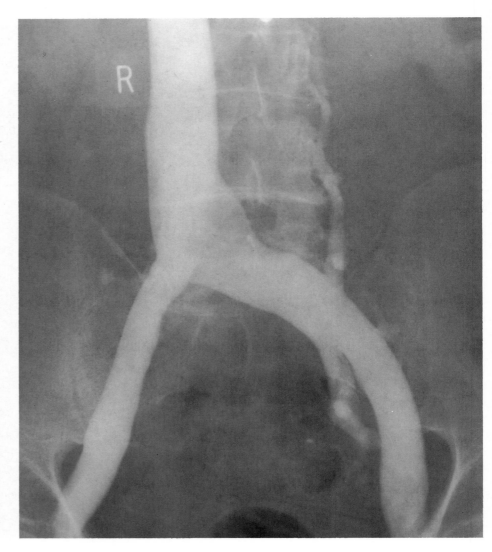

INFERIOR VENA CAVOGRAM

The inferior vena cava is demonstrated by catheterization of both femoral veins with simultaneous injection of contrast medium. The vein is formed from the junction of the two common iliac veins at the level of L5 and ascends, terminating in the lower posterior part of the right atrium. The inferior vena cava receives the following veins: lumbar, right testicular or ovarian, renal, right suprarenal, inferior phrenic and hepatic. The two main in-dications for performing this technique are, first, to check for evidence of venous thrombosis and, secondly, to look for extrinsic indentations due to lymph node enlargement (e.g. reticulosis). The entrance of the renal and hepatic veins can be seen. It is possible, however, to get some retrograde flow of contrast medium into the orgins of these veins by performing a Valsalva manoeuvre at the time of injection.

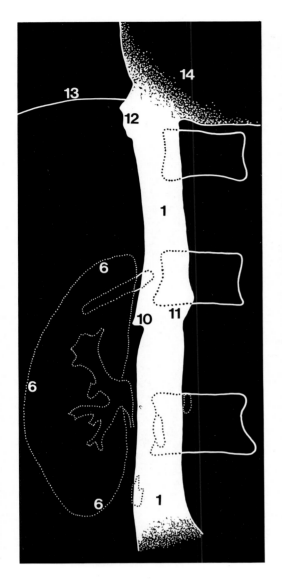

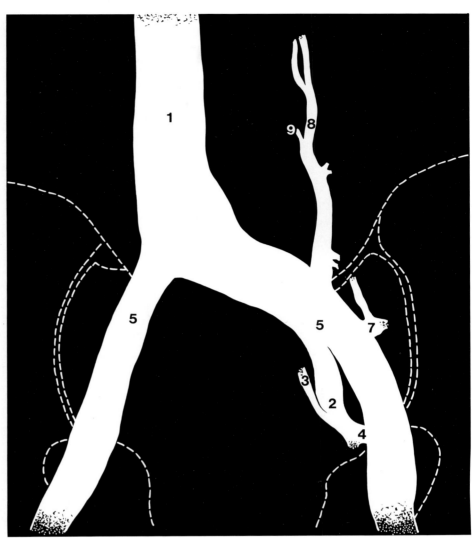

1	Inf. vena cava	6	Renal outline	11	Entrance of l. renal v.
2	Internal iliac v.	7	Iliolumbar v.	12	Entrance of hepatic vv.
3	Lat. sacral v.	8	Ascending lumbar v.	13	Diaphragm
4	Gluteal v.	9	Lumbar v.	14	R. atrium
5	Common iliac v.	10	Entrance of r. renal v.		

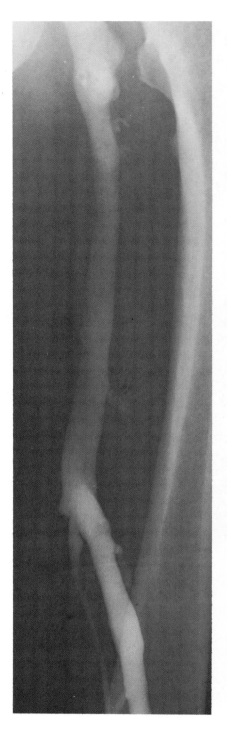 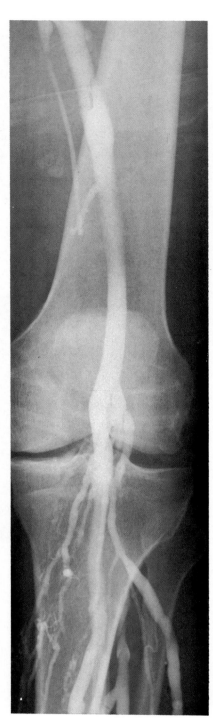 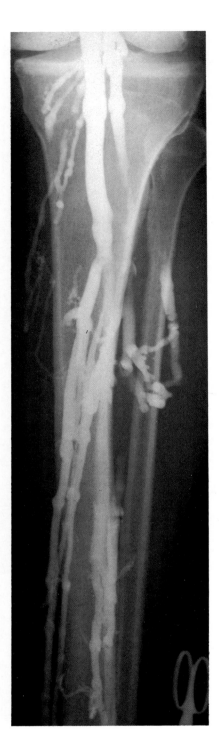

VEINS OF THE LOWER LIMB

These three films demonstrate the deep veins of the lower limb from ankle to hip. A superficial vein on the dorsum of the foot was injected by direct needle technique with constrictive bands placed above the ankle and below the knee. These bands cause the deep venous system to fill by occluding the superficial veins. There is a wide variation in the distribution of calf veins, but they are mainly grouped into the anterior and posterior tibial veins. These veins join to form the popliteal vein at the lower border of the popliteus muscle. The femoral vein accompanies the femoral artery and begins at the hiatus in the adductor magnus muscle. The termination of the superficial long saphenous vein can be seen in the saphenous opening, about 4 cm below and lateral to the pubic tubercle. A lateral film of the calf veins is often useful to show recent thrombosis which can be missed on a single anteroposterior view. A perforating vein can be seen going from the superficial to the deep venous system in the calf and these can become considerably enlarged and varicose.

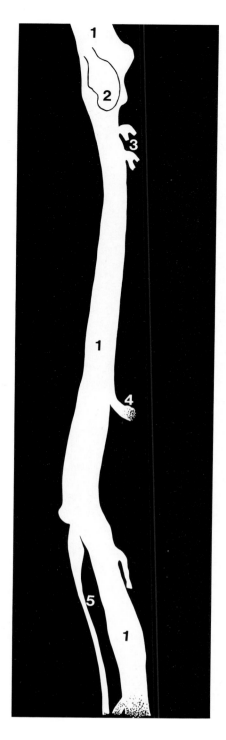
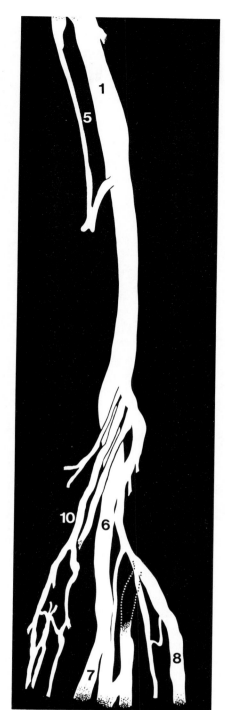
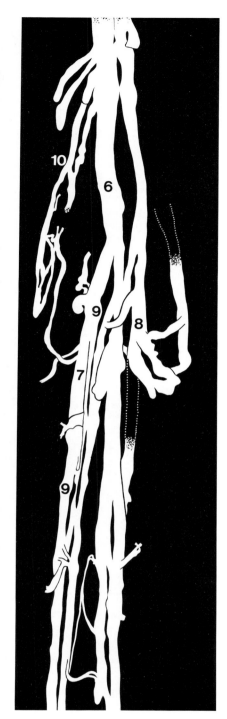

1	Femoral vv.	4	Perforating v.	8	Post. tibial v.
2	Termination of long saphenous v.	5	Muscular tributary of femoral v.	9	Venous valves
3	Lat. circumflex femoral v.	6	Popliteal v.	10	Veins draining gastrocnemius
		7	Ant. tibial v.		

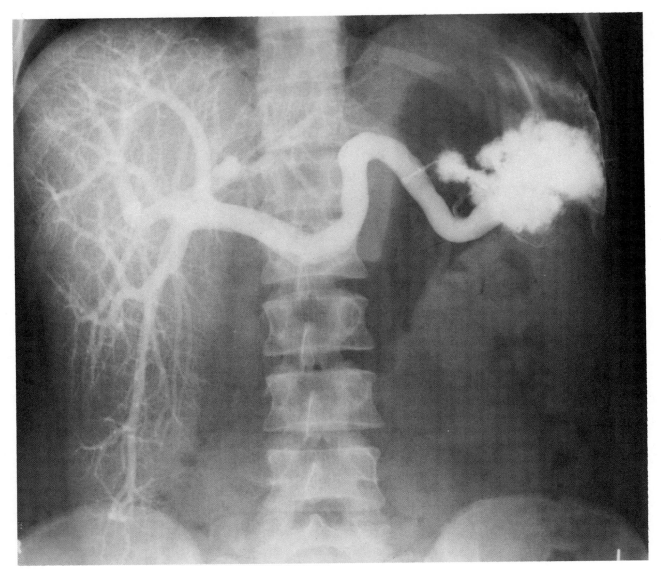

SPLENOPORTOGRAM

The portal circulation can be visualized by three techniques: percutaneous splenic puncture as shown here, operative mesenteric venogram and selective splenic arteriogram. In percutaneous splenic puncture, the needle is introduced into the tenth or eleventh intercostal space in the mid-axillary line. At the same time the splenic pulp pressure is measured by manometry. The majority of splenic venograms are performed for the investigation of portal hypertension. The tributaries of the portal vein are the splenic, superior mesenteric, left gastric, right gastric, paraumbilical and cystic veins. The portal system includes all the veins which drain blood from the intestine and from the spleen, pancreas and gall bladder. The portal vein and its tributaries have no valves in the adult but this is not so in the fetus. Note on this radiograph the large Riedel's lobe reaching as far as the iliac crest.

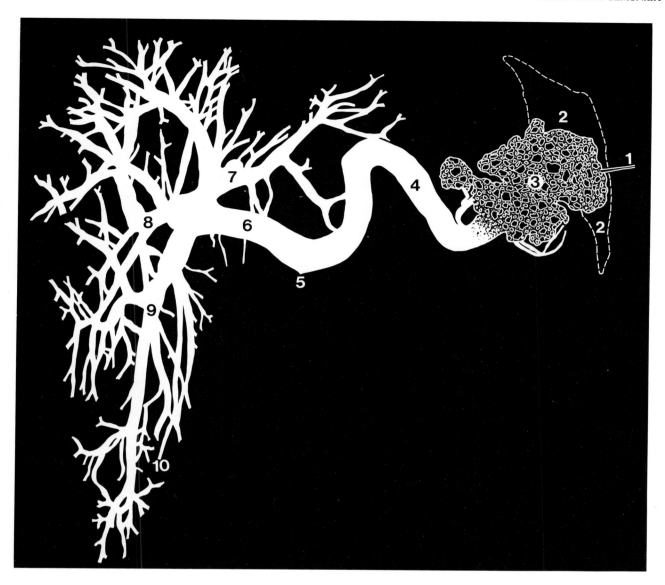

1 Needle in splenic pulp

2 Subcapsular contrast medium
   (leakage)

3 Contrast medium within splenic
   pulp

4 Splenic v.

5 Point of entrance of sup.
   mesenteric v.

6 Portal v.

7 L. portal v.

8 R. portal v.

9 Abnormally large segmental v. to
   Riedel's lobe

10 Riedel's lobe

SUPRARENAL VENOGRAMS

Suprarenal venography has become an increasingly important technique in the past few years and one of the most reliable methods for demonstrating small tumours such as occur in primary hyperaldosteronism. The right suprarenal vein is very short and drains directly into the inferior vena cava just above the upper pole of the right kidney. It may occasionally drain via the hepatic vein. The left suprarenal vein is longer and drains into the left renal vein. This vein may occasionally have some drainage via the inferior phrenic vein. The catheters used in this technique are both preshaped. There is commonly a higher success rate on the left. Considerable care must be taken in the amount of contrast injected because of the risk of suprarenal infarction. On the left side approximately 5 ml and on the right side 2 ml are usually sufficient. With selective catheterization it is possible to take blood samples for hormone analysis.

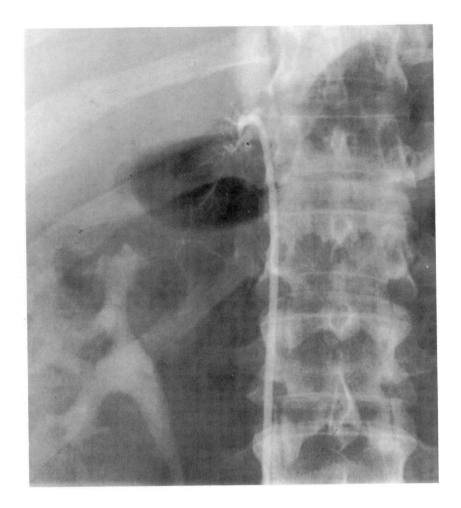

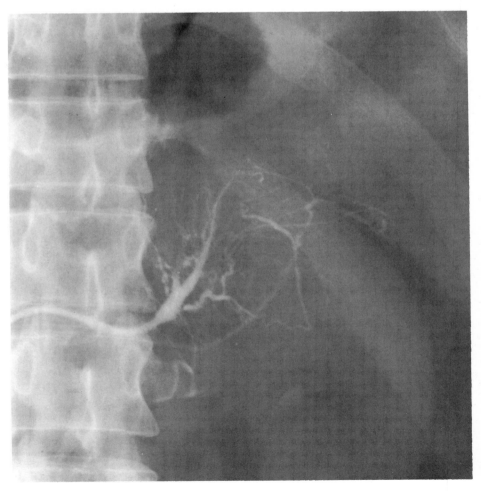

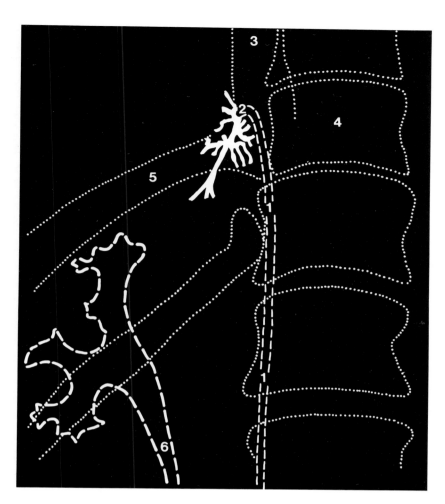

1 Catheter in inf. vena cava

2 Catheter tip in r. suprarenal (adrenal) v.

3 Contrast medium in inf. vena cava

4 Eleventh thoracic vertebral body

5 Eleventh rib

6 Ureter

7 Catheter in l. suprarenal (adrenal) v.

8 Capsular v.

9 Renal outline

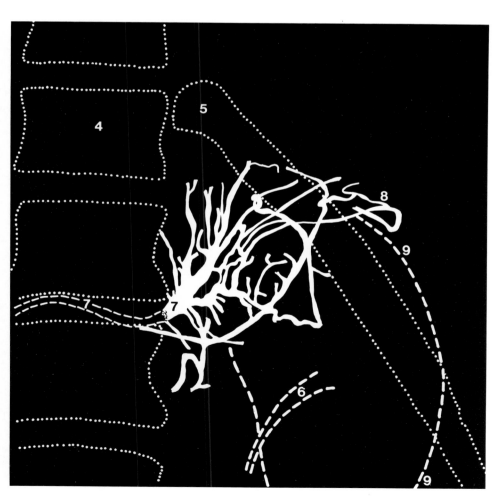

LYMPHATIC SYSTEM

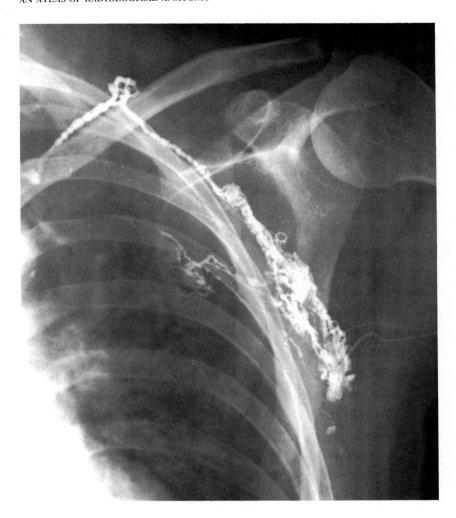

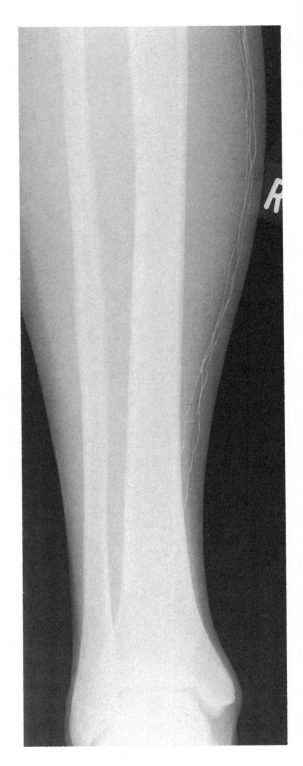

LYMPHANGIOGRAMS OF AXILLA AND LOWER LEG

Lymphangiography is performed in the upper and lower limb by the cannulation of lymph vessels which have been rendered visible by the subcutaneous injection of patent blue dye. The contrast used is iodized oil fluid injection (Lipiodol Ultra Fluid). This accumulates in the glands and shows their internal structure. If injection is too rapid or too forceful, extravasation can occur, particularly in the upper limb. There are normally one to four channels in the lower leg, following the course of the long saphenous vein. The beaded appearance is due to valves. The usual indication for axillary lymphography is oedema secondary to a mastectomy. As many as 40 nodes may occur in the axilla and they are best seen with a 30°–40° abduction of the humerus. Beware mistaking normal fibrofatty deposits for metastases in the axillary nodes.

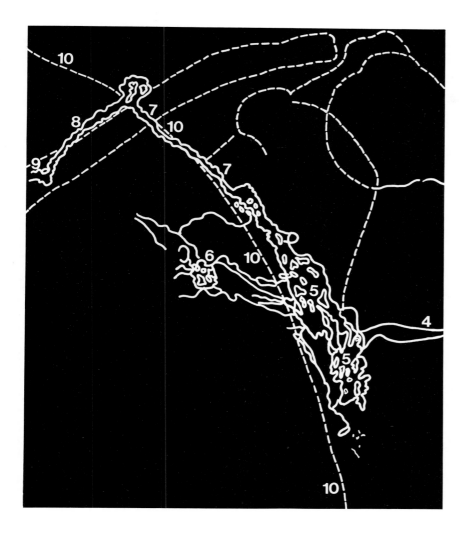

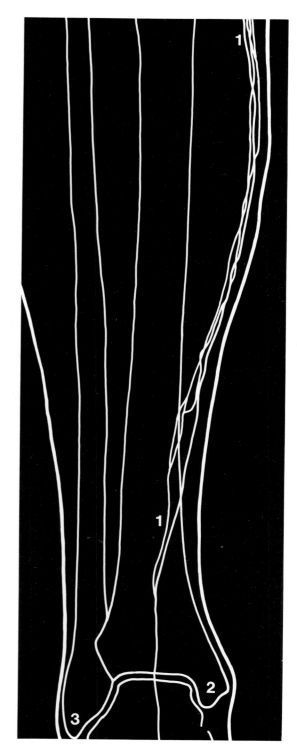

1 Superficial medial lymph vss.

2 Med. malleolus

3 Lat. malleolus

4 Brachial efferent lymph vss.

5 Site of central collecting nodes

6 Pectoral lymph node (anterior)

7 Subclavian duct

8 Normal 'beaded' efferent vs.

9 Termination of subclavian duct

10 Lat. border of thoracic cage

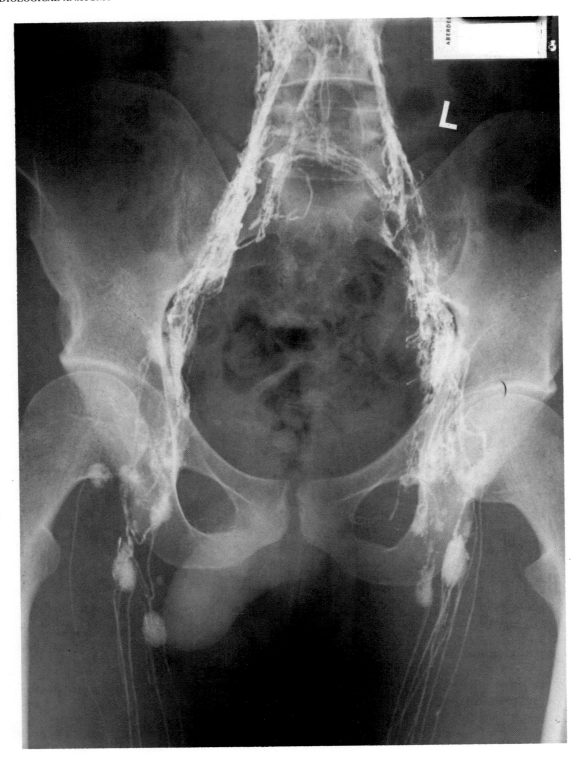

LYMPHANGIOGRAM (FIRST DAY)

The lymphatic system of the pelvis and abdomen is demonstrated by bilateral injections of contrast medium into the lymphatics of the feet. The importance of the first day or immediate films is to show the position of the afferent and efferent vessels as they enter and leave the nodes respectively. This is important if one is to avoid making false positive diagnoses of metastases in later films. Once the contrast medium has reached the thoracic duct then the injection should be stopped, because any more contrast given will go straight to the thoracic duct and hence into the left subclavian vein to end up as oil emboli in the lungs. One of the contraindications of this technique is when the patient has severe respiratory disease with a decreased transfer factor. The indications include investigation of lymphoedema, the detection of metastases (e.g. from kidney, cervix, testicle and bladder), and in the diagnosis and staging of the reticuloses.

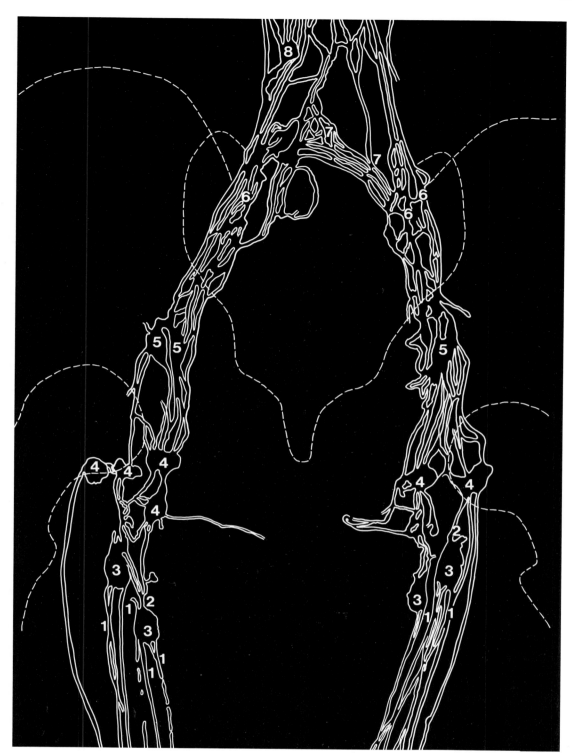

1 Numerous afferent lymph vss. in groin

2 Efferent lymph vss.

3 Superficial inguinal lymph nodes (lower group—subinguinal)

4 Superficial inguinal lymph nodes (upper group)

5 External iliac lymph vss.

6 Common iliac lymph vss.

7 Lumbar crossover of iliac vss.

8 Lower para-aortic node (lat. aortic)

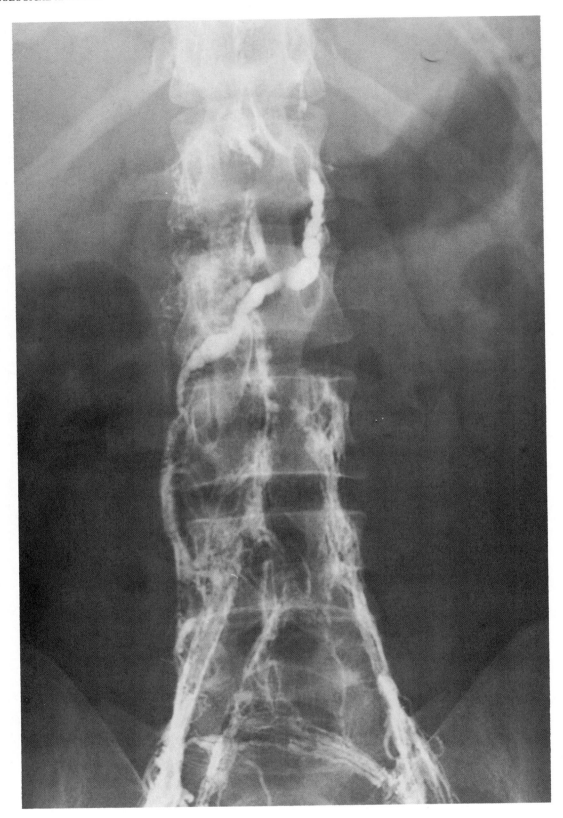

LYMPHANGIOGRAM (FIRST DAY)

The lumbar crossover of iliac vessels can be seen clearly on this film. Numerous crossflow channels exist between the two sides, and if there is obstruction these channels increase significantly. There are four sets of nodes around the aorta: the right and left para-aortic, the retro-aortic and the pre-aortic. The cisterna chyli is situated in front of the bodies of L1 and L2 and it receives vessels from the para-aortic group of glands and the intestinal lymphatic trunks. It gives off the thoracic duct, which ascends on the posterior thoracic wall to open into the left subclavian vein.

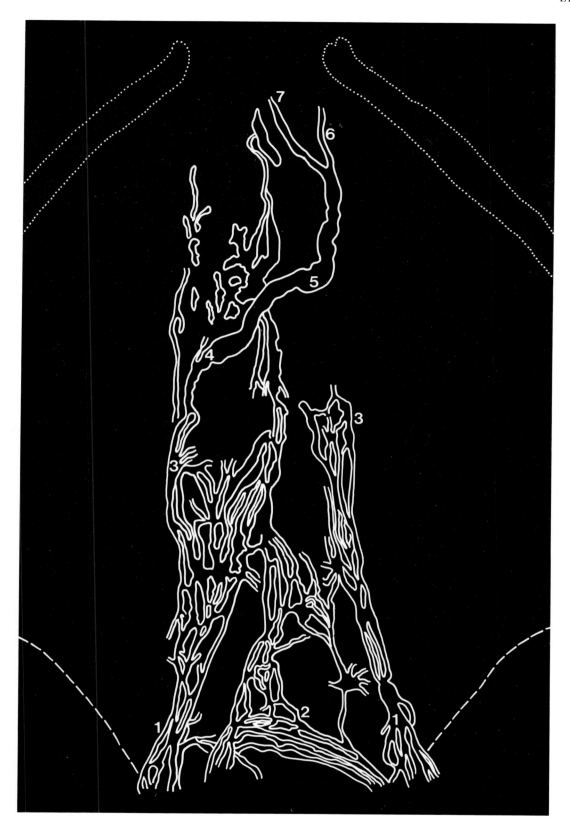

1 Common iliac lymph vss.

2 Lumbar crossover of lymph vss.

3 Para-aortic lymph vss.
   (paralumbar or lateral aortic)

4 Formation of cisterna chyli at L2

5 Cisterna chyli

6 Intercostal lymph vs.

7 Origin of thoracic duct

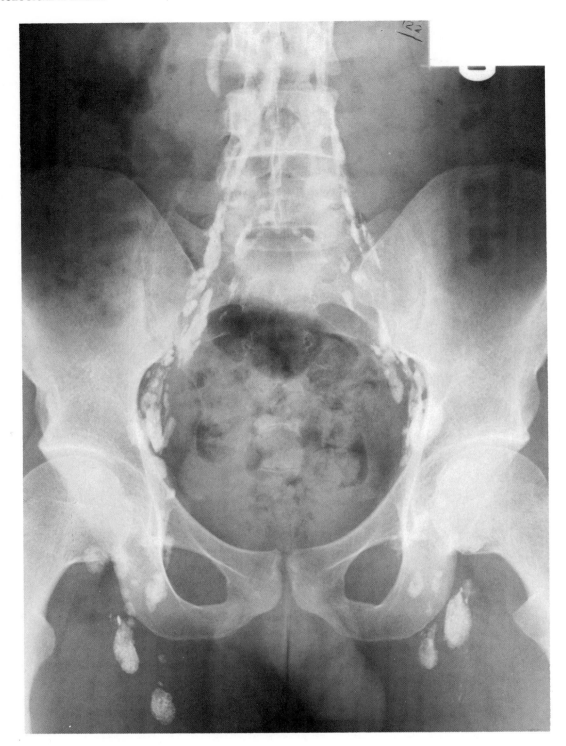

LYMPHANGIOGRAM (SECOND DAY)

This and the following film have been taken at 24 hours after the injection of contrast medium. Note how all the vessels are now clear of contrast medium and radiolucent areas are seen in the nodes where the afferent and efferent vessels enter and depart. The lymph node has a normal mottled appearance with the radiolucenies approximately 2 mm wide. Metastases, therefore, have to be larger than about 3 mm before they can be diagnosed. As the nodes of the pelvis lie along the lateral borders, near the iliac vessels, oblique views of the pelvis are required to see these nodes clearly. Signs of lymphatic obstruction include: stasis, dermal backflow, the filling of abnormal collateral channels and the opening of lymphaticovenous channels.

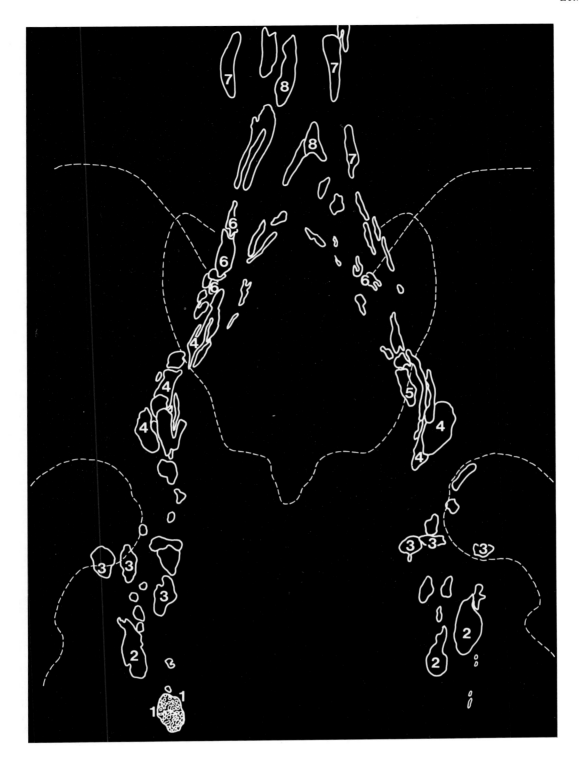

1 Normal follicular appearance of lymph nodes

2 Superficial inguinal lymph nodes (lower group)

3 Superficial inguinal lymph nodes (upper group)

4 External iliac lymph nodes

5 Internal iliac lymph nodes

6 Common iliac lymph nodes

7 Lower para-aortic nodes (lat. aortic)

8 Pre-aortic lymph nodes

LYMPHANGIOGRAM (SECOND DAY)

This AP film of the abdomen shows the normal position of the para-aortic lymph nodes. Note that the normal para-aortic nodes should not lie outside a line formed by the tips of the transverse processes. Signs of metastases in the nodes include: filling defects, failure of severely involved nodes to fill, obstruction of a normal lymphatic pathway, and distortion and displacement by a nodal mass. The place of lymphangiography in reticulosis is now well established but it is not possible to distinguish the various pathological types. As contrast medium remains in the lymphatic nodes for up to 18 months, it is a useful technique to x-ray again following treatment to show remission or recurrence of disease.

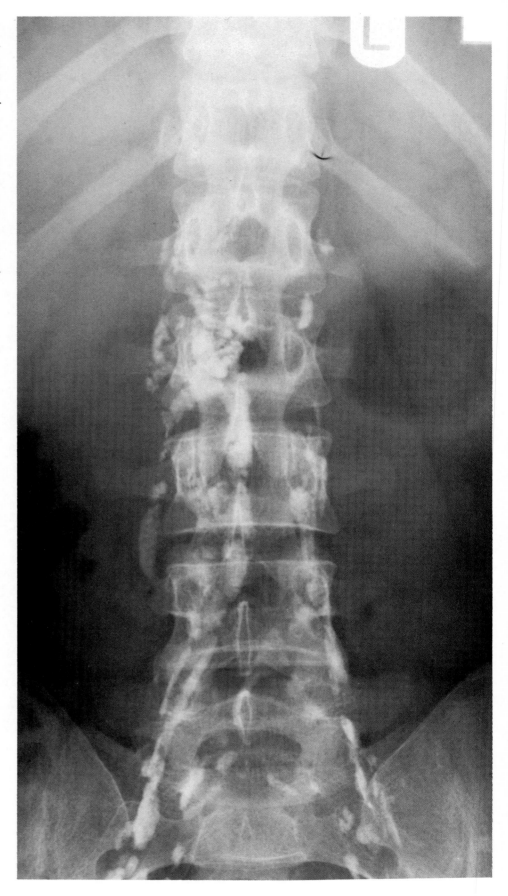

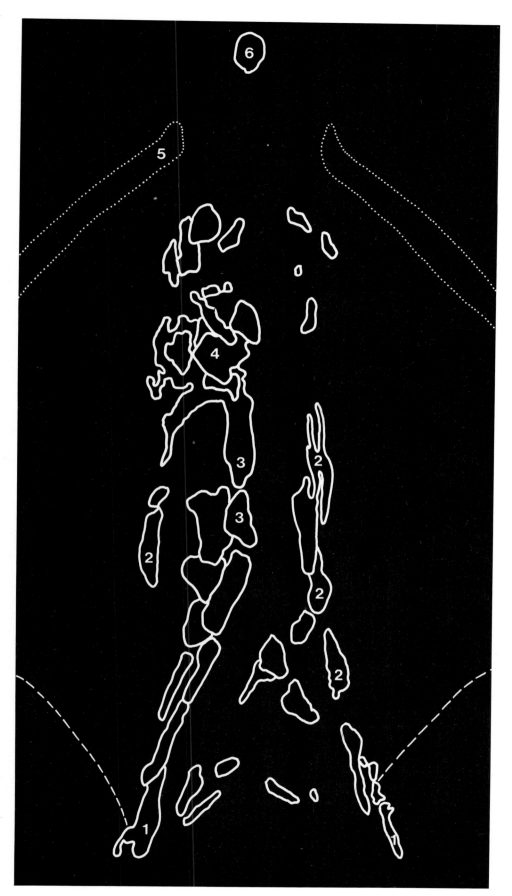

1   Common iliac lymph nodes

2   Para-aortic lymph nodes (lat. aortic or lumbar)

3   Central aortic lymph nodes

4   Coeliac group of nodes

5   Twelfth rib

6   Post. mediastinal lymph node

GASTROINTESTINAL TRACT

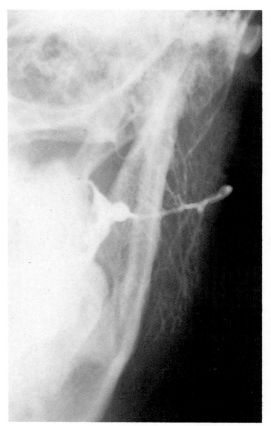

A

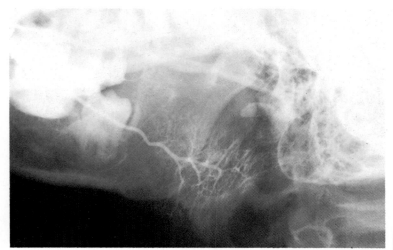

B

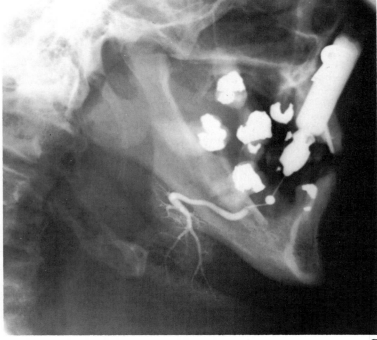

C

PAROTID AND SUBMANDIBULAR SIALOGRAMS

Water-soluble contrast medium of high iodine density has been used in these examinations but it is possible to use oil-based media instead. The parotid gland is the largest of the salivary glands and lies below the external auditory meatus, between the mandible and the sternomastoid muscle. The structures contained in the parotid gland include the external carotid artery, the retromandibular vein and, more superficially, the facial nerve. The parotid duct is about 5 cm in length and opens into the mouth opposite the second upper molar tooth. The submandibular gland lies in the floor of the mouth, in the submandibular triangle; its duct is also about 5 cm in length and opens via a narrow orifice onto the frenulum of the tongue. Conditions such as calculi, infection, trauma and neoplasia can be investigated by sialography.

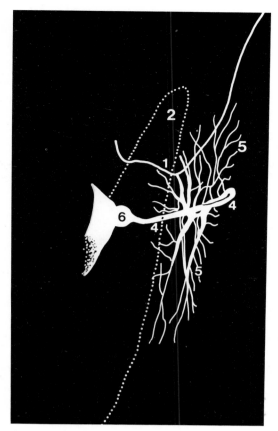

A

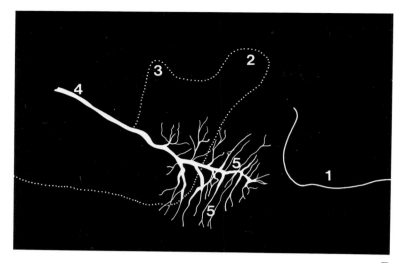

B

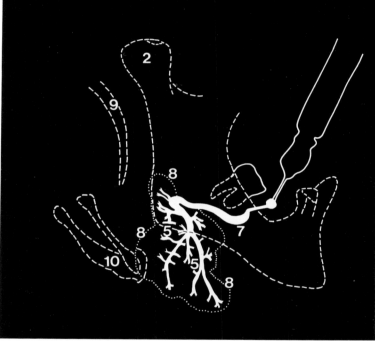

C

A   Parotid

B   Parotid

C   Submandibular

1   Mastoid process

2   Head of mandible (condylar
     process)

3   Coronoid process of mandible

4   Parotid duct (Stensen)

5   Secondary ductules

6   Catheter tip

7   Main submandibular duct
     (Wharton)

8   Borders of submandibular gland

9   Styloid process

10   Hyoid bone

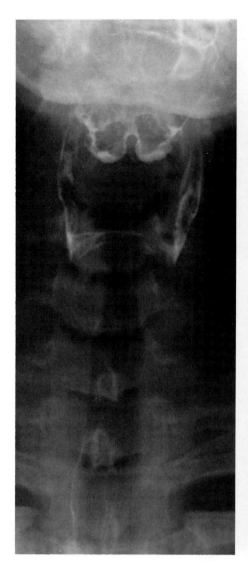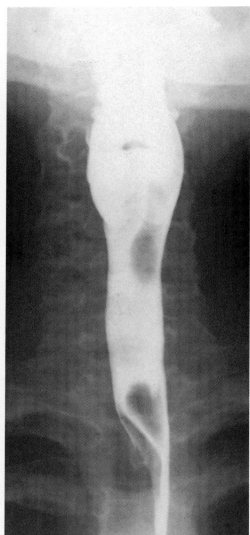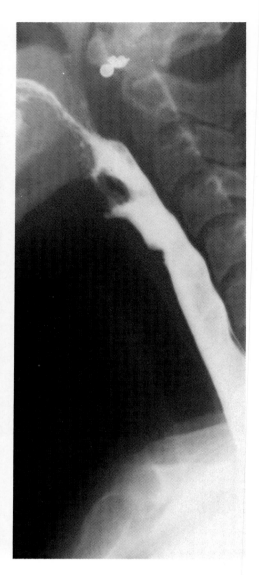

ANTEROPOSTERIOR AND LATERAL VIEWS OF UPPER OESOPHAGUS

The hypopharynx and the upper oesophagus are seen on these films. On swallowing, the larynx moves upwards and is closed off by the epiglottis. A peristaltic wave causes the barium to pass from the pharynx into the oesophagus. On the lateral film the narrowest portion of the oesophagus is at the level of the cricoid, and an impression on the anterior wall at this point is caused by the postcricoid venous plexus. This is a normal finding and should not be confused with the oesophageal webs which occur on the same anterior wall but are lower and thinner. Webs are also seen on the AP film whereas the venous impression is not. The crico-pharyngeus muscle impression occurs at the same level as the cricoid and shows as a posterior indentation into the barium column. Note the position of the epiglottis, valleculae and piriform sinuses.

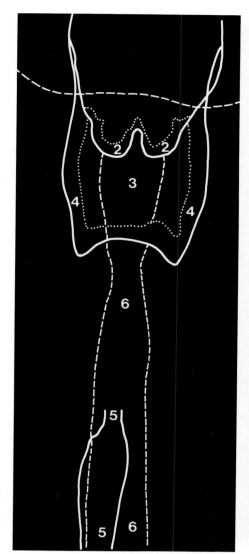
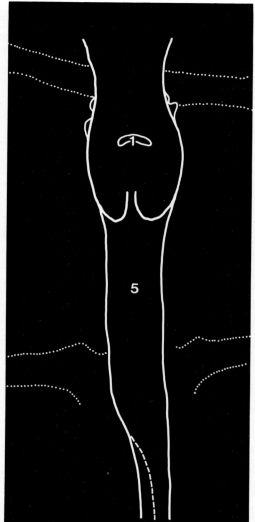
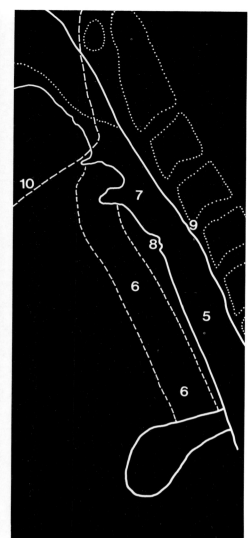

1	Epiglottis	5	Oesophagus	9	Site of cricopharẏngeus m.
2	Vallecula	6	Trachea	10	Mandible
3	Vestibule	7	Hypopharynx		
4	Piriform fossa (sinus)	8	Postcricoid venous plexus		

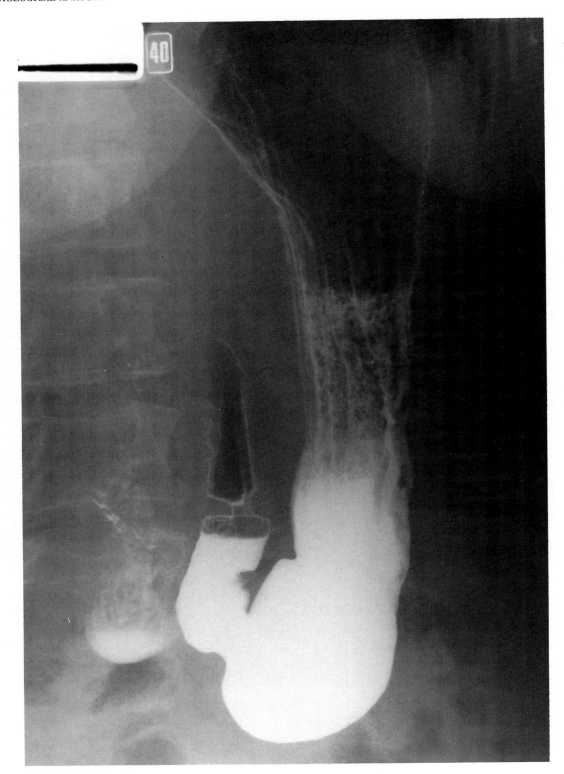

RIGHT ANTERIOR OBLIQUE BARIUM STUDY OF STOMACH AND DUODENUM

The duodenum is about 25 cm long, is in a fixed position, has no mesentery and is only partially covered with peritoneum. The C-shaped curve of the duodenum encloses the head of the pancreas. The duodenum is divided into four parts: the first or superior part begins at the pylorus and ends at the neck of the gall bladder; the descending or second part runs down the right side of the vertebral column to L3 and is crossed by the transverse colon. The common bile duct and pancreatic duct join to open into the medial side of this part of the duodenum. The third or horizontal part crosses the L3 vertebra anterior to the inferior vena cava and ends in the fourth part which lies in front of the abdominal aorta. The ascending or fourth part turns upwards to L2 where the duodenojejunal flexure occurs. This flexure is fixed by a fibromuscular band, called the suspensory ligament of the duodenum (Treitz), which arises from the diaphragm. Various projections and techniques in different positions are used to demonstrate the whole of the stomach and duodenum on a barium meal examination.

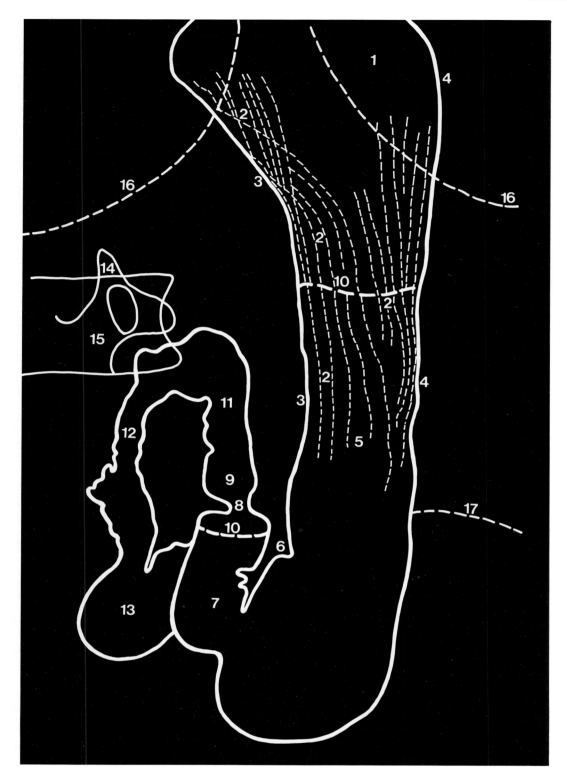

1	Fundal gas bubble	
2	Longitudinal ridges of mucous membrane (rugae)	
3	Lesser curvature	
4	Greater curvature	
5	Body of stomach	
6	Incisura angularis	
7	Antrum	
8	Pyloric canal	
9	Duodenal cap (bulb)	
10	Contrast medium fluid level	
11	First part of duodenum	
12	Second part of duodenum (descending)	
13	Third part of duodenum (horizontal)	
14	Sup. articular process of L3	
15	Pars interarticularis of L3	
16	Breast shadow	
17	Iliac crest	

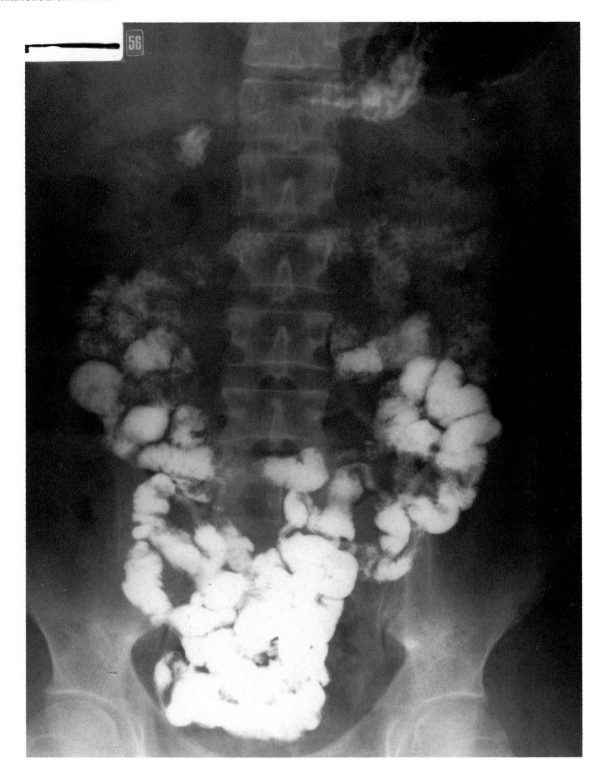

ANTEROPOSTERIOR BARIUM FOLLOW-THROUGH

This film and the next show a normal follow-through examination using barium alone. The length of the small intestine is approximately 5–7 m, with arbitrary divisions into jejunum and ileum. The diameter of the jejunum is around 25 mm and that of the ileum 20 mm. The plicae circulares begin in the second part of the duodenum and their maximum size and number occur in the middle portion of jejunum. They then diminish and finally disappear about the middle of the ileum. When performing follow-through examinations, it is important to know the characteristics of the barium used so that physiological abnormalities can be recognized in addition to any gross pathology.

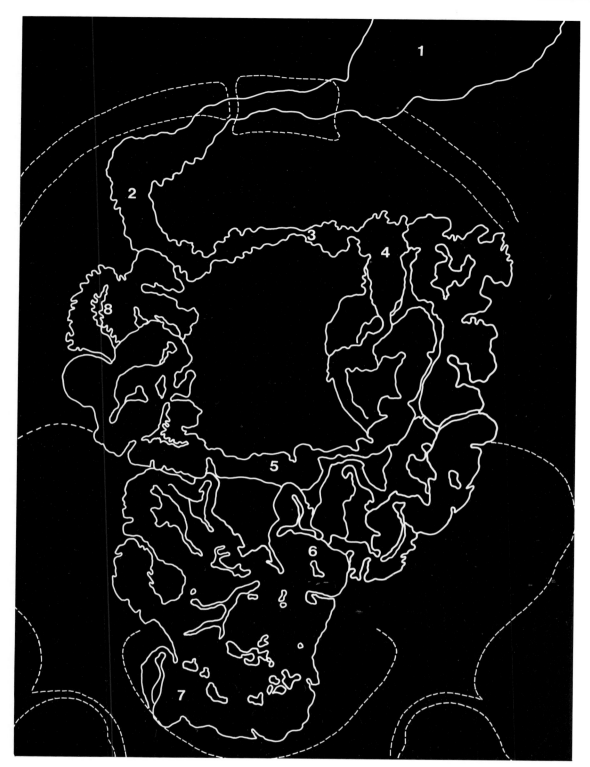

1   Stomach

2   Duodenal loop

3   Duodenojejunal flexure

4   Upper jejunum

5   Lower jejunum

6   Upper ileum

7   Lower ileum

8   Valvulae conniventes (plicae circulares)

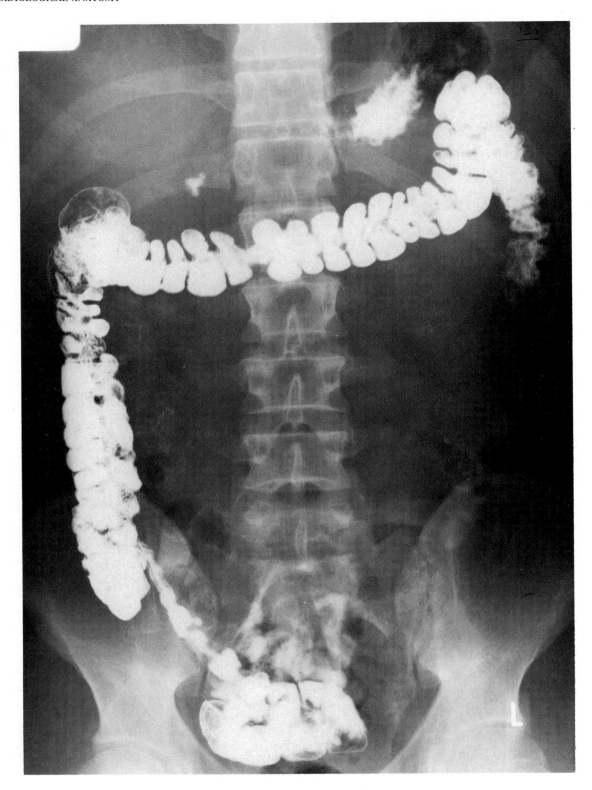

ANTEROPOSTERIOR BARIUM FOLLOW-THROUGH

This second film shows the ileum and the ileocaecal region. The ileocaecal valve often protrudes into the caecum and may produce a filling defect which can be mistaken for a tumour. The terminal ileum may manifest diseases such as regional enteritis (Crohn's disease). Malabsorption can also be investigated by a follow-through examination and two main groups are found: the first group with radiological features due mainly to steatorrhoea and the second group with disease-specific radiological features. Points to look for are dilution of contrast, rapid transit time, dilatation of small bowel and abnormalities of the circular folds. To test for lactose intolerance (disaccharide deficiency), lactose can be added to the barium and the resulting changes noted.

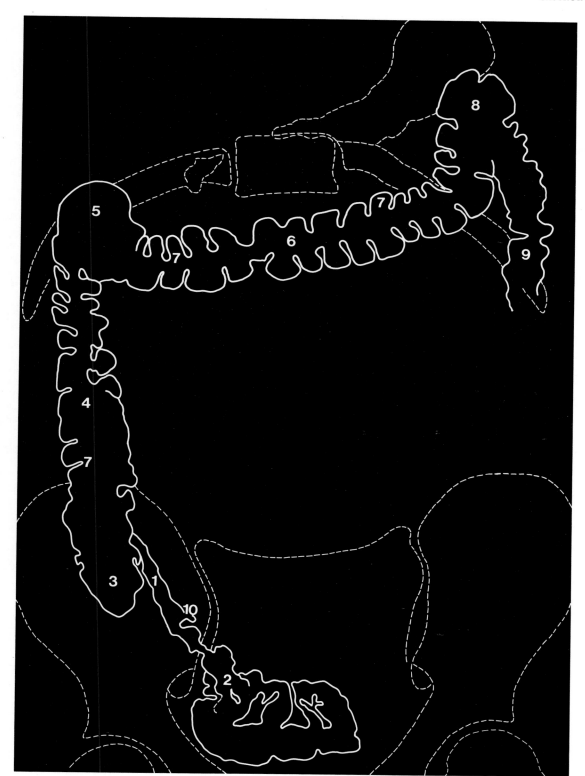

1 Terminal ileum	4 Ascending colon	7 Normal haustral pattern
2 Ileum	5 R. colic (hepatic) flexure	8 L. colic (splenic) flexure
3 Caecum	6 Transverse colon	9 Descending colon
		10 Small Meckel's diverticulum

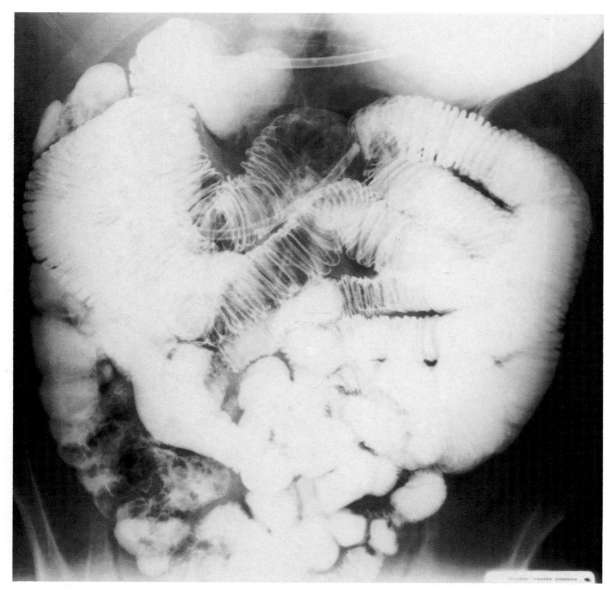

SMALL BOWEL ENEMA—DOUBLE AIR CONTRAST

This procedure is performed by intubating the duodenum, filling the intestine with barium, fluid and air, and giving a muscular relaxant drug to abolish peristalsis. The patient is asked to have a special low residue diet for 2–3 days prior to the examination so that the small bowel is relatively empty. The anatomy of the mucosal folds is seen more clearly than on the conventional follow-through examination and this allows a higher diagnostic accuracy rate. The detail of the terminal ileum can also be visualized and very early lesions can be diagnosed. Note the reflux of contrast medium into the stomach.

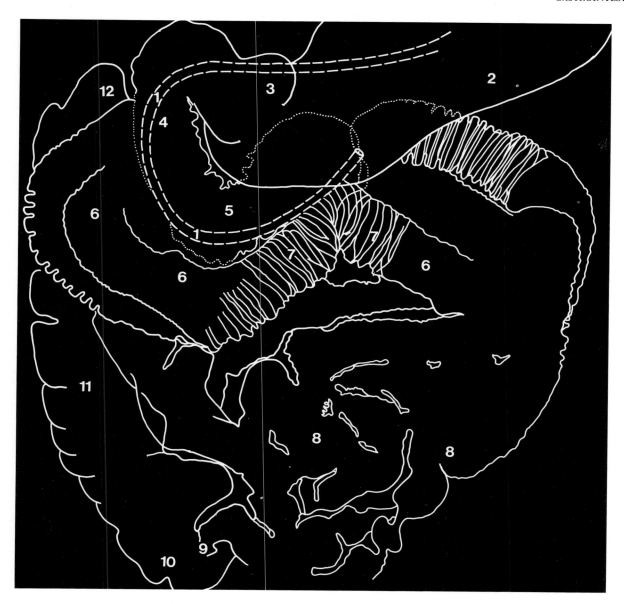

1	Catheter in C-shaped duodenum	5	Third part of duodenum	9	Ileocaecal valve
2	Contrast medium in stomach antrum	6	Jejunal coils	10	Caecum
3	First part of duodenum	7	Valvulae conniventes (plicae circulares)	11	Ascending colon
4	Second part of duodenum	8	Ileum	12	R. colic (hepatic) flexure

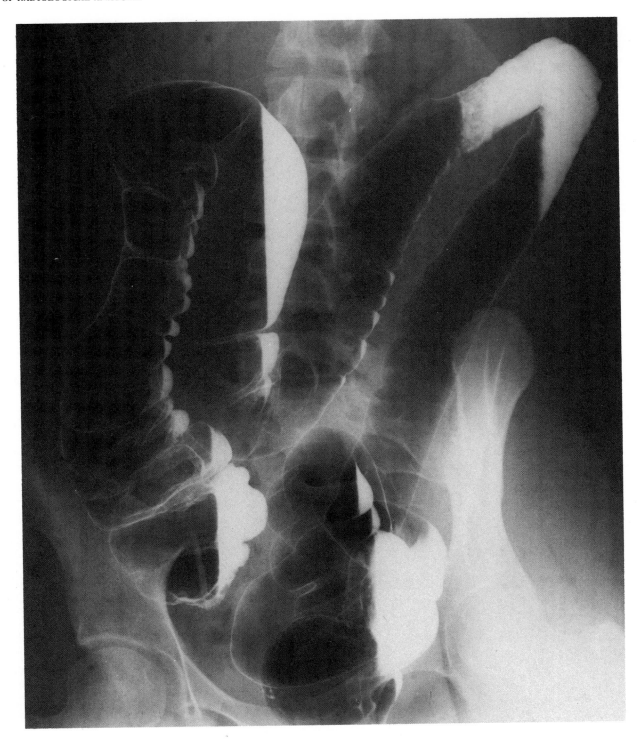

LARGE BOWEL ENEMA—DOUBLE AIR CONTRAST: LATERAL DECUBITUS VIEW

This shows the method of performing a barium enema examination by using air to distend the colon with a smaller volume of barium to coat the mucosa. This is a decubitus film taken with a horizontal beam and is one of the routine series of radiographs performed. The commonest area in which lesions (particularly polyps) are missed is in the sigmoid colon because of the position of its loops in the pelvis. Ideally, digital examination of the rectum and sigmoidoscopy should be performed prior to an enema examination as a high percentage of pathological lesions present in the last 20 cm of the large bowel.

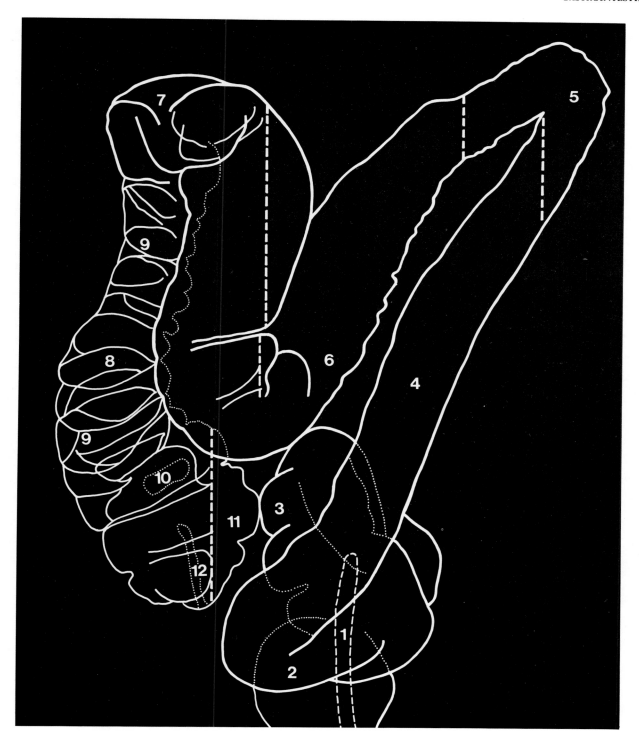

1   Catheter in rectum

2   Rectum

3   Sigmoid colon

4   Descending colon

5   L. colic (splenic) flexure

6   Transverse colon

7   R. colic (hepatic) flexure

8   Ascending colon

9   Haustrations (plicae semilunares)

10 Ileocaecal valve

11 Caecum

12 Vermiform appendix

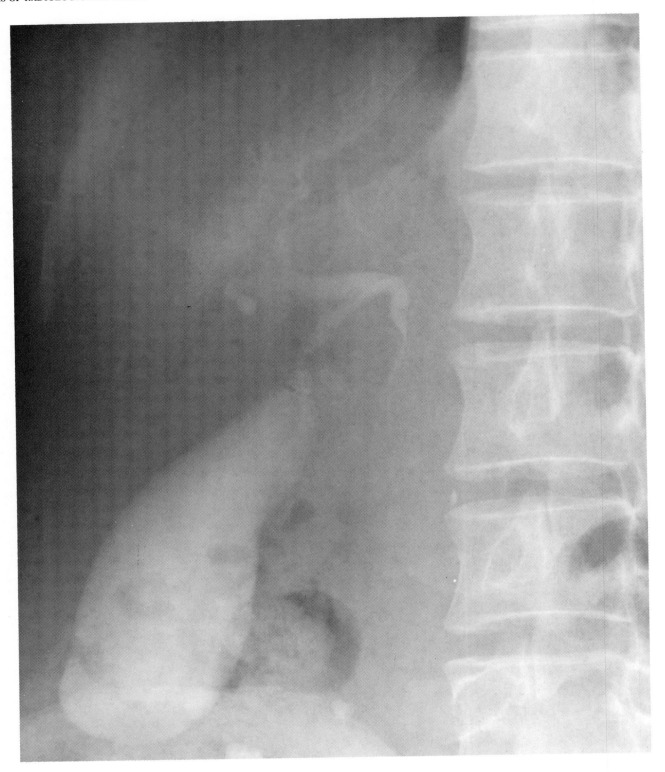

ORAL CHOLECYSTOGRAM—PRONE OBLIQUE VIEW

The contrast used here is calcium ipodate, given orally. It is absorbed from the intestine and concentrated in the gall bladder. Note the unusually well shown hepatic ducts which are not commonly seen in this examination. It is normally necessary to administer contrast intravenously (e.g. meglumine iodipamide) to demonstrate the detailed anatomy of the intra- and extrahepatic ducts. The gall bladder is situated under the right lobe of the liver and is attached to it by connective tissue. The inferior sur-face is covered with peritoneum continuous with the liver. The cystic duct joins the common hepatic duct to form the common bile duct just below the porta hepatis, but this junction may be considerably lower. If this occurs, the cystic duct will lie in the right free margin of the lesser omentum. The mucous membrane of the cystic duct is thrown into a series of folds, giving rise to the appearances of the so-called spiral valve of Heister.

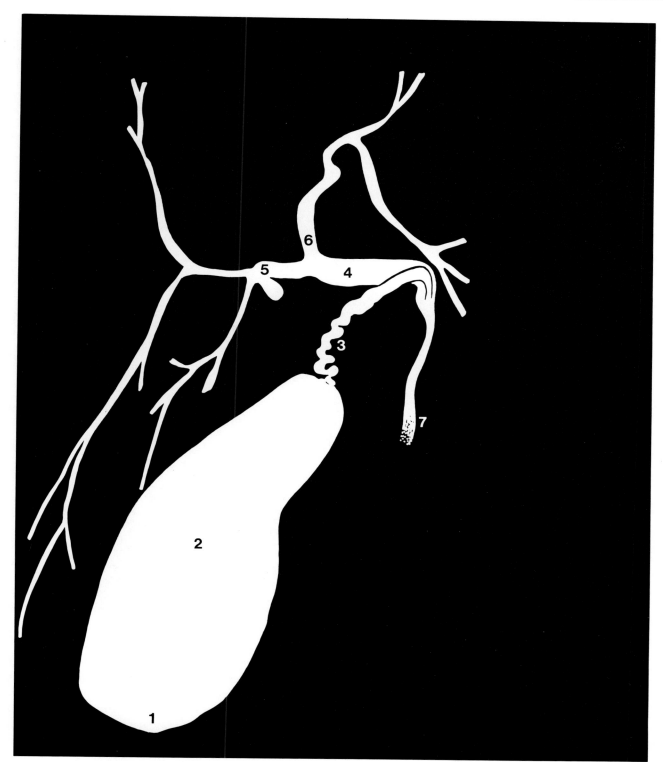

1	Fundus of gall bladder	3	Cystic duct	5	R. hepatic duct
2	Body of gall bladder	4	Common hepatic duct	6	L. hepatic duct
				7	Common bile duct

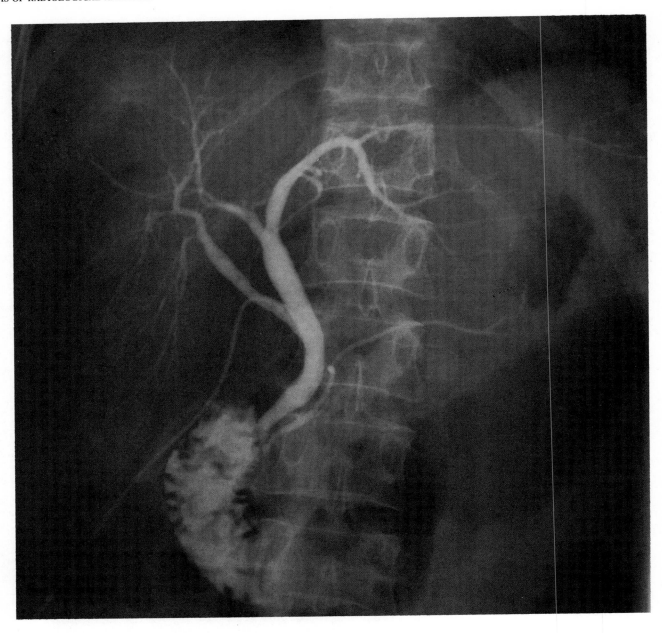

POSTOPERATIVE CHOLANGIOGRAM

This examination is performed by injecting water-soluble contrast medium into the biliary system via a tube left in situ after cholecystectomy and common bile duct exploration. The points to note are: the diameter of the common bile duct, which should be less than 12 mm; the free flow of contrast into the duodenum; the presence or absence of filling defects in the biliary system; and reflux into the pancreatic duct. Note that duodenal filling with contrast medium has no relevance in an intravenous cholangiogram examination, as its absence is not a sign of obstruction. Care must be taken when injecting the contrast into the common bile duct, to ensure that no air bubbles are introduced, and thus avoid false positive diagnoses of retained gallstones.

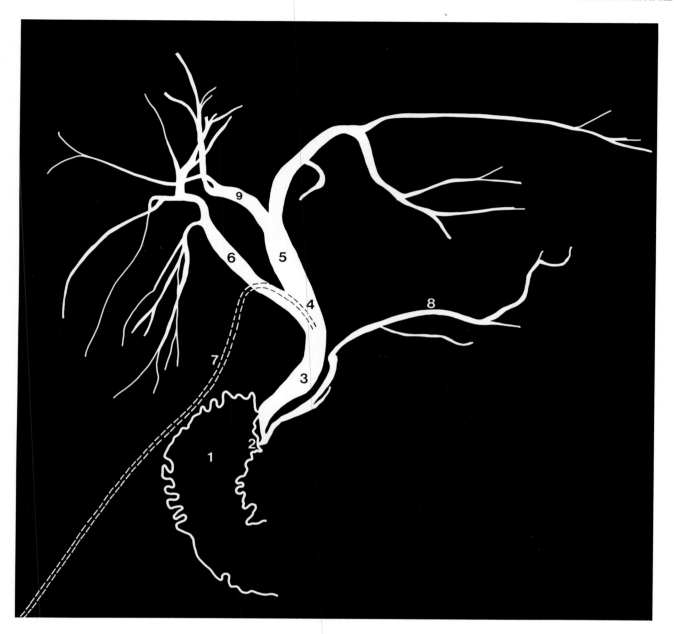

1 Contrast in descending part of
   duodenum

2 Hepatopancreatic ampulla (Vater)

3 Common bile duct

4 Common hepatic duct

5 L. hepatic duct

6 R. hepatic duct (ventral branch)

7 Catheter (T-tube)

8 Contrast reflux in pancreatic duct

9 R. hepatic duct (dorsal branch)

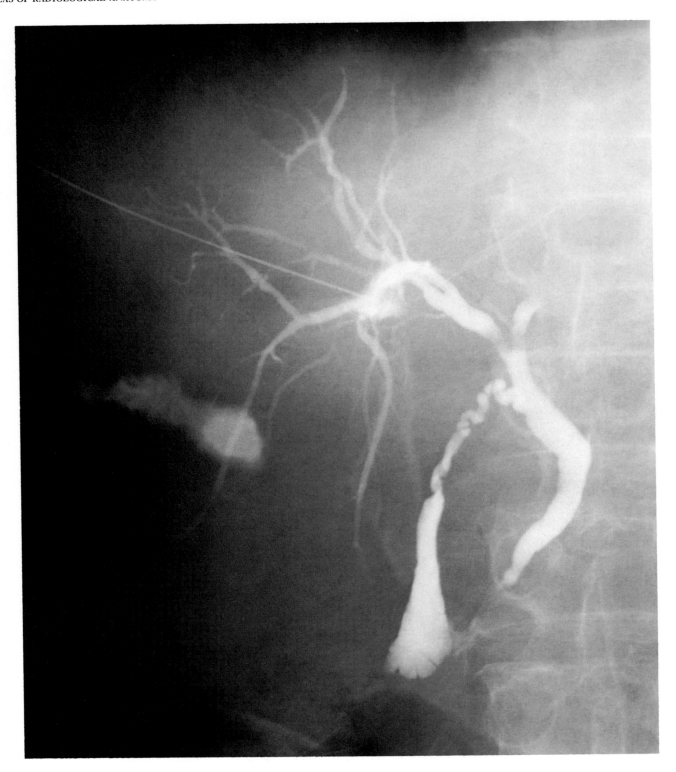

PERCUTANEOUS TRANSHEPATIC CHOLANGIOGRAM

This examination has been performed by introducing a needle from the right side of the abdomen into the substance of the liver, to enter the right hepatic duct. With this type of small gauge needle, it is possible to enter normal as well as dilated ducts and is thus a valuable diagnostic technique. Note that with this type of needle, no bile can be aspirated, hence contrast is injected while the needle is withdrawn until a bile duct is entered. The left hepatic duct is filled only at its origin—this is normal in a supine position as this duct runs anteriorly. A little contrast is seen entering the duodenum and there is narrowing of the lower end of the common bile duct as it enters the duodenal wall. In jaundiced patients this technique differentiates between obstructive and non-obstructive lesions and is of special use in the study of congenital biliary atresia. Complications include sepsis and biliary peritonitis, and some authorities say that this technique should be performed only when surgery is available immediately afterward for those cases with biliary obstruction.

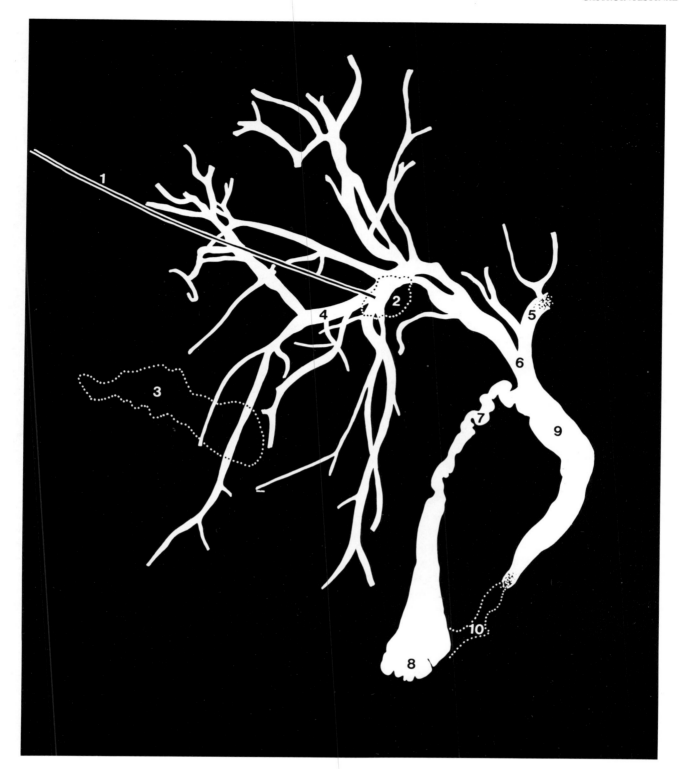

1 Thin needle entering r. hepatic duct

2 Parenchymal contrast medium leakage

3 Parenchymal contrast medium

4 R. hepatic duct

5 L. hepatic duct

6 Common hepatic duct

7 Spiral valve of cystic duct

8 Gall bladder fundus

9 Common bile duct

10 Contrast medium flowing into duodenum

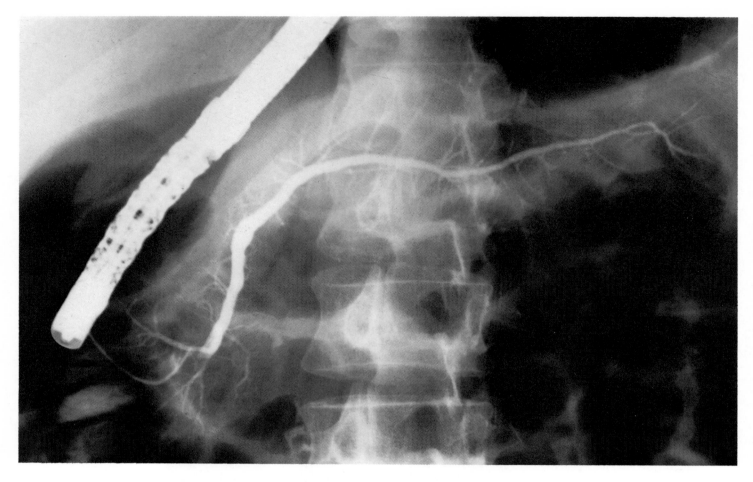

ENDOSCOPIC RETROGRADE CHOLANGIOPANCREATOGRAM

Endoscopy of the stomach and duodenum is performed and cannulation of the ampulla of Vater is attempted under direct vision. Water-soluble contrast is then gently introduced into the common bile duct from below and outlines the biliary and pancreatic ducts. The selectivity of the injection will depend on the position of the junction between the biliary and pancreatic ducts. The pancreatic duct lies closer to the posterior surfaces of the pancreas and runs right through the gland, giving small ducts at right angles. The body of the pancreas is separated from the stomach by the omental bursa and the tail lies in contact with the spleen between the two layers of the lienorenal ligament. The accessory pancreatic duct drains from the head of the pancreas and may join the main duct or open separately into the duodenum. Complications of this technique include fever, a rise in serum amylase and septicaemia.

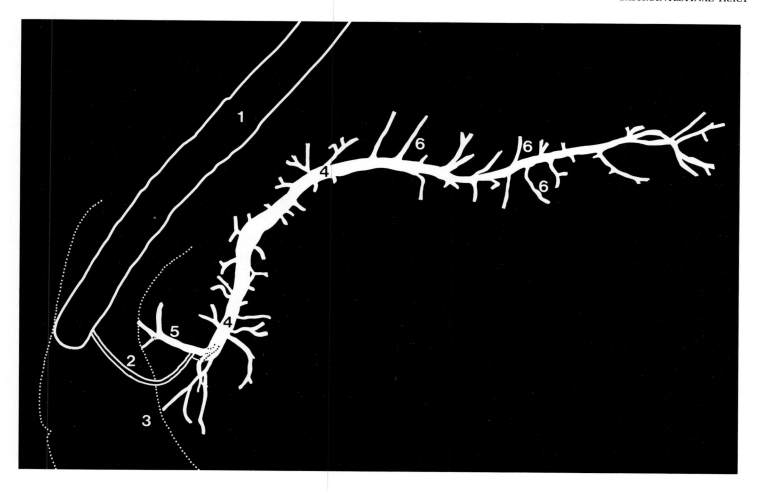

1   Fibreoptic endoscope in second part of duodenum

2   Cannula inserted into main pancreatic duct (Wirsung) via ampulla

3   Gas in second part of duodenum

4   Main pancreatic duct

5   Accessory duct (Santorini)

6   Intralobular ducts in 'herring-bone' pattern

GENITOURINARY SYSTEM

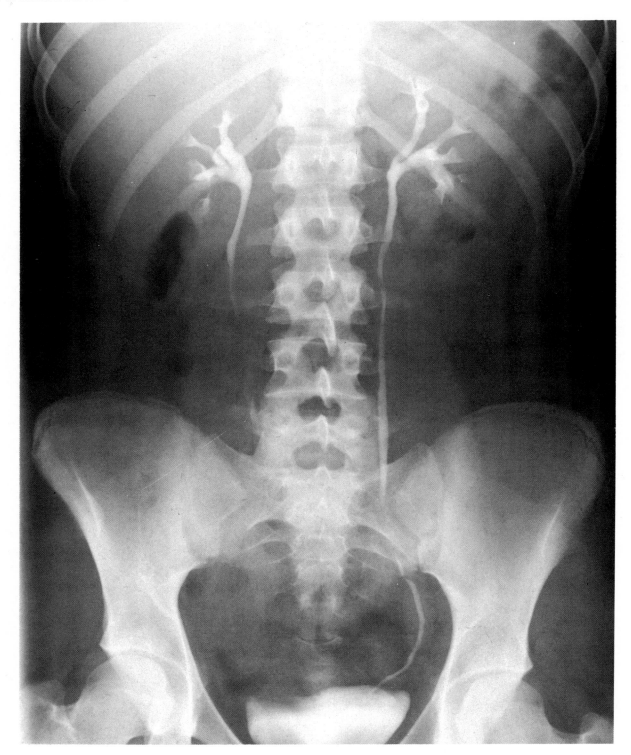

INTRAVENOUS PYELOGRAM (UROGRAM)

The right kidney is usually smaller, further from the midline and lower than the left kidney. This film was taken at 20 minutes following an intravenous injection of water-soluble contrast medium (40 ml of contrast with iodine content of 420 mg/ml). Ureteric compression had just been released so that the full length of the ureters is visualized with contrast. Note this patient's age by the epiphyseal lines of the iliac crests, which fuse at approximately 25 years. The splenic hump on the left kidney is just a variant of normal and should not be confused with a mass. The papillae indent the minor calyces and are the site for the termination of the collecting tubules (ducts of Bellini). High dose urography often with nephrotomography is used in the investigation of renal failure, ureteric obstruction, emergency examination following trauma and for the differential diagnosis of renal masses.

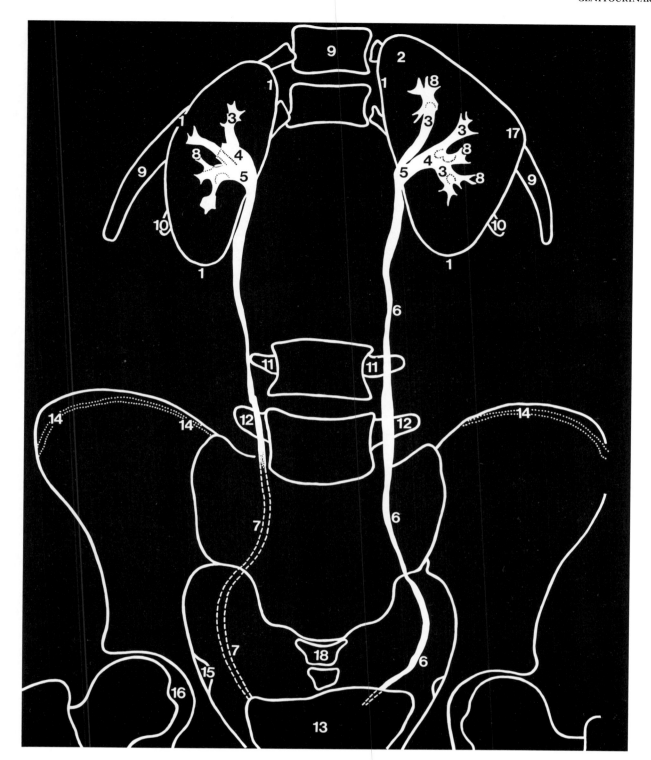

1	Renal outline	7	Position of r. ureter	13	Bladder
2	Sup. lobe of renal cortex	8	Position of renal papilla	14	Epiphyseal line
3	Minor calyx	9	Eleventh thoracic vertebral body and rib	15	Ischial spine
4	Major calyx	10	Twelfth rib	16	Fovea
5	Pelvis of kidney	11	Transverse process of L4	17	Splenic hump
6	L. ureter	12	Transverse process of L5	18	Coccyx

MALE URETHROGRAM AND SEMINAL VESICULOGRAM (VASOGRAM)

Indications for male urethrography include demonstration of urethral strictures, false passages, injuries or fistulae. Viscous contrast medium is injected in a retrograde direction and, using a clamp, the urethra is outlined. Anatomically it is divided into three parts: the prostatic urethra, the membranous urethra which is the site of the external sphincter and the penile urethra. Injection is made under screen control taking films at different angles so that short strictures are not missed. The seminal vasogram was performed under general anaesthetic and demonstrates the proximal vas deferens and the seminal vesicles, both of which drain via the ejaculatory ducts on the colliculus seminalis (verumontanum). As this study is performed under non-physiological conditions, there is reflux of contrast into the bladder which would not occur during ejaculation as the bladder neck is then closed.

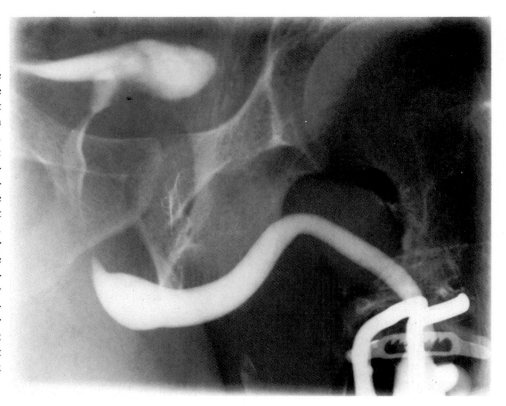

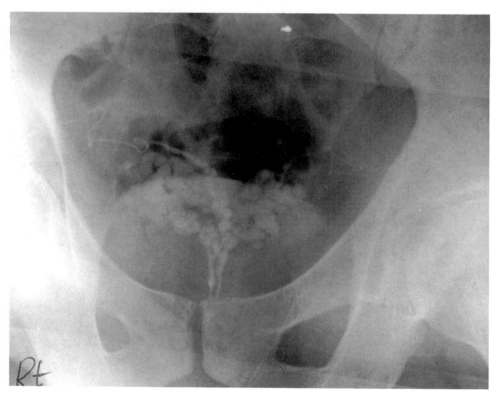

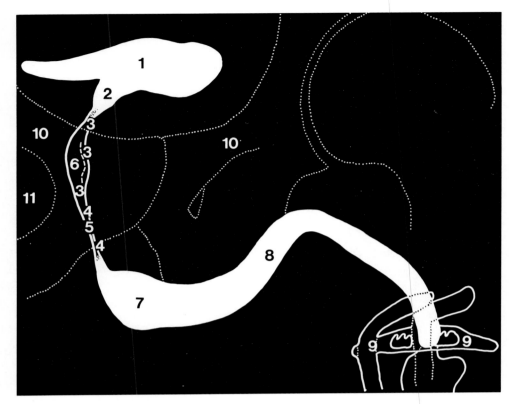

1 Contrast medium in urinary bladder

2 Bladder neck

3 Prostatic urethra

4 Membranous urethra

5 Site of sphincter urethrae (external sphincter)

6 Site of colliculus seminalis (verumontanum)

7 Bulbous urethra

8 Spongy urethra (penile)

9 Penile clamp (Knuttson's)

10 Sup. ramus of pubis

11 Obturator foramen

12 Ductus deferens (vas deferens)

13 Ampulla of ductus deferens

14 Seminal vesicle

15 Ejaculatory duct

16 Phlebolith

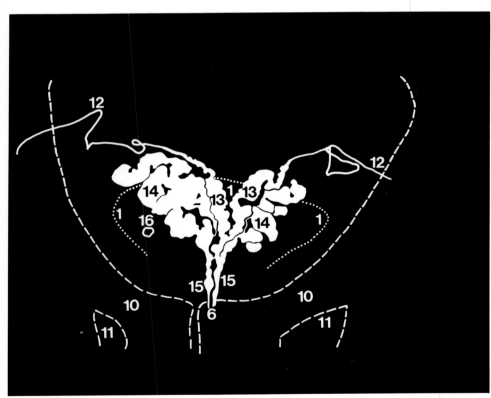

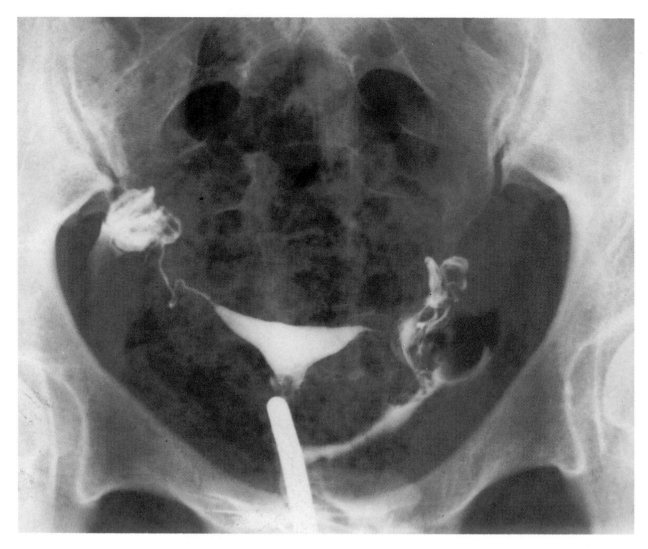

HYSTEROSALPINGOGRAM

The two main indications for this examination are infertility and recurrent abortion. Watertight cannulation of the cervix is performed and aqueous contrast medium is injected to outline the uterus and uterine tubes. Some authorities use oil-based contrast but granuloma formation and a flare-up of any pelvic infection may result. The narrowest point of the fallopian or uterine tube is at the entrance to the uterine cavity. The widest point is at the abdominal end, the infundibulum, before it opens into the peritoneal cavity. Free spillage of contrast into the pelvic cavity is an important sign and should be distinguished from loculated spill due to pelvic inflammatory disease. When possible this examination should be performed 7–10 days following menstruation as earlier in the cycle, venous intravasation may result, and later on in the cycle accidental fetal irradiation may occur.

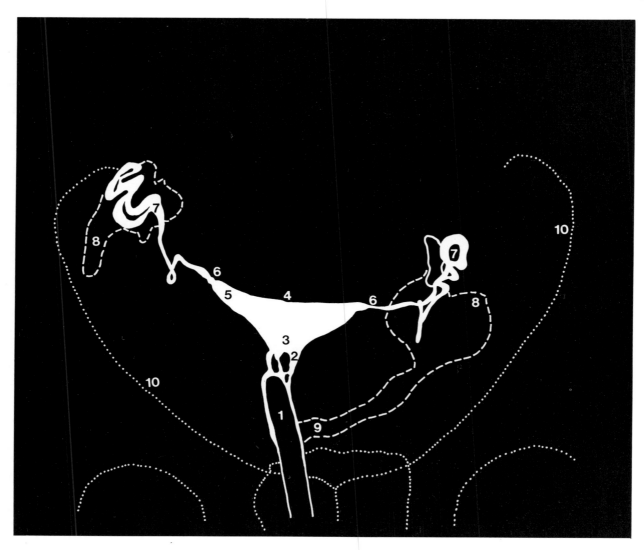

1	Vaginal cannula	5	Cornu	8 'Overspill' into peritoneal cavity
2	Cervix uteri	6	Isthmus of uterine tube (fallopian tube)	9 'Overspill' in rectouterine pouch (Douglas)
3	Body of uterus filled with contrast medium	7	Ampulla of uterine tube	10 Pelvic brim
4	Fundus of uterus			

MISCELLANEOUS

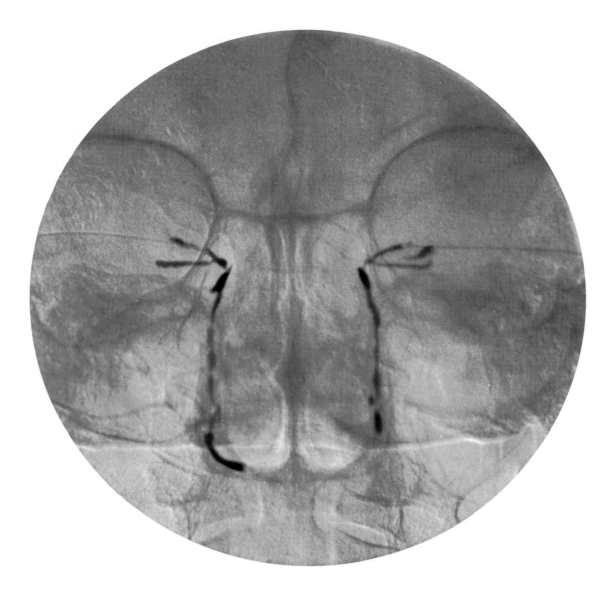

SUBTRACTION MACRODACRYOCYSTOGRAM

The inferior canaliculus is cannulated, having first dilated the punctum. The superior punctum is normally outlined by reflux of contrast but can be injected separately if necessary. Oil-based contrast medium is used and 2 ml usually suffices to show the whole duct system. The two canaliculi join to form the common canaliculus before entering the lacrimal sac. The sac is approximately 12 mm long and shows a slight constriction at its lower end which is said to be due to the orbicularis oculi muscle. This corresponds to the valve of Krause. The lacrimal duct extends downwards to open into the nasal cavity in the inferior meatus. The anatomists describe a second constriction in the intraosseous part of the duct and this is caused by a fold of mucosa (valve of Taillefer). At the site of opening into the inferior meatus, there is a slightly expanded orifice with another valve of mucous membrane called the lacrimal fold (valve of Hasner). Indications for this technique include obstruction (either partial or complete), diverticula, sinuses, fistulae, polyps and tumours.

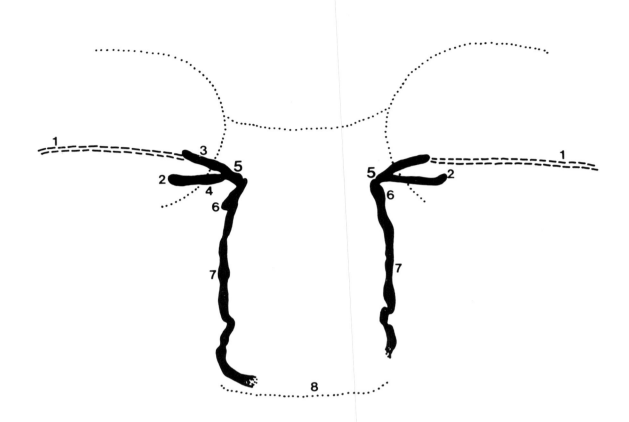

1	Lacrimal catheters	4	Inf. canaliculus	7	Nasolacrimal duct
2	Site of puncta lacrimalia	5	Common canaliculus	8	Hard palate
3	Sup. canaliculus	6	Lacrimal sac		

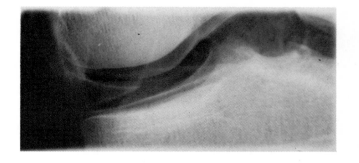
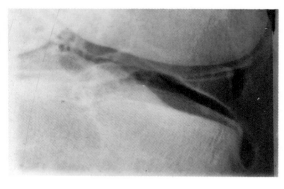
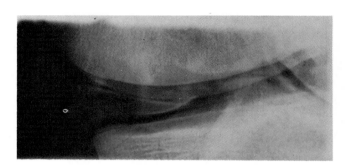
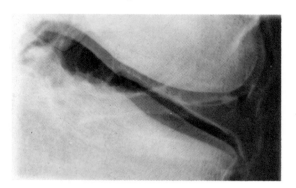

DOUBLE CONTRAST ARTHROGRAMS OF KNEE JOINT

This technique is performed by inserting a needle laterally behind the patella, into the joint space; 30 ml of air is injected followed by 5 ml of aqueous contrast medium. The knee joint is then distended with carbon dioxide and the needle is removed. Valgus or varus stress on the knee is performed while films are taken so that the relative compartment under examination is opened up and the meniscus is separated from the condyles by gas. The medial meniscus is wedge shaped and is larger than the lateral meniscus. The most characteristic feature of the lateral meniscus is the separation of the posterior part by the popliteus tendon sheath. The two cruciate ligaments in the intercondylar area are intracapsular but extra-articular. Indications for knee arthrography include acute injury, recurrent joint effusion, popliteal cyst formation, cruciate ligament injury and persistent symptoms following meniscectomy. Absolute contraindications are acute infection of the joint or overlying skin.

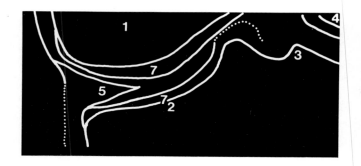
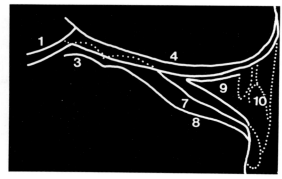
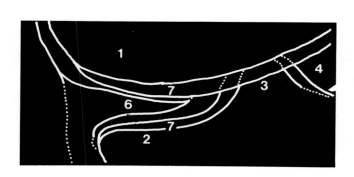
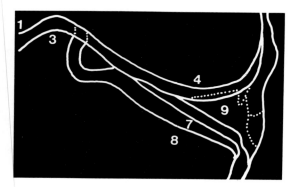

1   Med. femoral condyle

2   Med. tibial condyle

3   Intercondylar eminence

4   Lat. femoral condyle

5   Middle third of med. meniscus (semilunar cartilage)

6   Post. horn of med. meniscus (semilunar cartilage)

7   Articular cartilage

8   Lat. tibial condyle

9   Lat. meniscus (semilunar cartilage)

10   Site of popliteus t.

ARTHROGRAMS OF SHOULDER AND KNEE

The bursae of the shoulder joint can be shown by injecting aqueous contrast medium through a needle inserted just anterior to the acromioclavicular joint. Two main extensions to the synovial cavity are noted, one along the sheath of biceps muscle and the other a subscapular bursa extending beneath the coracoid process. Rotator cuff injuries with leakage into the supraspinatus bursa can be shown and injuries to the long head of biceps tendon can also be demonstrated.

The lateral knee arthogram shows the cruciate ligaments to their best advantage. Damage is rare but anterior cruciate ligament tears may occur with or without meniscal injury. This may be shown by anterior tibial traction films.

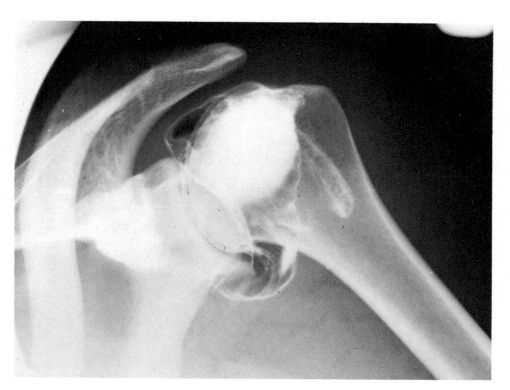

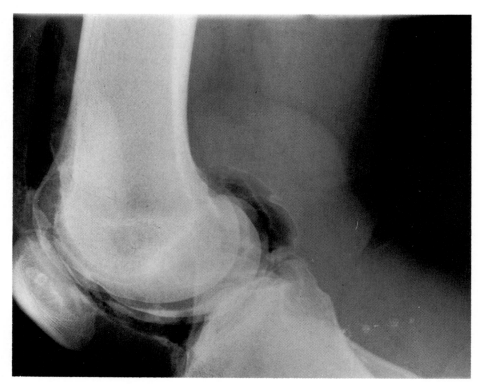

240

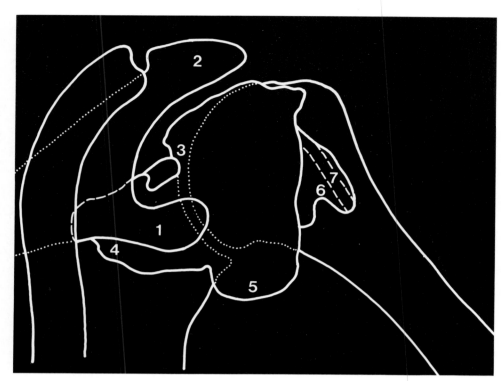

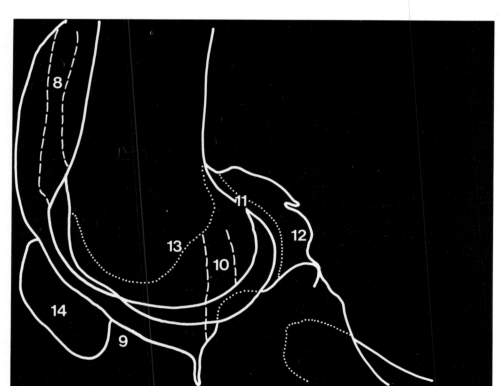

1   Coracoid process

2   Acromion

3   Glenohumeral joint

4   Subcoracoid bursa

5   Axillary pouch

6   Synovial sheath of intertubercular sulcus

7   T. of long head of biceps

8   Suprapatellar bursa

9   Infrapatellar pad of fat

10 Ant. cruciate ligament

11 Articular cartilage

12 Post. extension of synovial cavity

13 Position of intercondylar fossa (notch)

14 Patella

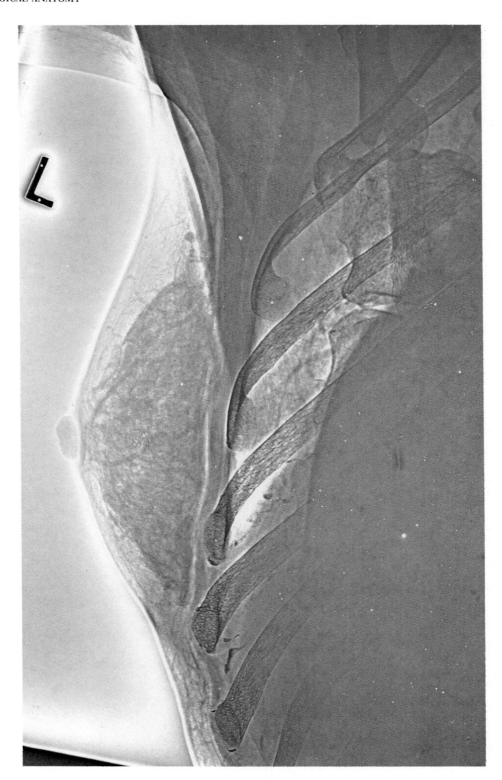

XEROMAMMOGRAM

Xeroradiography is performed using an aluminium–selenium plate which is electrostatically charged. Some advantages of this technique over conventional mammography are that a higher power of 40–45 kV can be used, exposure times are shorter and finer detail is said to be seen. The radiation dosage to the breast is much the same as a conventional radiographic examination. The main indication for mammography is in the investigation of a breast mass. It is usually possible to distinguish between a benign and malignant lesion, but it is not always possible to distinguish between benign lesions. Carcinomata of the breast can be recognized by the appearance of the mass itself. Secondary changes in other parts of the breast can also be very useful in this diagnosis. The breast structure varies considerably, depending on the age of the patient—an adolescent breast is very different from a postmenopausal breast. Note that xeromammography shows muscle boundaries very clearly.

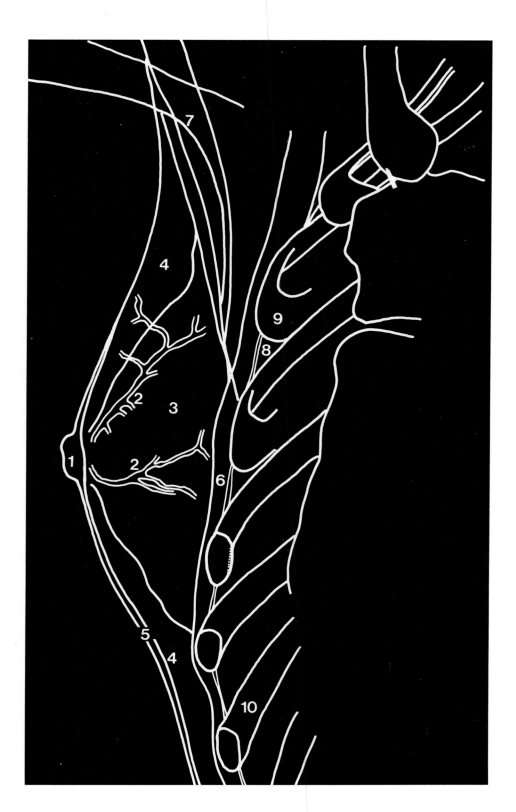

1   Nipple

2   Veins

3   Glandular tissue

4   Adipose tissue

5   Epidermis

6   Intercostal muscles

7   Lat. border of pectoralis major

8   Edge of pleura

9   Second rib

10   Sixth rib

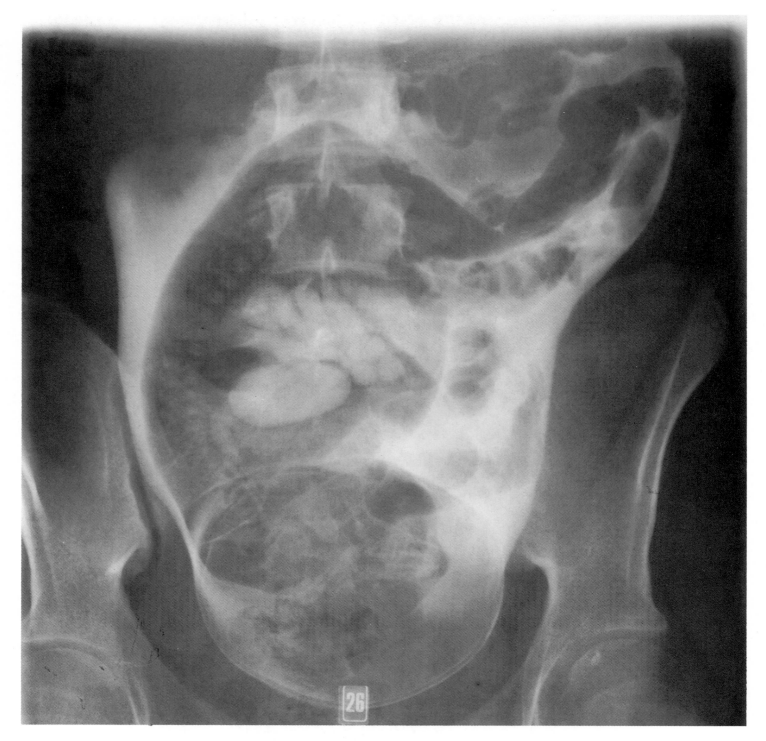

ANTEROPOSTERIOR AMNIOGRAM IN THIRD TRIMESTER

Amniography is performed by introducing a needle through the maternal abdominal wall into the amniotic cavity. It is best performed well away from the placenta to avoid haemorrhage! About 25 ml of aqueous contrast medium is injected and films are taken between 30 minutes and 6 hours. Apart from fetal irradiation the risks include premature labour, placental haemorrhage and fetal injury. This procedure is undertaken to help diagnose placental site, fetal death or abnormalities and as a guide prior to intrauterine fetal blood transfusion. It is also useful in detecting premature rupture of membranes by showing contrast medium in the vagina; rarely, it may diagnose an extrauterine pregnancy. Normally the fetus swallows contrast from within the amniotic fluid and demonstrates the gastrointestinal tract. In cases of intrauterine death, there is no gastrointestinal uptake of contrast medium. This examination is now rarely performed, ultrasound having replaced it. The amniogram is retained here only to demonstrate fetal anatomy.

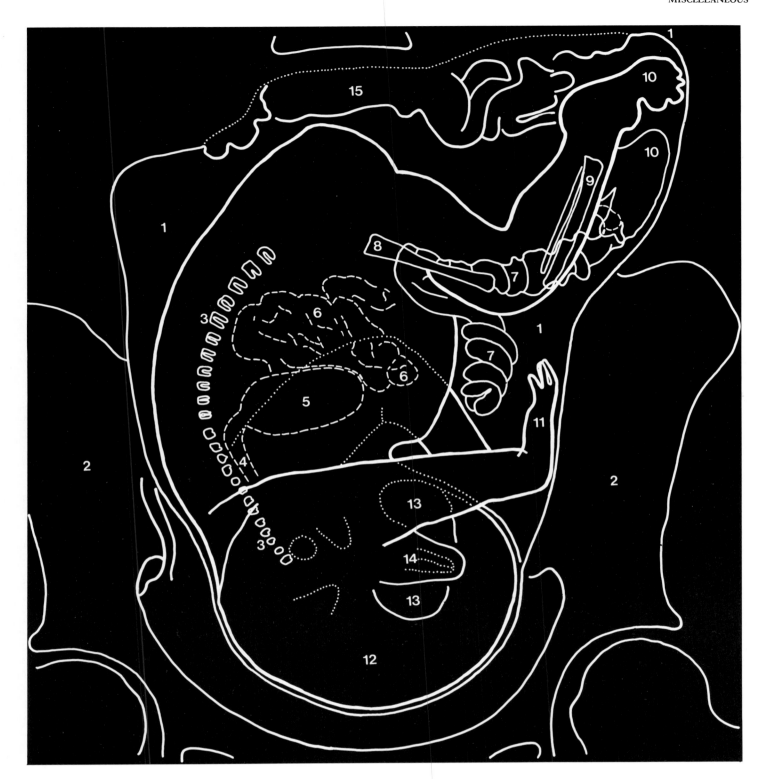

1   Contrast medium in amniotic cavity

2   Maternal ilium

3   Fetal vertebral column

4   Contrast medium in oesophagus

5   Contrast medium in stomach

6   Contrast medium in small bowel

7   Umbilical cord

8   Developing femur

9   Developing tibia

10   Outlined fetal feet

11   Outlined fetal hand

12   Fetal skull

13   Orbit

14   Nasal cavity

15   Placenta

COMPUTED TOMOGRAPHY

The following section deals with the body from the base of the skull through to the pelvis and includes views of the arm and leg. All the sections are in the transverse axial plane, the patients lying supine and with suspended respiration (inspiration) where necessary. All slices are 10 mm thick except where stated. The top slice is shown at upper left, the second slice is upper right, the third slice is bottom left and the fourth slice is bottom right. 'Left' and 'right' markers, and window settings are given only on the first slice on a page to avoid unnecessary labelling. No definitive vertebral levels are given, nor are any scanograms (planograms) included. This is deliberate policy as vertebral levels vary considerably with the build of the patient and with respiratory movement.

It is more appropriate to describe structures in relation to other structures and to note their position. Thus slice increments in millimetres are given in all the following scans and can be related to important anatomical landmarks. If desired, vertebral levels can be readily assessed by this method.

By convention, the head and upper neck are viewed from above, and the rest of the body from below, hence the 'left' and 'right' markers' positions. A double window facility is used on the sections through the chest to allow the soft tissues to be shown on one setting and the lung fields on the other. This saves duplication but does produce a highlighting artefact around the pleura and the trachea.

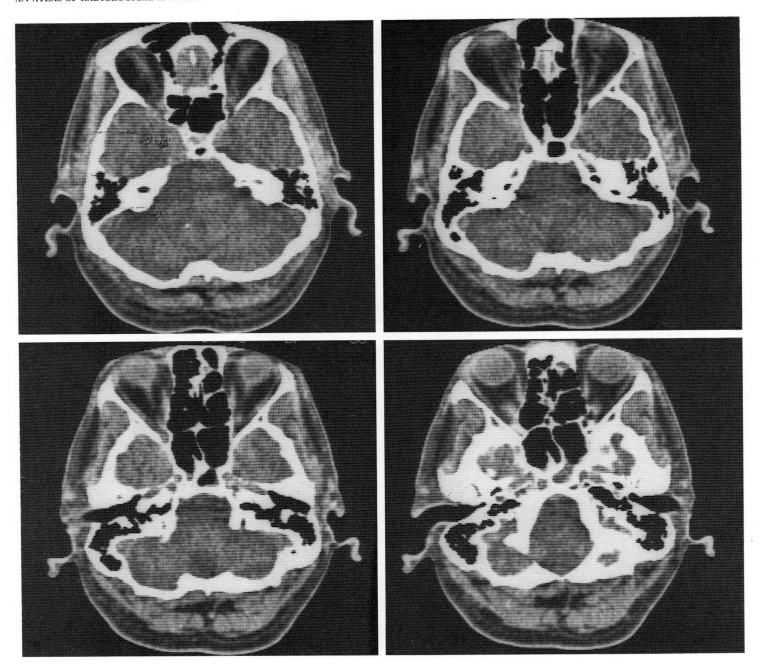

UPPER NECK: 1

This group and the following eight sections show 4 mm incremental slices from the levels of the pons and posterior fossa to the vertebral body of C2. These twelve sections are labelled in the traditional way for viewing cranial CT; that is, the images are viewed from above with the patient's left side on the left of the page. In the mid-cervical region the convention changes so that the left side of the patient is on the right-hand side of the page, the scans being viewed from below. The precise point of the changeover is variable. This originated so that neurosurgeons would be able to compare the radiographs directly with the operating field at craniotomy. (Slice increments 4 mm)

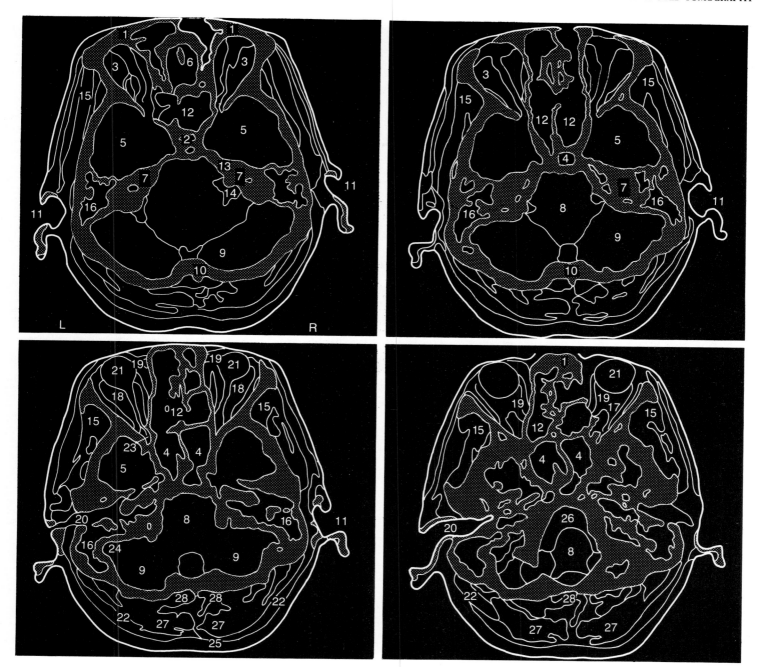

1	Frontal bone	11	Pinna	20	External auditory meatus
2	Pituitary fossa	12	Ethmoid sinus	21	Globe
3	Orbital fat	13	Petrous ridge	22	Sternomastoid m.
4	Sphenoid sinus	14	Cerebellopontine angle	23	Optic canal
5	Temporal lobe	15	Temporalis m.	24	Sigmoid sinus
6	Crista galli	16	Mastoid air cells	25	Trapezius m.
7	Petrous temporal bone	17	Lat. rectus m.	26	Site of basilar a.
8	Pons	18	Optic n.	27	Semispinalis capitis m.
9	Cerebellum	19	Sup. oblique m.	28	Rectus capitis post. m.
10	Occiput				

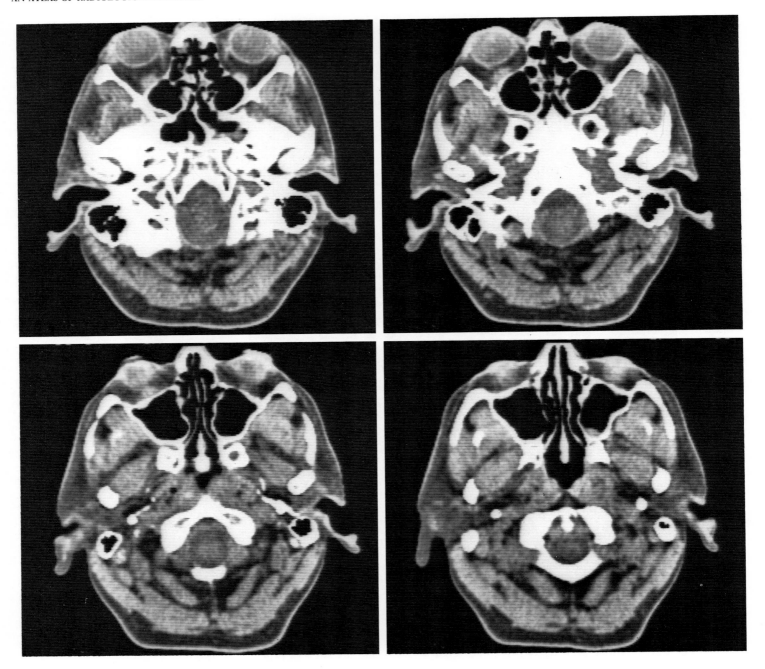

UPPER NECK: 2

The maxillary sinus is pyramidal, with its apex formed by the zygomatic process laterally and its base medially by the lateral wall of the nose. The sinus opens high on the medial wall, into the middle meatus—a poor position for drainage. The posterior wall of the sinus is pierced by the dental canals, through which pass the superior dental vessels and nerves to the molar teeth. The floor of the sinus is formed by the alveolar process, and may be penetrated by the roots of the canine and molar teeth. (Slice increments 4 mm)

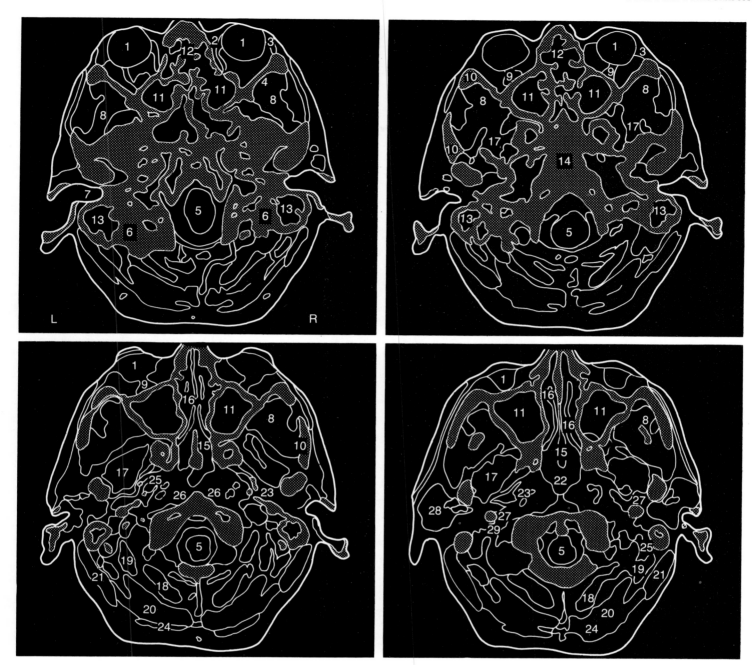

1	Globe	11	Maxillary sinus	21	Sternomastoid m.
2	Med. rectus m.	12	Ethmoid sinus	22	Nasopharynx
3	Lat. palpebral lig.	13	Mastoid antrum	23	Auditory tube
4	Greater wing of sphenoid	14	Clivus	24	Trapezius m.
5	Medulla	15	Vomer	25	Post. belly digastric m.
6	Petrous temporal bone	16	Conchae	26	Long. capitis m.
7	External auditory meatus	17	Lat. pterygoid m.	27	Styloid process
8	Temporalis m.	18	Rectus capitis post. m.	28	Parotid gland
9	Inf. rectus m.	19	Sup. oblique m.	29	Carotid sheath
10	Zygomatic arch	20	Semispinalis capitis m.		

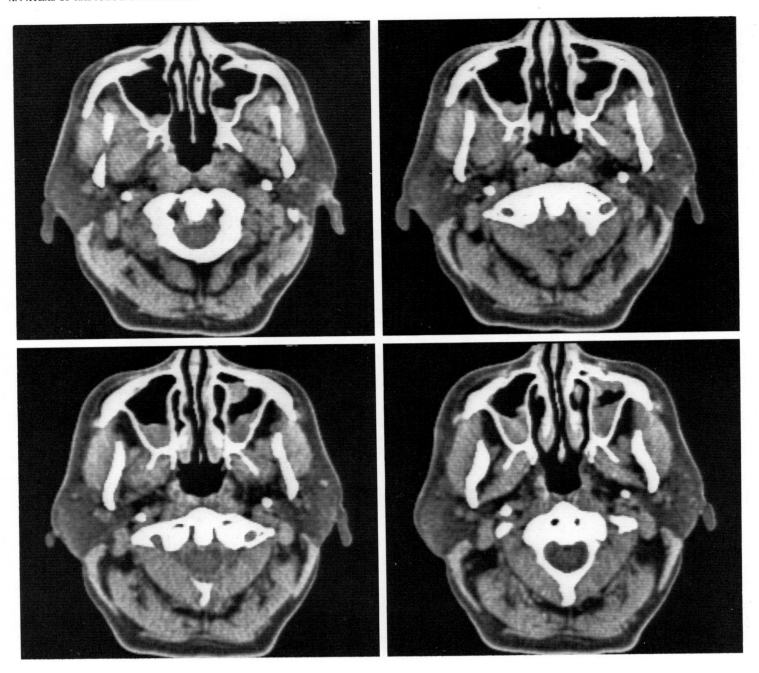

UPPER NECK: 3

The parotid gland is a low-density structure of irregular shape. It contains within its structure the facial nerve and its five terminal branches, the external carotid artery and the posterior facial vein. The external carotid artery divides into its terminal branches, the maxillary and superficial temporal, as it emerges from the gland, behind the neck of the mandible. The parotid gland also contains lymph nodes. The superficial group drain the ear, scalp and upper face, whilst the deep group receive lymph from the middle ear, nose, palate and cheek. (Slice increments 4 mm)

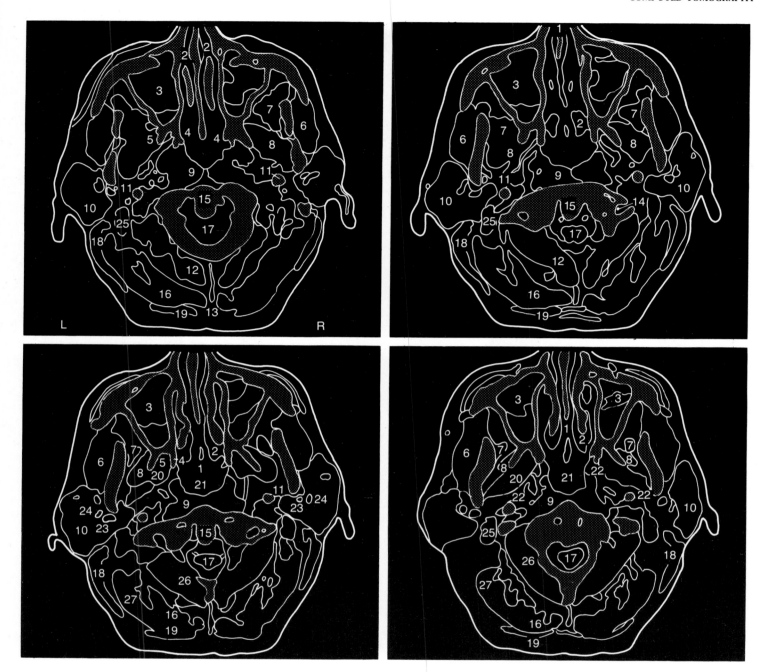

1 Nasal septum	10 Parotid gland	19 Trapezius m.
2 Conchae	11 Styloid process	20 Med. pterygoid m.
3 Maxillary sinus	12 Rectus capitis post. m.	21 Nasopharynx
4 Med. pterygoid plate	13 Ligamentum nuchae	22 Eustachian tube
5 Lat. pterygoid plate	14 Foramen transversarium	23 Retromandibular v.
6 Masseter m.	15 Dens of axis (odontoid peg)	24 Superficial temporal a.
7 Temporalis m.	16 Semispinalis capitis m.	25 Post. belly digastric m.
8 Lat. pterygoid m.	17 Spinal cord	26 Inf. oblique m.
9 Long. capitis m.	18 Sternomastoid m.	27 Splenius capitis m.

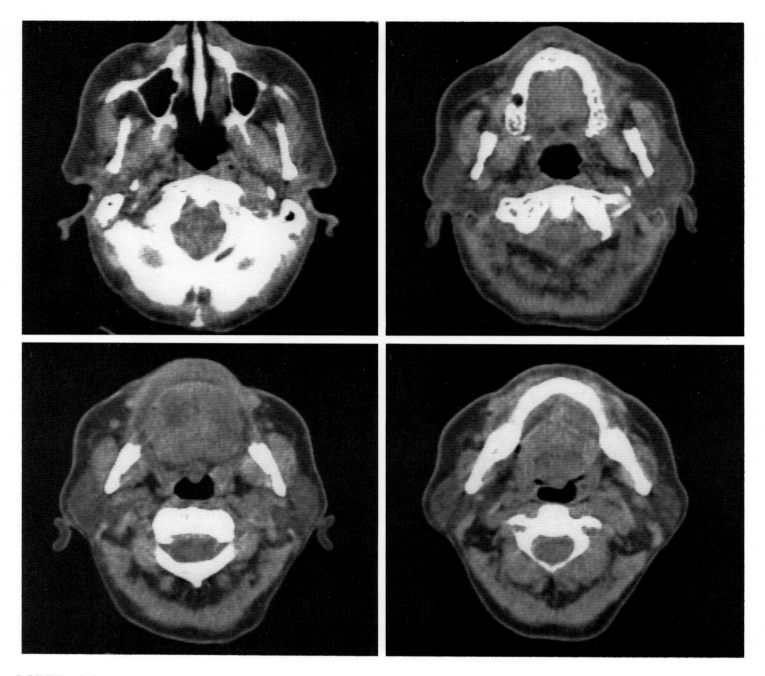

LOWER NECK: 1

This group and the following eight sections are shown at 10 mm slice increments with conventional labelling of left and right sides. The pterygoid processes of the sphenoid descend from the junction of the greater wings and the body. The pterygoid fossa formed by the two processes contains the medial pterygoid and tensor palati muscles. The parotid duct, which is about 5 cm long, passes across the masseter, turns 90°, pierces the buccinator and opens into the mouth opposite the second upper molar tooth. (Slice increments 10 mm)

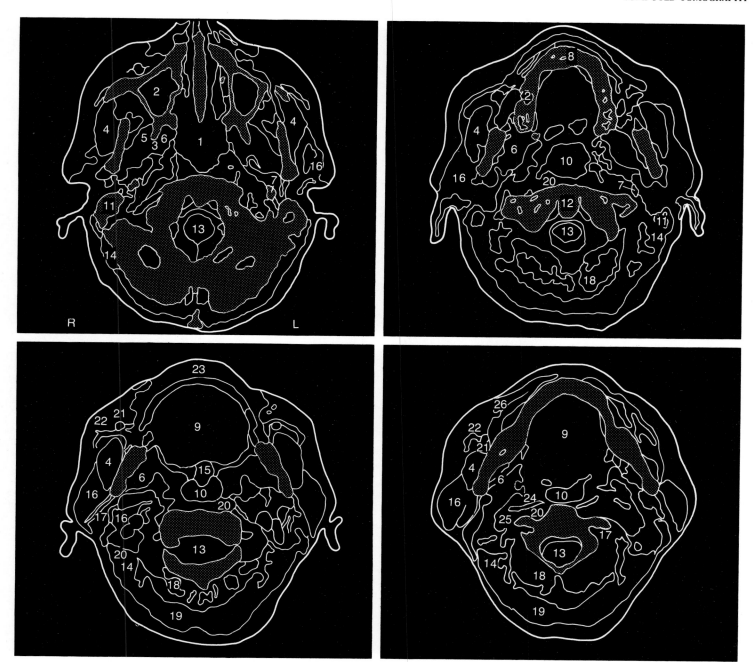

1	Nasopharynx	10	Oropharynx	19	Splenius capitis m.
2	Maxillary sinus	11	Tip of mastoid	20	Long. capitis m.
3	Lat. pterygoid plate	12	Dens of axis (odontoid peg)	21	Depressor anguli oris m.
4	Masseter m.	13	Spinal cord	22	Parotid duct
5	Lat. pterygoid m.	14	Sternomastoid m.	23	Lower lip
6	Med. pterygoid m.	15	Uvula	24	Internal carotid a.
7	Styloid process	16	Parotid gland	25	Internal jugular v.
8	Maxilla	17	Foramen transversarium	26	Orbicularis oris m.
9	Tongue m.	18	Semispinalis capitis m.		

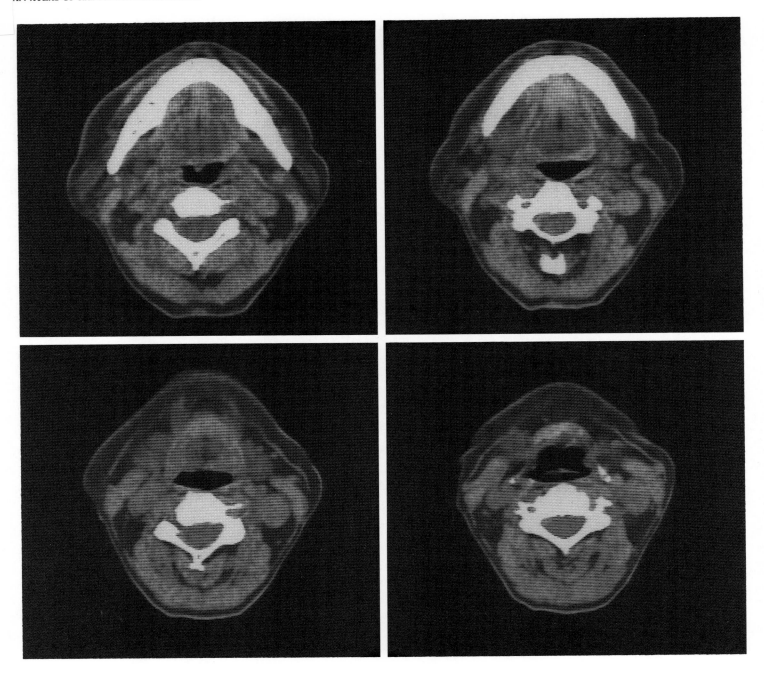

LOWER NECK: 2

The submandibular gland is formed of superficial and deep parts, lying hooked around the mylohyoid muscle. The submandibular duct is 5 cm long and is thinner than the parotid duct. It runs between the mylohyoid and the hyoglossus muscles, passes close to the sublingual gland and opens out onto the sublingual papilla at the side of the frenulum of the tongue. Note a congenital anomaly of the left internal jugular vein, which is dilated but otherwise normal. (Slice increments 10 mm)

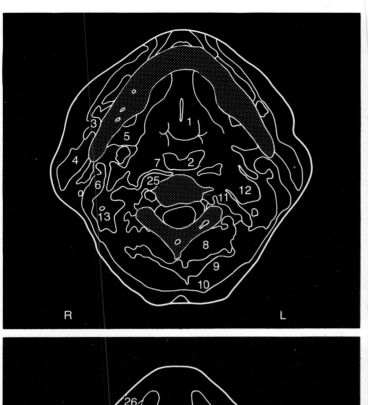
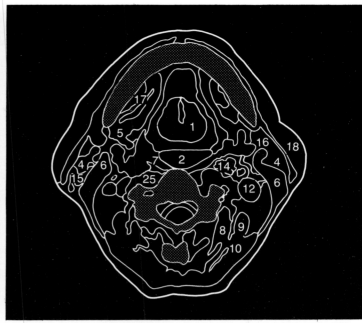
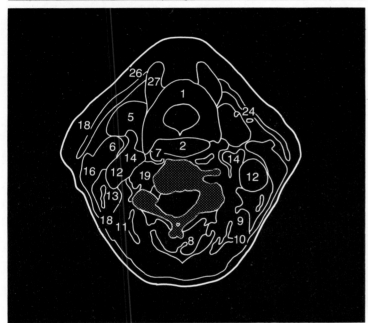
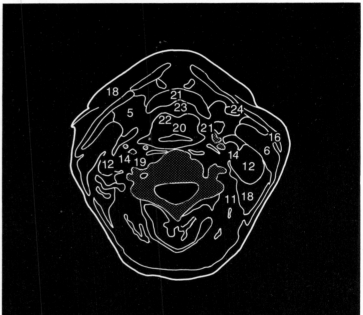

1 Tongue	10 Splenius capitis m.	19 Scalenus ant. m.
2 Oropharynx	11 Levator scapulae m.	20 Epiglottis
3 Masseter m.	12 Internal jugular v.	21 Hyoid bone
4 Parotid gland	13 Spinal accessory n.	22 Valleculae
5 Submandibular gland	14 Internal carotid a.	23 Median glossoepiglottic fold
6 Sternomastoid m.	15 Facial n. and retromandibular v.	24 Lingual a.
7 Pharyngeal constrictor m.	16 External jugular v.	25 Long. coli m.
8 Semispinalis cervicis m.	17 Submandibular duct	26 Platysma m.
9 Semispinalis capitis m.	18 Deep cervical fascia	27 Ant. belly digastric m.

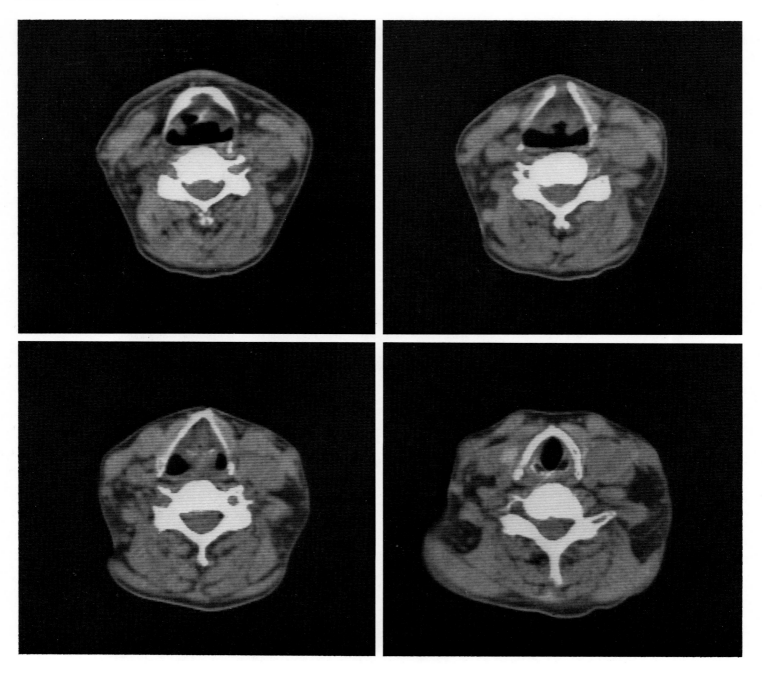

LOWER NECK: 3

The congenital dilatation of the left internal jugular vein is more obvious in these sections.

The larynx is formed of three single cartilages, thyroid, cricoid and epiglottis, and three paired cartilages, two arytenoids, two corniculates and two cuneiforms. The vocal folds or true cords stretch from the middle of the angle of the thyroid cartilage to the vocal processes of the arytenoid cartilages. When examining the larynx by CT, quiet respiration is preferred to breath holding because the laryngeal anatomy is less distorted. (Slice increments 10 mm)

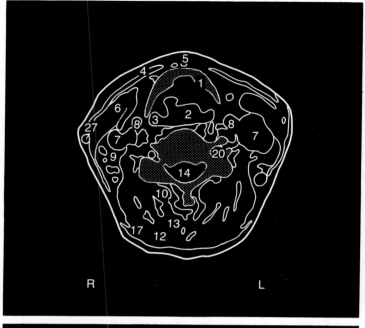
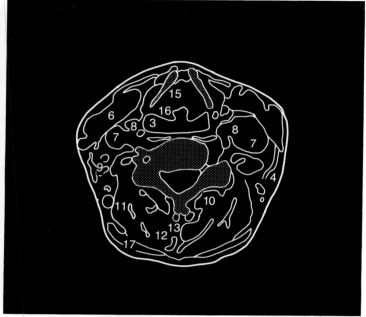
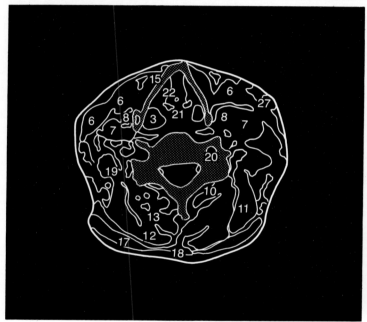
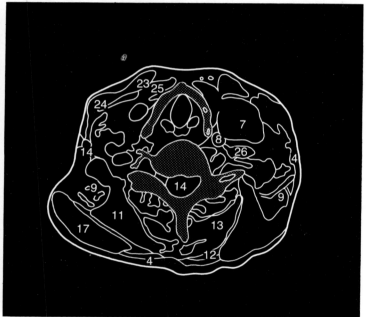

1	Hyoid bone	10	Multifidus m.	19	Scalenus medius m.
2	Vestibule	11	Levator scapulae m.	20	Vertebral a.
3	Piriform fossa	12	Splenius capitis m.	21	Arytenoid cartilage
4	Deep cervical fascia	13	Semispinalis capitis m.	22	Vocal folds
5	Ant. jugular v.	14	Spinal cord	23	Sternal head of sternomastoid m.
6	Sternomastoid m.	15	Thyroid laminae	24	Clavicular head of sternomastoid m.
7	Internal jugular v.	16	Aryepiglottic folds	25	Sternothyroid and sternohyoid m.
8	Internal carotid a.	17	Trapezius m.	26	Scalenus ant. m.
9	Cervical plexus	18	Ligamentum nuchae	27	External jugular v.

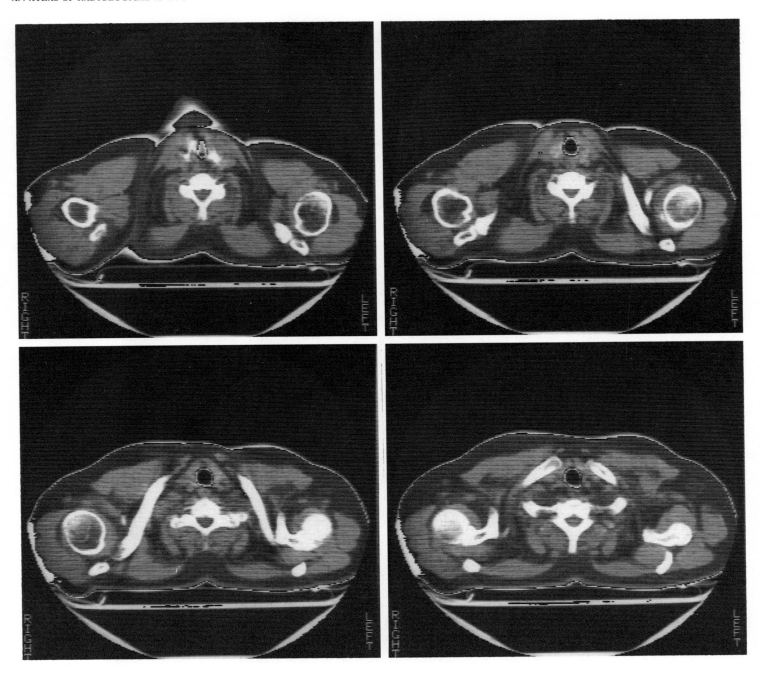

UPPER CHEST: 1

In this chest section and those which follow, the patient is in the supine position with the arms placed above the head. This brings the sternomastoid and the pectoralis major muscles into the same sectional plane. Inferior to the cricoid cartilage lies the thyroid gland, appearing as a denser (higher CT number) structure than the surrounding soft tissue. The two lobes and isthmus are clearly seen. The posterior triangle is roofed by the deep cervical fascia, which splits to enclose the trapezius muscle posteriorly and the sternomastoid muscle anteriorly. The spinal accessory nerve lies adjacent to the inferior surface of the deep fascia.

The pectoralis minor muscle is an important landmark in relations of the brachial plexus and axillary vessels. The muscle arises from the costochondral junctions of the third, fourth and fifth ribs and is inserted into the coracoid process. It is this muscle which divides anatomically the axillary artery into its three parts. (Slice increments 12 mm)

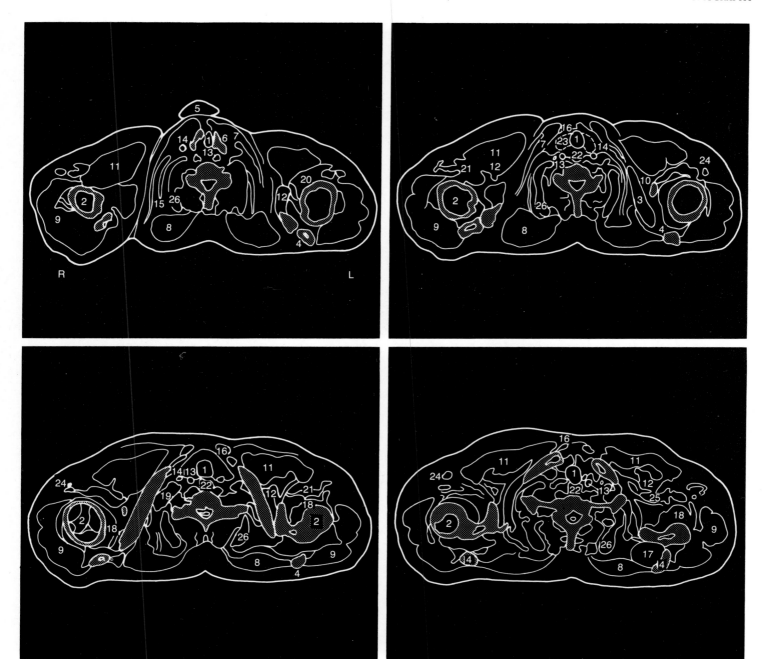

1	Trachea	10	Coracoid process	19	Scalenus ant. m.
2	Humerus	11	Pectoralis major m.	20	Coracobrachialis m.
3	Clavicle	12	Pectoralis minor m.	21	Brachial plexus
4	Acromion	13	Common carotid a.	22	Oesophagus
5	Chin	14	Internal jugular v.	23	Thyroid gland
6	Cricoid cartilage	15	Deep cervical fascia	24	Cephalic v.
7	Strap m.	16	Sternomastoid m.	25	Axillary vss.
8	Trapezius m.	17	Supraspinatus m.	26	Levator scapulae m.
9	Deltoid m.	18	Subscapularis m.		

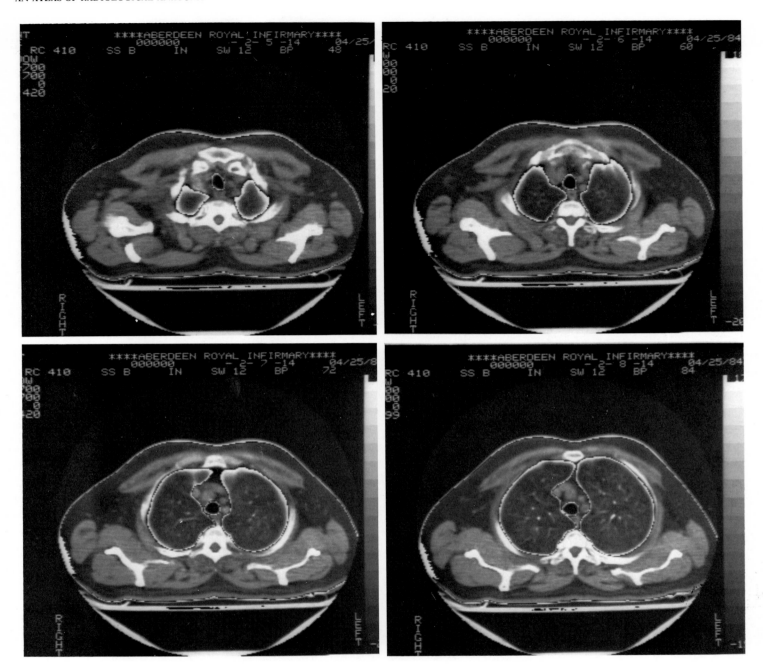

UPPER CHEST: 2

The apices of the lung fields are visible in the first section. The anatomy of the muscles related to the scapula is also well demonstrated. The important anatomical features at these levels are the relationships of the vessels in the mediastinum. The left brachiocephalic vein crosses from the left arm anterior to the great arteries to join the right brachiocephalic vein, forming the superior vena cava. Between the left brachiocephalic vein and the trachea lies the first branch of the aorta, the brachiocephalic (innominate) artery. To its left, and slightly posterior, lie the second and third branches, the left common carotid artery and the left sub-

clavian artery. The oesophagus lies posterior and slightly to the left of the trachea, on the anterior aspect of the vertebral bodies.

In the anterior mediastinum of adults the pleural surfaces of the two upper lobes are almost in apposition. The small space contains mainly fat but is a common site for lymph node enlargement, particularly in Hodgkin's disease. The anterior mediastinum can also move laterally, with herniation of the lung across the midline. This phenomenon may occur after thoracic surgery with lung resection and with other conditions involving changes in lung volume. (Slice increments 12 mm)

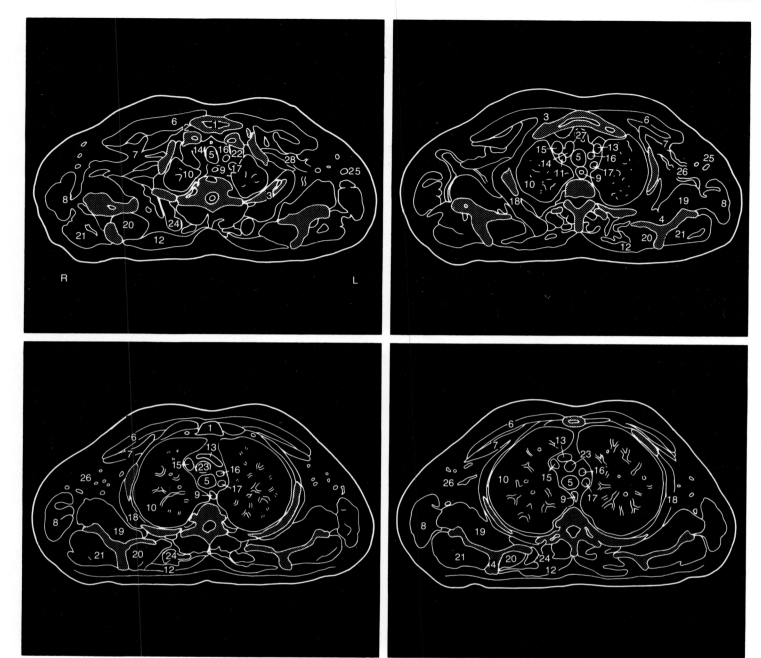

1	Manubrium	11	R. subclavian a.	20	Supraspinatus m.
2	Clavicle	12	Trapezius m.	21	Infraspinatus m.
3	Second rib	13	L. brachiocephalic v.	22	L. internal jugular v.
4	Scapula	14	R. carotid a.	23	Brachiocephalic a.
5	Trachea	15	R. brachiocephalic v.	24	Rhomboid m.
6	Pectoralis major m.	16	L. carotid a.	25	Cephalic v.
7	Pectoralis minor m.	17	L. subclavian a.	26	Axillary nodes
8	Deltoid m.	18	Serratus ant. m.	27	Inf. thyroid v.
9	Oesophagus	19	Subscapularis m.	28	Axillary vss.
10	Lung				

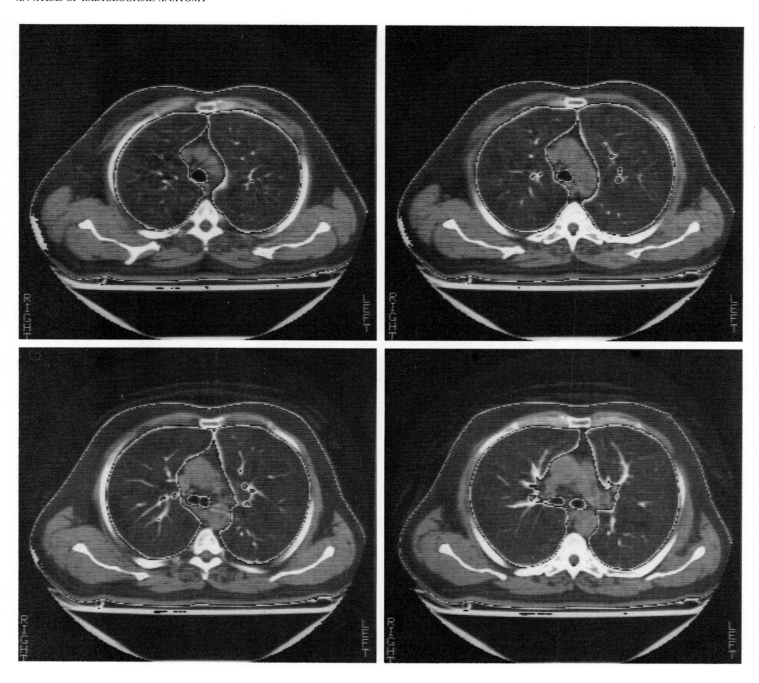

UPPER CHEST: 3

The trachea divides at the level of the T4/5 disc, but in deep inspiration this landmark may be seen at a lower vertebral level. The left recurrent laryngeal nerve lies in the angle formed by the trachea and the oesophagus.

The thoracic duct arises from the cisterna chyli, enters the thorax through the aortic opening in the diaphragm, ascends, crosses to the left at T4–7 and drains into the junction of the left subclavian and internal jugular veins. The azygos system develops from the paired posterior cardinal and supracardinal veins. The main azygos vein ascends lateral to the thoracic duct, arches anteriorly at the level of the carina and enters the superior vena cava. In the supine position with deep inspiration the venous return to the heart is increased and the azygos vein dilates. This is the reason for the prominent azygos vein seen in a supine chest radiograph and on CT.

A few small lymph nodes are noted in the right paratracheal and subcarinal area. Lymph node enlargement can be accurately assessed by CT but, because the technique is not tissue specific, the cause of the enlargement cannot be defined. CT has become the best method for the assessment and definition of mediastinal structures. (Slice increments 12 mm)

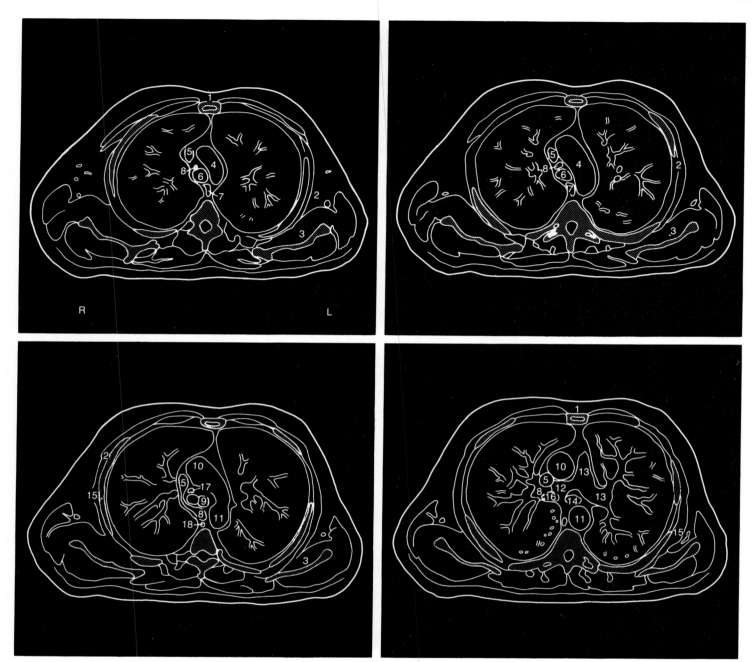

1	Sternum	7	Oesophagus	13	L. pulmonary a.
2	Rib	8	Azygos v. and arch	14	L. main bronchus
3	Scapula	9	Carina	15	Serratus ant. m.
4	Aortic arch	10	Ascending aorta	16	R. main bronchus
5	Sup. vena cava	11	Descending aorta	17	R. paratracheal lymph nodes
6	Trachea	12	Subcarinal area	18	Thoracic duct

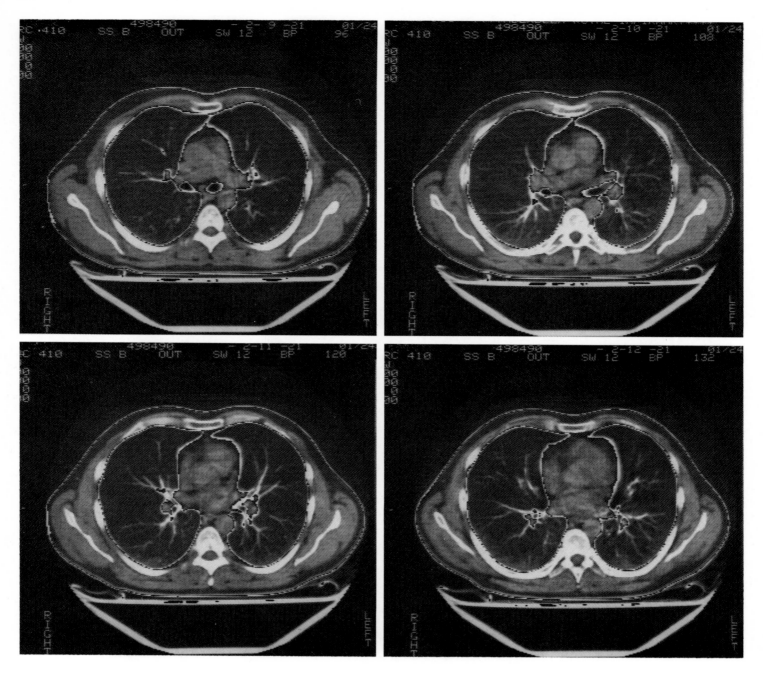

LOWER CHEST: 1

The pulmonary trunk divides under the aortic arch, with the right pulmonary artery passing horizontally between the superior vena cava and the right main bronchus. The pulmonary arteries form the hilar shadows on a PA chest radiograph and are clearly seen in the upper left section. Both pulmonary arteries divide into branches which follow the course of the segmental bronchi, usually on the posterolateral or superior aspects.

The coronary arteries pass forwards one on either side of the pulmonary artery, to run in the interventricular and atrioventricular sulci.

The pulmonary veins drain into the centrally placed left atrium. There are two pulmonary veins on each side. The inferior veins drain the lower lobes, the left superior drains the upper lobe and the right superior the upper and middle lobes.

There is a characteristic 'bare' area in the right lung, seen in the upper right section, due to the position of the horizontal fissure and hence the lack of blood vessels. (Slice increments 12 mm)

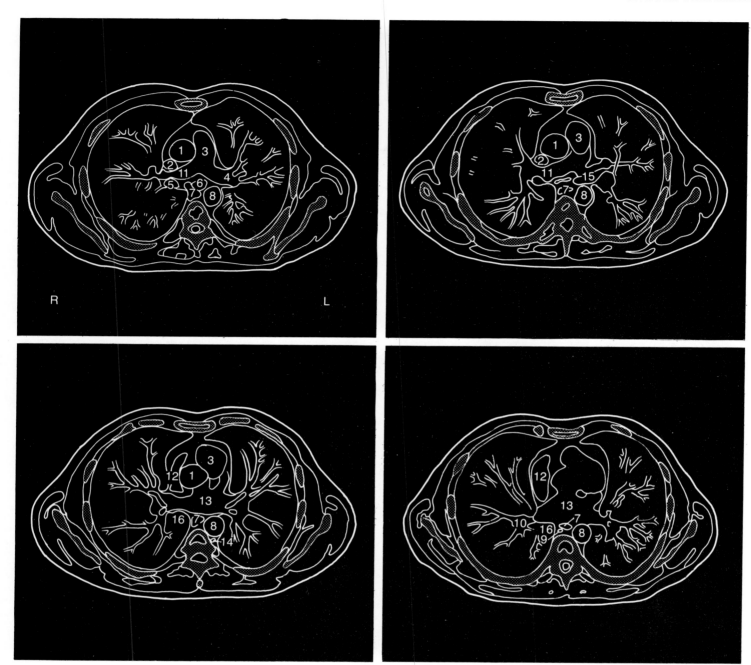

1	**Ascending aorta**	
2	**Sup. vena cava**	
3	**Pulmonary trunk**	
4	**L. pulmonary a.**	
5	**R. main bronchus**	
6	**L. main bronchus**	

7	**Oesophagus**
8	**Descending aorta**
9	**Azygos v.**
10	**Pulmonary v.**
11	**R. pulmonary a.**

12	**R. atrium**
13	**L. atrium**
14	**Hemiazygos v.**
15	**L. upper lobe of bronchus**
16	**Azygo-oesophageal recess**

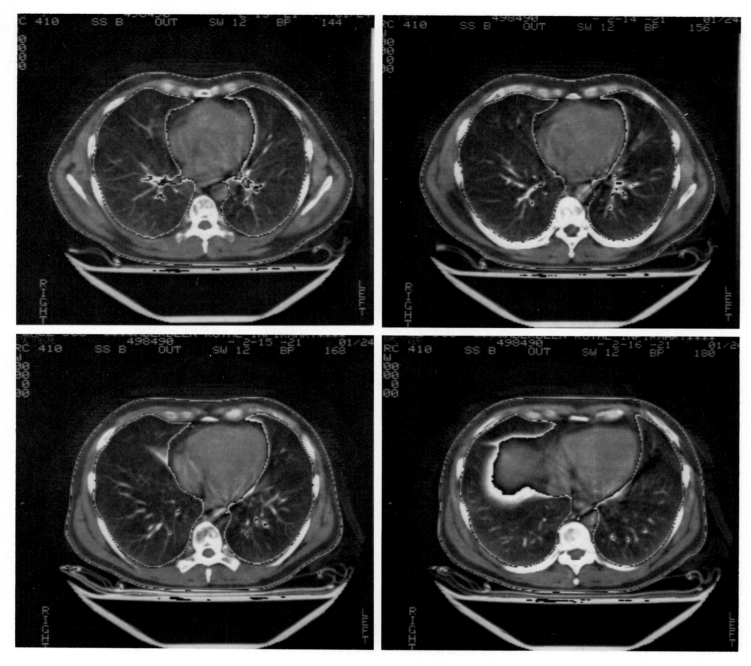

LOWER CHEST: 2

The cardiac chambers are poorly seen with computerized tomography unless ECG gating with high doses of intravenous contrast is used. Most of the CT sections in this atlas were taken at the scan speed of around 10 seconds, resulting in cardiac movement artefacts. The internal architecture and wall characteristics of the cardiac chambers are better demonstrated using ultrasound or nuclear magnetic resonance (NMR).

Both the azygos and hemiazygos vessels are visible in these sections. The vagus nerve and the thoracic duct (unless opacified with contrast) are rarely seen clearly.

Note the relatively anterior position of the inferior vena cava, with the oesophagus and aorta lying posteriorly. This relationship explains the vertebral levels at which these three structures pass through the curved diaphragm: the inferior vena cava at T8/9, the oesophagus at T9/10 and the aorta at T11/12 depending on the phase of respiration. (Slice increments 12 mm)

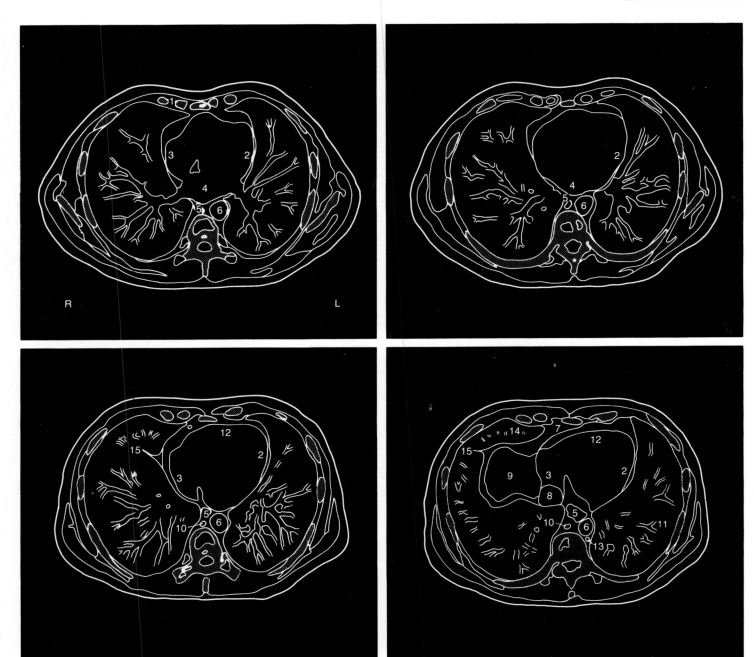

1	Costal cartilage	6	Descending aorta	11	Pulmonary vss.
2	L. ventricle	7	Pericardium	12	R. ventricle
3	R. atrium	8	Inf. vena cava	13	Hemiazygos v.
4	L. atrium	9	R. hemidiaphragm	14	Middle lobe of r. lung
5	Oesophagus	10	Azygos v.	15	Oblique fissure

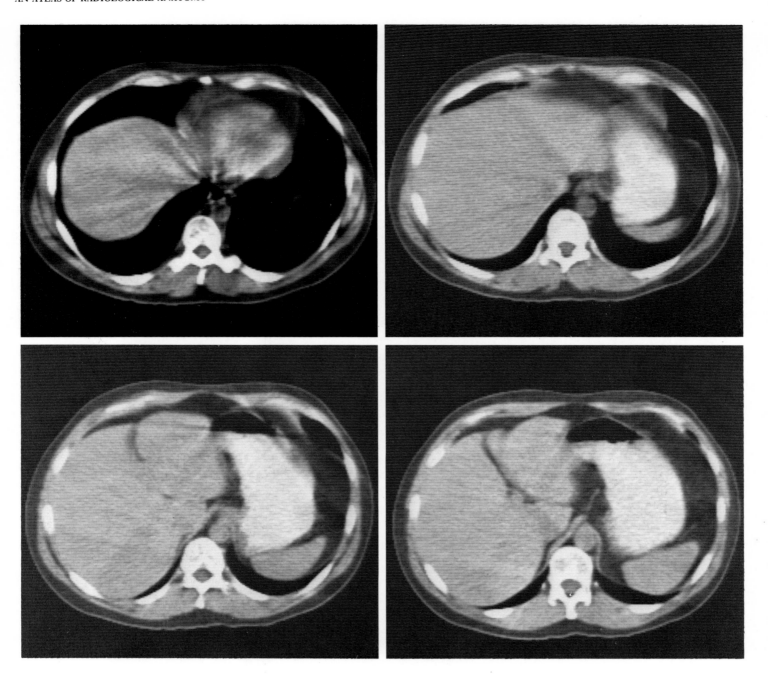

ABDOMEN: 1

The ligamentum teres (or round ligament) is the remnant of the left umbilical vein and runs in the free border of the falciform ligament. This ligament extends from the anterior abdominal wall and diaphragm to the convex surface of the liver. The ligamentum venosum is the true divider of the liver into its right and left lobes, and is the obliteration of the ductus venosus. The fissure for the ligamentum teres divides the left lobe into medial and lateral segments. The quadrate lobe lies anterior to the porta hepatis, the caudate lobe posterior. The lesser omentum is attached to the fissure for the ligamentum venosum and to the porta hepatis.

Little of the internal detail of the liver is visible on unenhanced scans. Intravenous contrast demonstrates the venous anatomy. Intrahepatic bile ducts may be seen when dilated or after cholangiography.

Although CT is not tissue specific, it is possible to show differences in density of the liver depending on the fat and water content. In fatty infiltration, the normal liver density (range approx 45–70 Hounsfield units (HU)) may be reduced considerably and lie below that of water (0 HU). (Slice increments 15 mm)

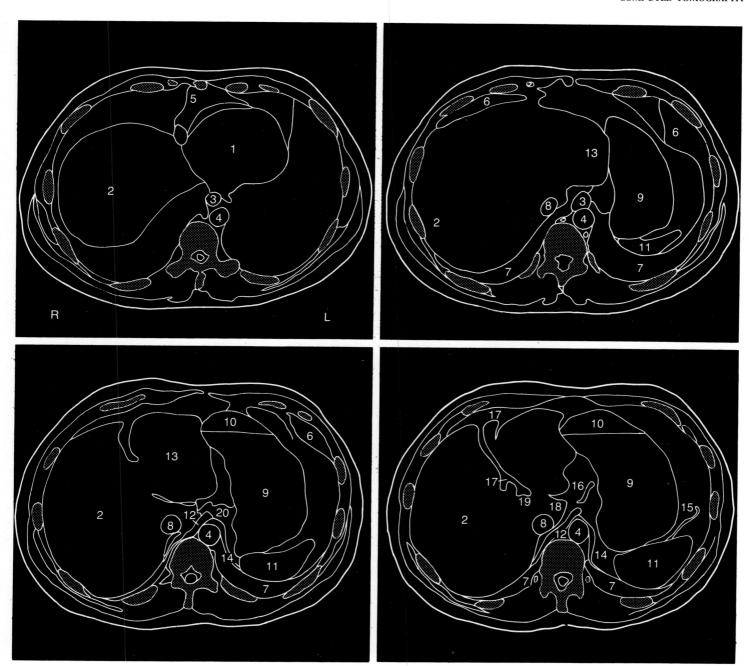

1 Heart	**8** Inf. vena cava	**15** L. gastroepiploic vss.
2 Liver, r. lobe	**9** Stomach	**16** L. gastric vss.
3 Oesophagus	**10** Stomach gas	**17** Fissure for ligamentum teres
4 Descending aorta	**11** Spleen	**18** Caudate lobe
5 Pericardial fat	**12** R. crus of diaphragm	**19** Porta hepatis
6 Ant. costophrenic recess	**13** Liver, l. lobe (med. segment)	**20** Oesophagogastric junction
7 Post. costophrenic recess	**14** L. crus of diaphragm	

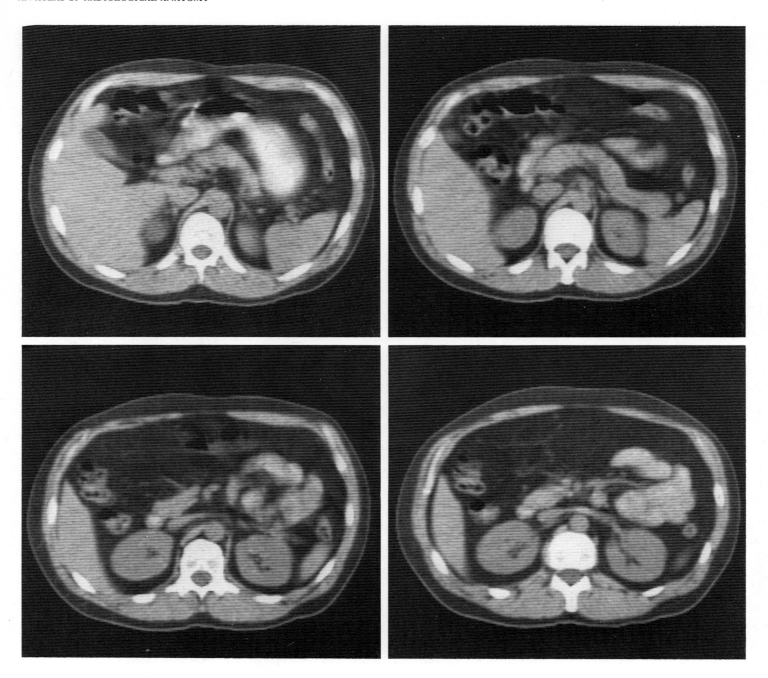

ABDOMEN: 2

The anatomy of the retroperitoneum is shown in these four sections. Both adrenal glands lie anteromedially to the upper poles of the kidneys. Their detailed anatomy is described on p. 304. The portal vein is formed from the splenic, superior mesenteric and inferior mesenteric, together with the left and right gastric veins. It ascends behind the neck of the pancreas to enter the lower omentum where the bile duct and hepatic artery lie anteriorly and the inferior vena cava lies posteriorly. The portal vein passes to the right end of the porta hepatis where it divides. The right branch enters the right lobe, and the left branch passes horizontally to enter the left, quadrate and caudate lobes.

Note the position of the left renal vein as it lies horizontally, anterior to the aorta, to drain into the inferior vena cava. Rarely, a congenital anomaly may occur where the left renal vein lies posterior to the aorta and may thus become obstructed. Note also the shape of the diaphragmatic crura throughout their length as they have a tendency to be mistaken for a variety of structures including intercostal arteries, enlarged nodes and anomalous veins! There is also variation in the thickness of the crura, particularly the right. (Slice increments 15 mm)

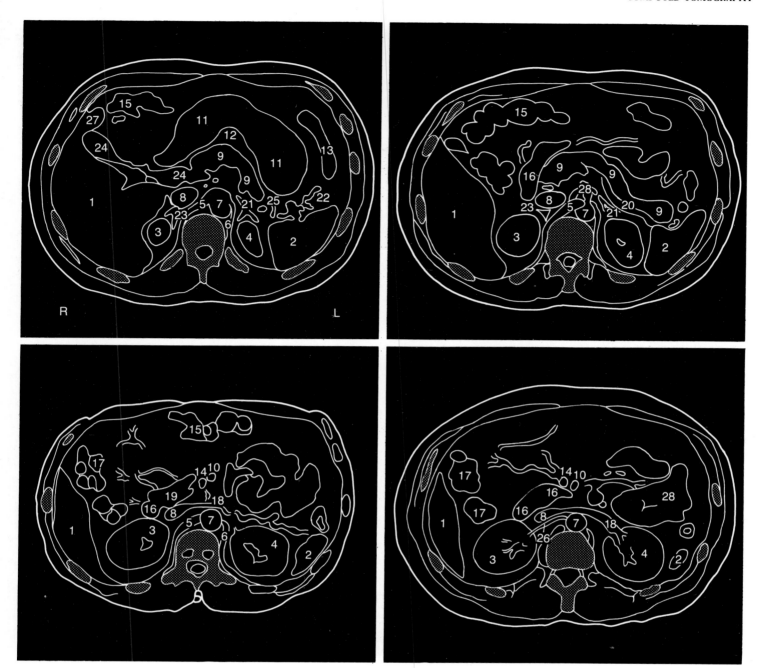

1	Liver, r. lobe	11	Stomach: a) body; b) antrum	20	Splenic v.
2	Spleen	12	Lesser sac (omental bursa)	21	L. adrenal gland
3	R. kidney	13	Splenic flexure	22	L. gastroepiploic vss.
4	L. kidney	14	Sup. mesenteric v.	23	R. adrenal gland
5	R. crus of diaphragm	15	Transverse colon	24	Gall bladder
6	L. crus of diaphragm	16	Duodenum	25	Splenic a.
7	Abdominal aorta	17	Ascending colon	26	R. renal a.
8	Inf. vena cava	18	L. renal v.	27	Liver, l. lobe
9	Pancreas: a) head; b) body; c) tail	19	Uncinate process of pancreas	28	Small intestine
10	Sup. mesenteric a.				

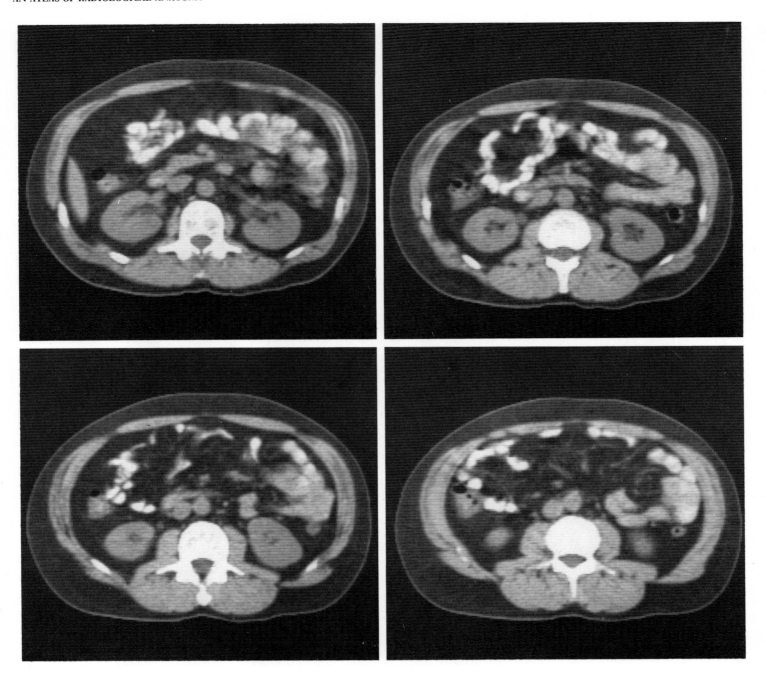

ABDOMEN: 3

The superior mesenteric vein lies anterior and to the right of the superior mesenteric artery. If the vein lies to the artery's left, then malrotation of the small bowel will be present.

The ureter can be seen lying on the psoas muscle, with the gonadal vessels anteriorly.

The duodenum is moulded to the head of the pancreas and is divided into four parts. The superior mesenteric artery and vein cross anterior to the third part in the root of the mesentery and may occasionally cause compression.

The inferior mesenteric artery originates deep to the third part of the duodenum at L3 vertebral level, the normal umbilicus being at the L3/4 disc level. (Slice increments 15 mm)

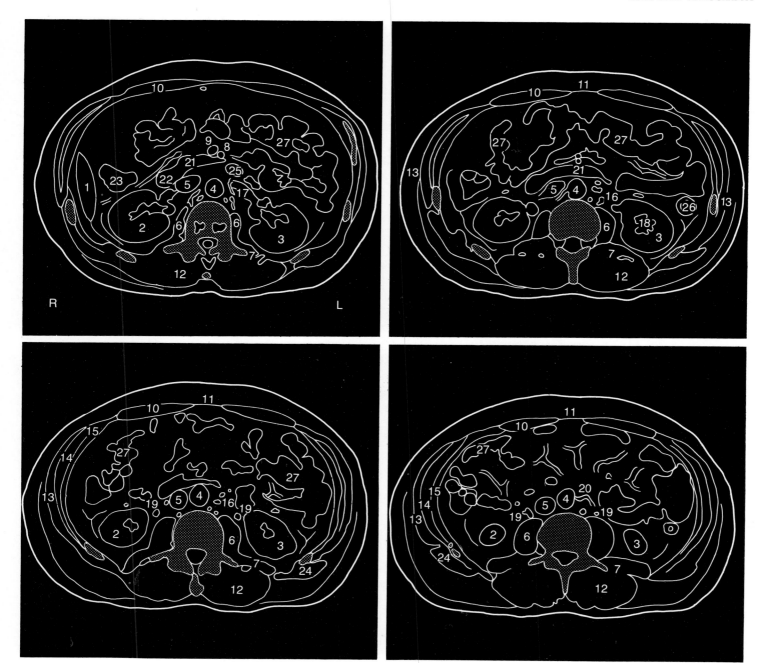

1	Liver, r. lobe	10	Rectus abdominis m.	19	Ureter
2	R. kidney	11	Linea alba	20	Lumbar a.
3	L. kidney	12	Erector spinae m.	21	Duodenum, third part
4	Abdominal aorta	13	External oblique m.	22	Duodenum, second part
5	Inf. vena cava	14	Internal oblique m.	23	Ascending colon
6	Psoas major m.	15	Transversus abdominis m.	24	Latissimus dorsi m.
7	Quadratus lumborum m.	16	Testicular vss.	25	Duodenum, fourth part
8	Sup. mesenteric a.	17	L. renal v.	26	Descending colon
9	Sup. mesenteric v.	18	Renal hilum	27	Small intestine

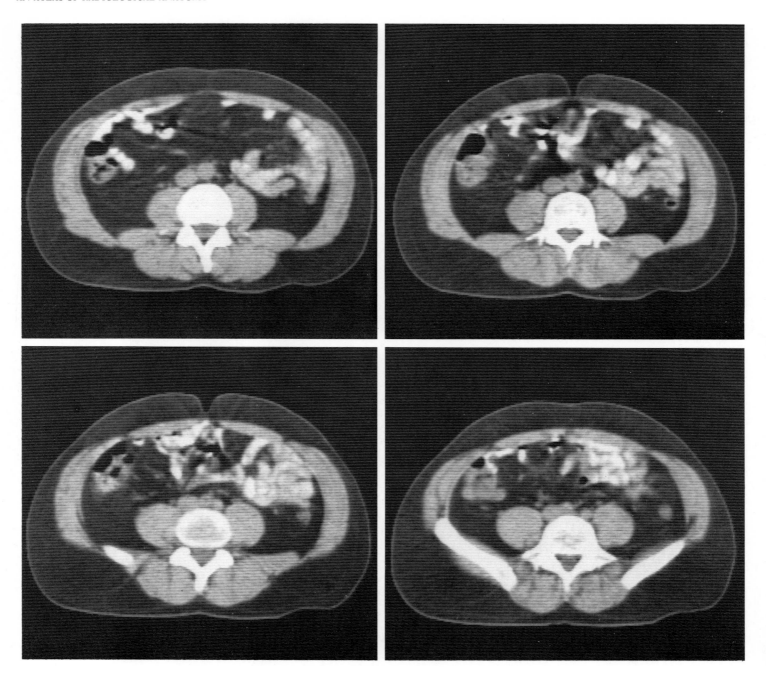

ABDOMEN: 4

In the thin 'normal' adult the umbilicus lies at the level of the L3/4 disc. It lies lower in the old because of the abdominal wall laxity and in the young because of pelvic undevelopment. The aorta divides at the level of L4 into the common iliac arteries, which in turn divide opposite the L5/S1 disc into the internal and external iliac arteries. At this point they are crossed by the ureters. The fan-shaped iliacus muscle arises from the upper aspect of the iliac fossa and inserts with the psoas major tendon into the lesser trochanter. (Slice increments 15 mm)

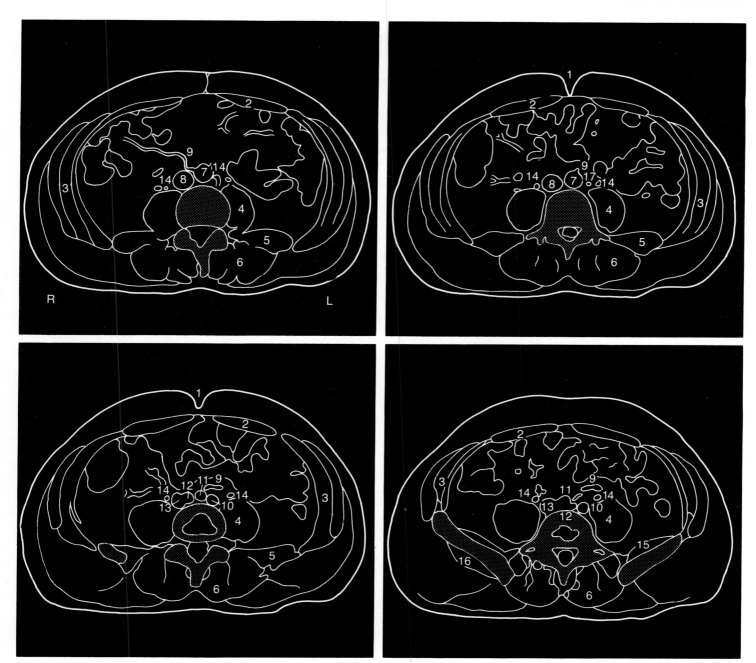

1	Umbilicus	6	Erector spinae m.	12	L. common iliac v.
2	Rectus abdominis m.	7	Abdominal aorta	13	R. common iliac v.
3	Oblique and transverse abdominal mm.	8	Inf. vena cava	14	Ureter
		9	Inf. mesenteric vss.	15	Iliacus m.
4	Psoas major m.	10	L. common iliac a.	16	Gluteus medius m.
5	Quadratus lumborum m.	11	R. common iliac a.		

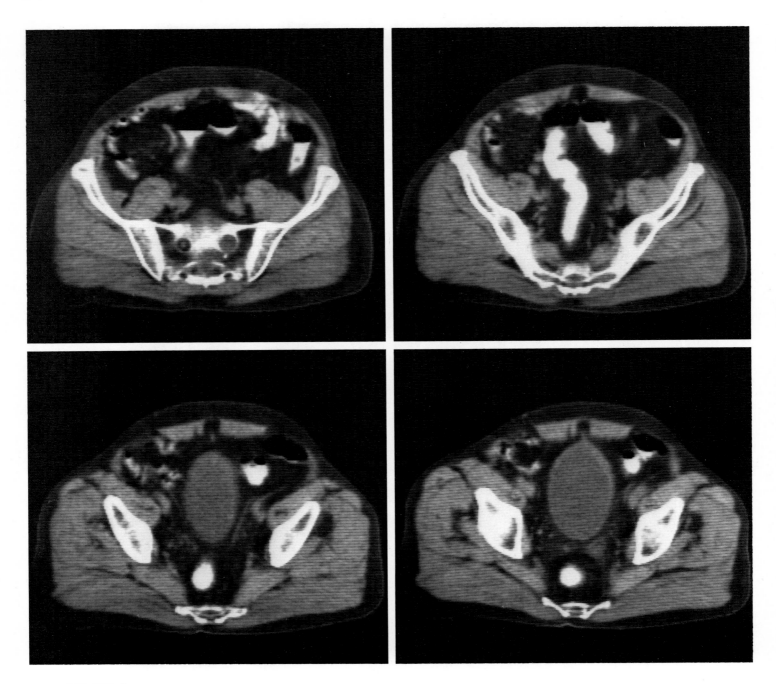

MALE PELVIS: 1

In this and the next group of sections through a male pelvis, the first three are at 20 mm increments, the remainder at 10 mm.

Bowel preparation is used routinely for all abdominal and pelvic examinations. A low-residue gas-free diet is employed for 2 days, to reduce gut contents and gas artefacts. The distal small bowel and proximal colon are opacified by the patient taking contrast medium such as 1.5% Gastrografin orally the night before the examination. Thirty minutes and 5 minutes prior to the scan, a further 1% Gastrografin in 500 ml of fluid is given to opacify stomach and upper small bowel. Rectal contrast is also used for pelvic examinations to outline the rectum and distal colon. A full bladder is also desirable. (Slice increments 20 and 10 mm)

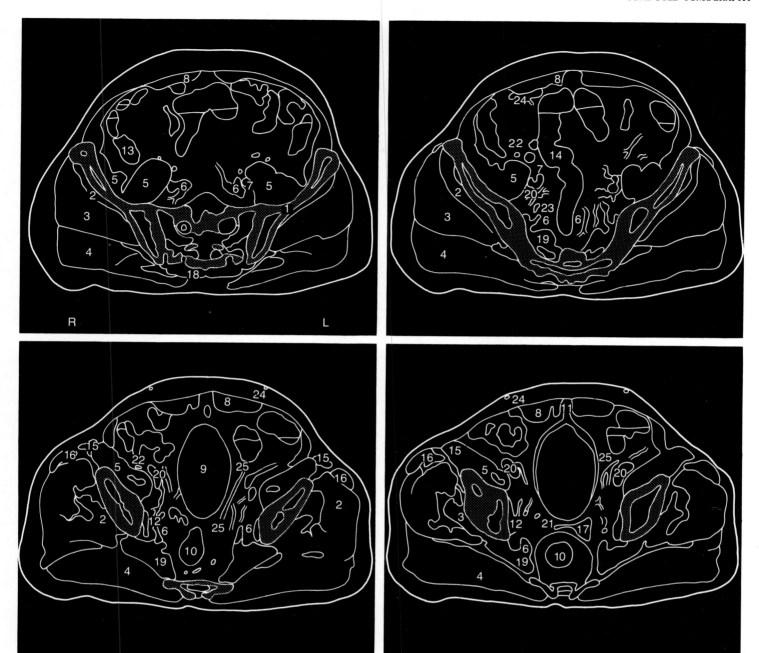

1	Ilium	9	Bladder	17	Seminal vesicle
2	Gluteus minimus m.	10	Rectum	18	Erector spinae m.
3	Gluteus medius m.	11	Urachus	19	Piriformis m.
4	Gluteus maximus m.	12	Obturator internus m.	20	External iliac vss.
5	Iliopsoas m.	13	Caecum	21	Ureter
6	Iliac vss.	14	Sigmoid colon	22	Femoral n.
7	External iliac a.	15	Sartorius m.	23	Obturator a.
8	Rectus abdominis m.	16	Tensor fasciae latae m.	24	Superficial epigastric vss.
				25	Ductus deferens

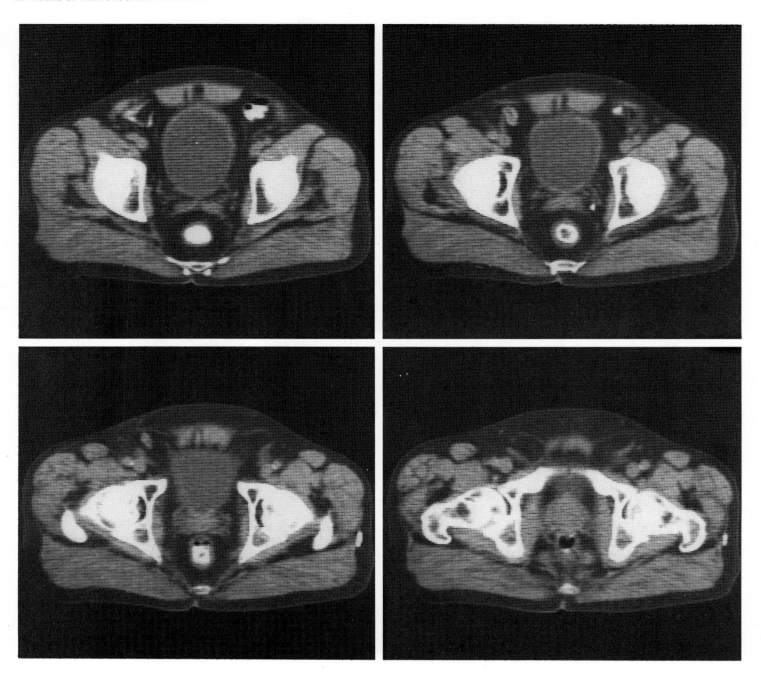

MALE PELVIS: 2

The vas deferens begins at the epididymis, passes upwards in the spermatic cord through the inguinal canal and enters the pelvis after crossing the external iliac vessels. It continues backwards between the perineum and the lateral pelvic wall, crosses the ureter and reaches the seminal vesicle, where it joins the duct from the vesicle to form the common ejaculatory duct.

The relationship of the femoral artery and vein should be noted because of the frequent use of these vessels for catheterization.

An interesting muscle on these sections is the obturator internus. This arises from the anterolateral wall of the pelvis and the obturator membrane. It forms tendinous bands which make a right-angled turn to exit the lesser sciatic foramen between the ischial spine and the tuberosity before inserting into the greater trochanter.

A little calcium is seen in the iliotibial tract following thickening and fibrosis of the fascia lata. (Slice increments 20 and 10 mm)

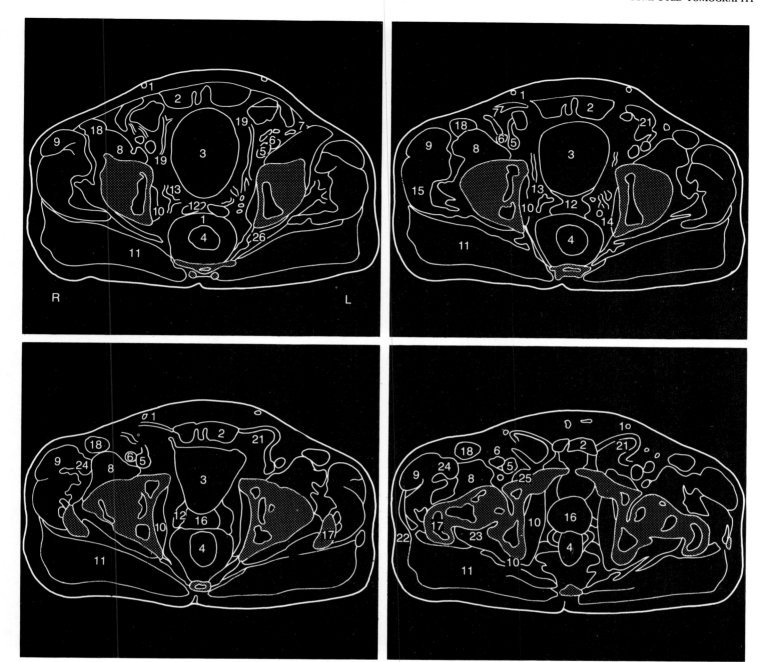

1 Superficial epigastric vss.	10 Obturator internus m.	19 Ductus deferens
2 Rectus abdominis m.	11 Gluteus maximus m.	20 Sacrospinous lig.
3 Bladder	12 Seminal vesicle	21 Spermatic cord
4 Rectum	13 Internal iliac vss.	22 Iliotibial tract
5 Femoral v.	14 Phlebolith	23 Gemellus m.
6 Femoral a.	15 Gluteus medius m.	24 Rectus femoris m.
7 Femoral n.	16 Prostate gland	25 Pectineus m.
8 Iliopsoas m.	17 Greater trochanter	26 Piriformis m.
9 Tensor fasciae latae m.	18 Sartorius m.	

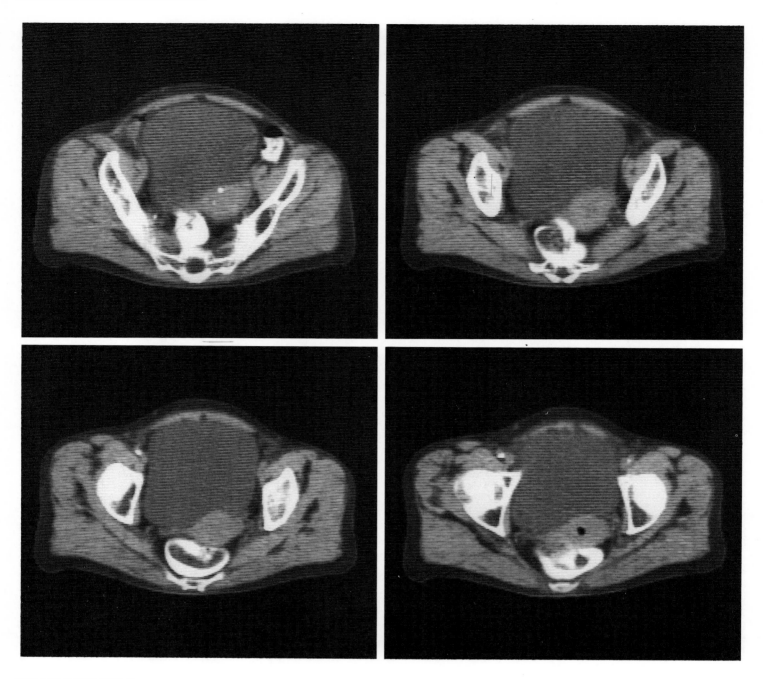

FEMALE PELVIS: 1

The female pelvis in this group and the next is shown in sections of 12 mm increments. Bowel preparation is the same as previously described on p. 278, with the addition of a tampon inserted into the vagina. This allows the vaginal walls to be seen, together with the position of the cervix. In this patient there is a small calcified fibroid visible in the fundus of the uterus.

The piriformis muscle arises from the front of the sacrum and leaves the pelvis via the greater sciatic foramen to insert into the greater trochanter, close to or with the tendon of obturator internus. (Slice increments 12 mm)

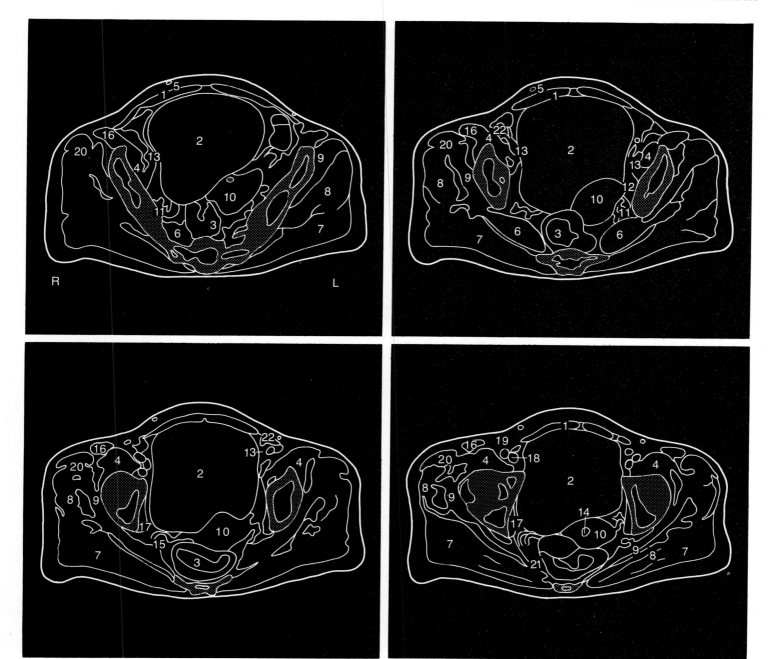

1	Rectus abdominis m.	9	Gluteus minimus m.	16	Sartorius m.
2	Bladder	10	Uterus	17	Obturator internus m.
3	Rectum	11	Internal iliac vss.	18	Femoral v.
4	Iliopsoas m.	12	Ureter	19	Femoral a.
5	Superficial epigastric vss.	13	External iliac vss.	20	Tensor fasciae latae m.
6	Piriformis m.	14	Cervix	21	Sacrospinous lig.
7	Gluteus maximus m.	15	Uterine tube (fallopian)	22	Round lig. of uterus
8	Gluteus medius m.				

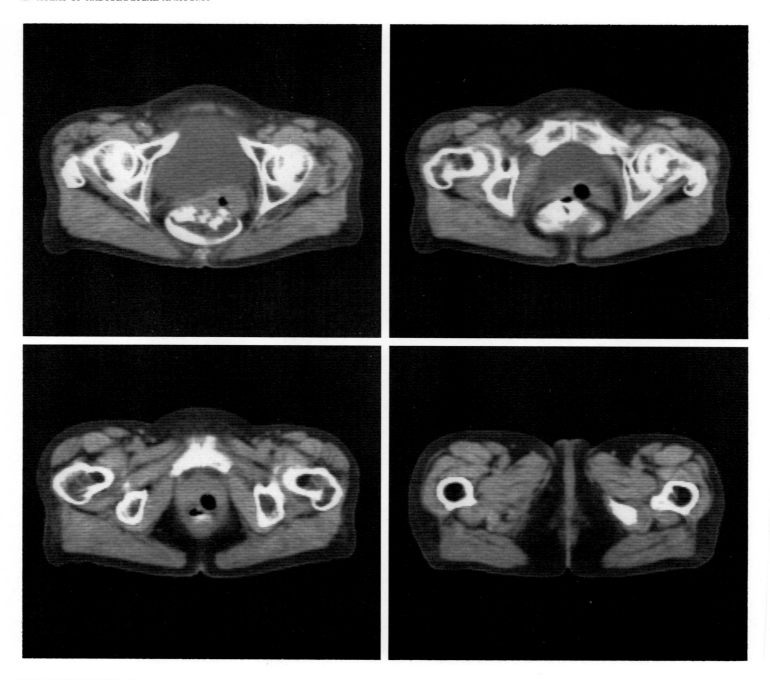

FEMALE PELVIS: 2

The ischiorectal (ischioanal) fossa is formed medially by the sphincter ani, laterally by the obturator internus, posteriorly by the gluteus maximus, anteriorly by the perineal membrane and superiorly by the levator ani. Within the fossa lie the internal pudendal vessels and pudendal nerve in the pudendal canal, the inferior rectal vessels and nerve and branches of the sacral plexus. (Slice increments 12 mm)

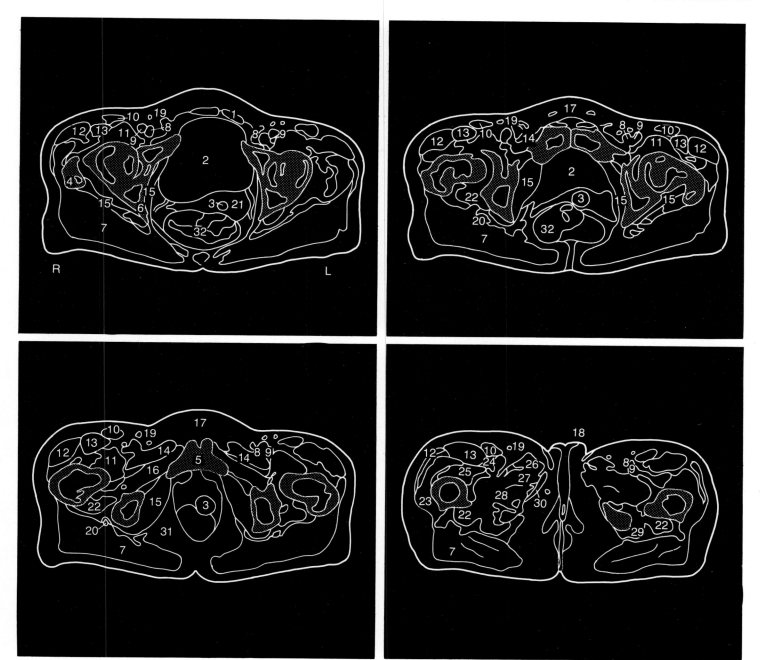

1	Rectus abdominis m.	12	Tensor fasciae latae m.	23	Vastus lateralis m.
2	Bladder	13	Rectus femoris m.	24	Subsartorial canal
3	Vagina	14	Pectineus m.	25	Vastus intermedius m.
4	Greater trochanter	15	Obturator internus m.	26	Adductor long. m.
5	Pubic symphysis	16	Obturator externus m.	27	Adductor brev. m.
6	Ischium	17	Mons pubis	28	Adductor magnus m.
7	Gluteus maximus m.	18	Labia major	29	Hamstrings origin
8	Femoral v.	19	Long saphenous v.	30	Gracilis m.
9	Femoral a.	20	Sciatic n.	31	Ischiorectal fossa
10	Sartorius m.	21	Cervix	32	Rectum
11	Iliopsoas m.	22	Quadratus femoris m.		

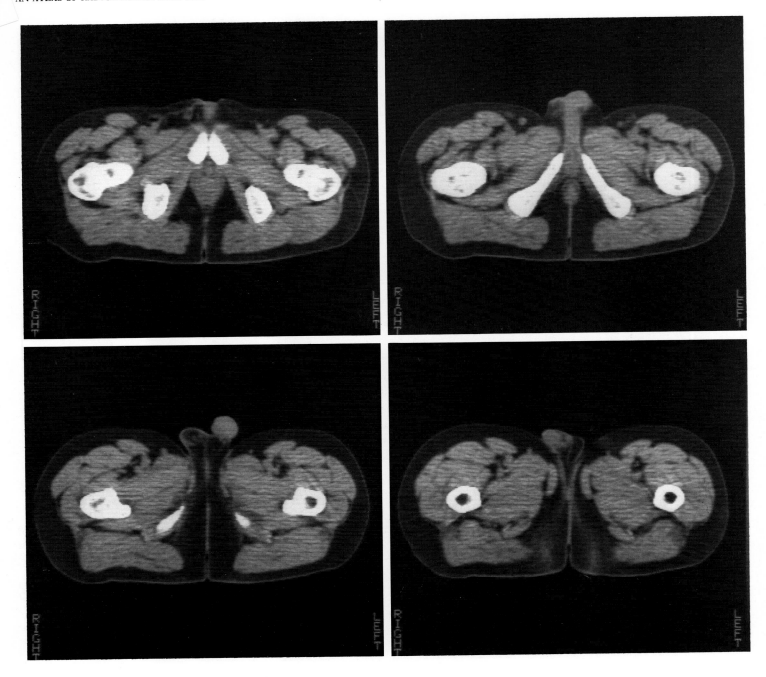

THIGH TO KNEE: 1

These sections through a male pelvis are in 20 mm increments. The muscles of the male urogenital region are difficult to show anatomically, but are well seen above. The superficial transverse perineal muscles run from the ischial tuberosities to the perineal body and fix it when they contract.

The largest nerve in the body, the sciatic nerve, lies between the gluteus maximus and the quadratus femoris. It divides into the tibial and common peroneal nerves in the lower thigh. The sciatic nerve is accompanied by the posterior cutaneous nerve of the thigh and the inferior gluteal artery. (Slice increments 20 mm)

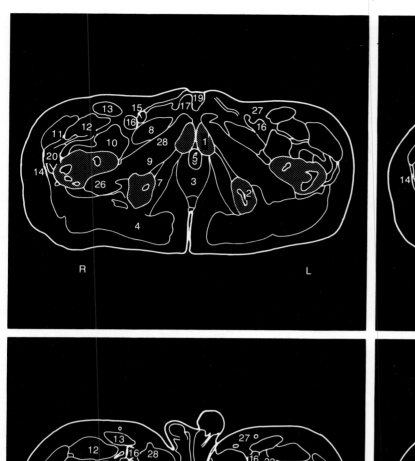
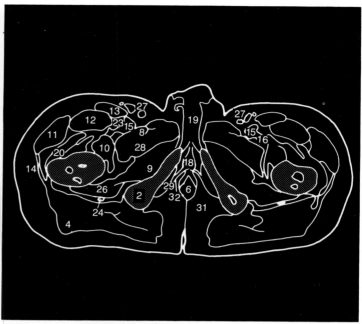
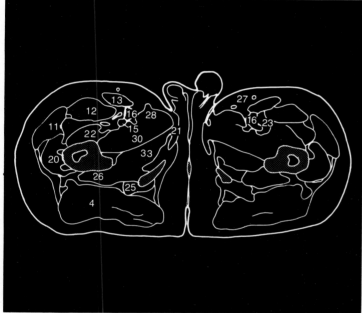
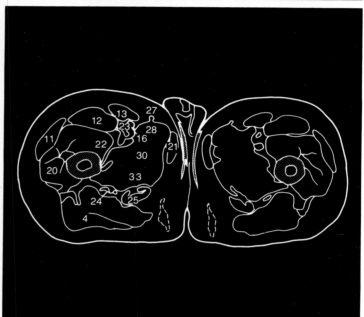

1	Pubis	12	Rectus femoris m.	23	Subsartorial canal
2	Ischium	13	Sartorius m.	24	Sciatic n.
3	Prostate	14	Iliotibial tract	25	Hamstring mm.
4	Gluteus maximus m.	15	Femoral v.	26	Quadratus femoris m.
5	Urethra	16	Femoral a.	27	Long saphenous v.
6	Anus	17	Spermatic cord	28	Adductor long. m.
7	Obturator internus m.	18	Penile bulb	29	Ischiocavernosus m.
8	Pectineus m.	19	Penile shaft	30	Adductor brev. m.
9	Obturator externus m.	20	Vastus lateralis m.	31	Ischiorectal fossa
10	Iliopsoas	21	Gracilis m.	32	Superficial transverse peroneal m.
11	Tensor fasciae latae m.	22	Vastus medialis m.	33	Adductor magnus m.

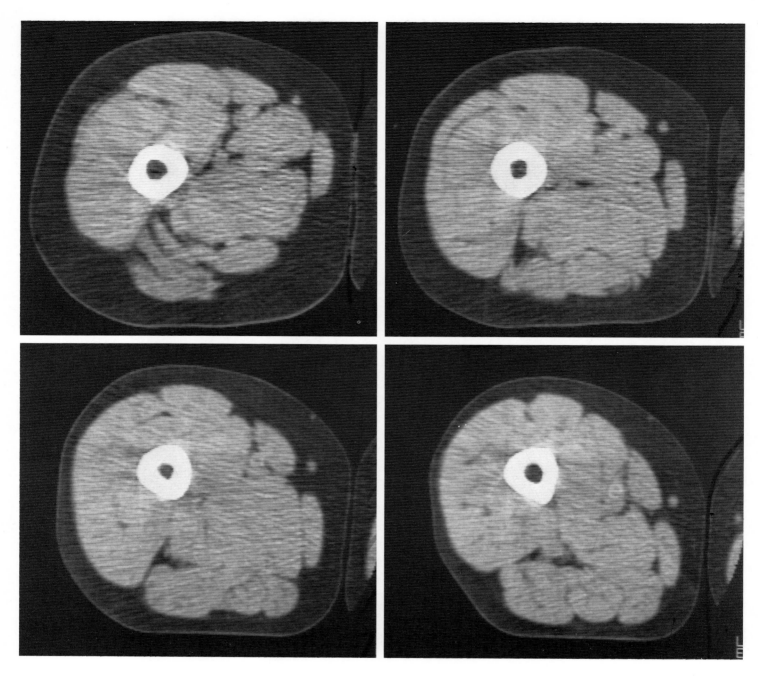

THIGH TO KNEE: 2

In this group and the next, the sections are at increments of 40 mm down the length of the femur.

The femoral artery begins at the inguinal ligament and ends where it passes through the hiatus in adductor magnus to become the popliteal artery. The femoral sheath is a continuation inferiorly of abdominal fasciae and contains the femoral artery and vein, the femoral nerve lying lateral to and outside the sheath. The branches of the femoral artery are the superficial epigastric arising 1 cm below the inguinal ligament, the superficial circumflex iliac, the superficial and deep external pudendal arteries and the profunda femoris. (Slice increments 20 mm)

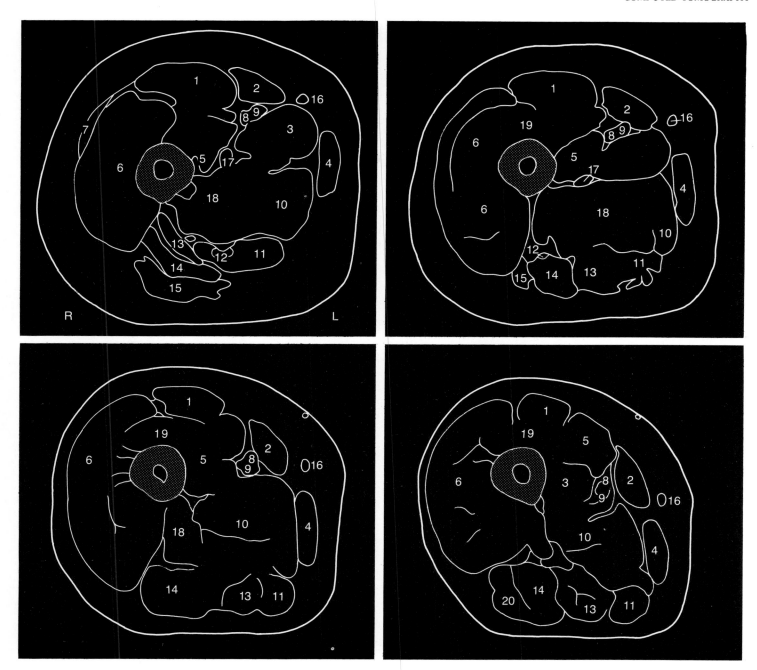

1	Rectus femoris m.	8	Femoral a.	15	Gluteus maximus m.
2	Sartorius m.	9	Femoral v.	16	Long saphenous v.
3	Adductor long. m.	10	Adductor magnus m.	17	Profunda femoris vss.
4	Gracilis m.	11	Semimembranosus m.	18	Adductor brev. m.
5	Vastus medialis m.	12	Sciatic n.	19	Vastus intermedius m.
6	Vastus lateralis m.	13	Semitendinosus m.	20	Short head of biceps femoris m.
7	Tensor fasciae latae m.	14	Biceps femoris m.		

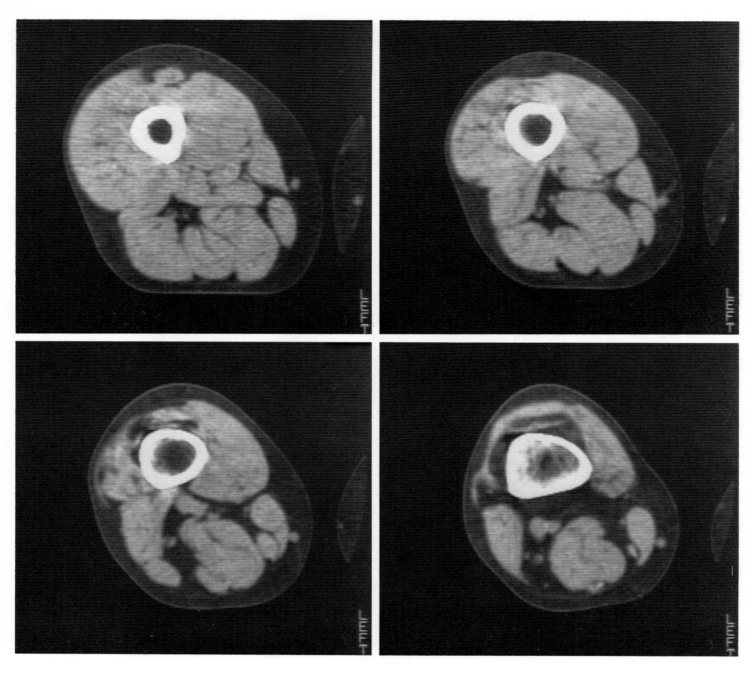

THIGH TO KNEE: 3

The ability of CT to demonstrate muscular and vascular structures in limbs makes it a useful tool in the investigation of soft tissue and bony masses. The high spatial and density resolutions allow fat and fatty masses to be readily assessed.

However, fibrous masses, including fibrosarcoma, may be indistinguishable from infection or haemorrhage. In the staging of primary bone tumours, CT is helpful in the assessment of marrow and soft tissue infiltration, although it is difficult to separate tumour invasion from oedema and inflammation. (Slice increments 20 mm)

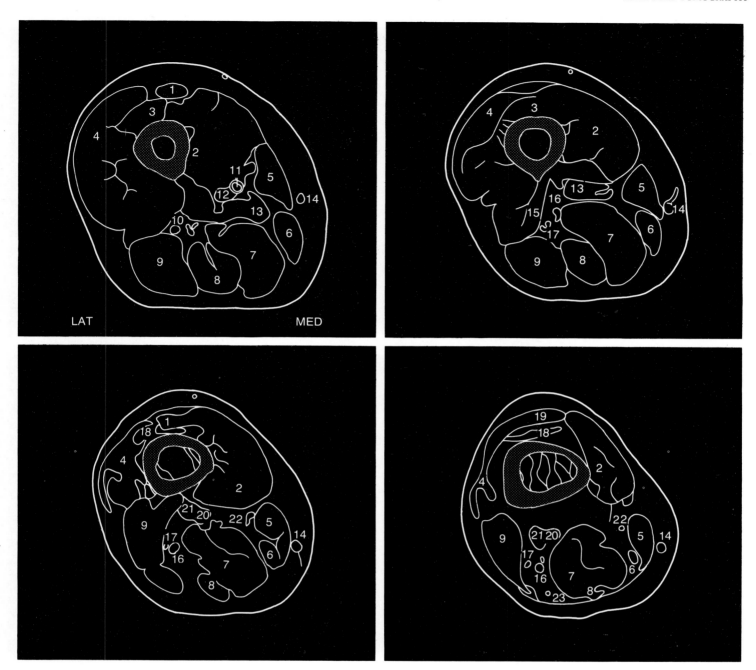

LAT   MED

1	Rectus femoris m.	9	Biceps femoris m.	17	Common peroneal n.
2	Vastus medialis m.	10	Sciatic n.	18	Suprapatellar bursa
3	Vastus intermedius m.	11	Femoral a.	19	Quadriceps t.
4	Vastus lateralis m.	12	Femoral v.	20	Popliteal a.
5	Sartorius m.	13	Adductor magnus m.	21	Popliteal v.
6	Gracilis m.	14	Long saphenous v.	22	Saphenous n.
7	Semimembranosus m.	15	Short head of biceps femoris m.	23	Short saphenous v.
8	Semitendinosus m.	16	Tibial n.		

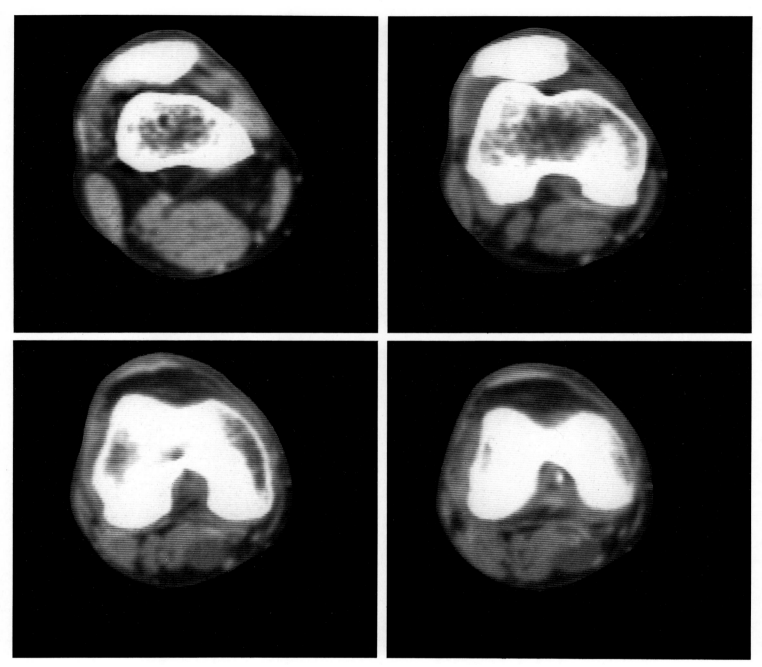

KNEE AND LOWER LEG: 1

A Baker's cyst is included in this 'normal' anatomy atlas purely because the patient's scans showed excellent anatomical detail! The cyst is formed when the popliteal bursa becomes inflamed and swelling develops. A high pressure may be present inside the cyst and rupture may occur on flexion. The cyst may be long and have a valve-like action allowing fluid to enter from the knee joint but not to return. When rupture occurs, the resulting acute inflammation simulates the signs of acute thrombophlebitis. (Slice increments 10 and 20 mm)

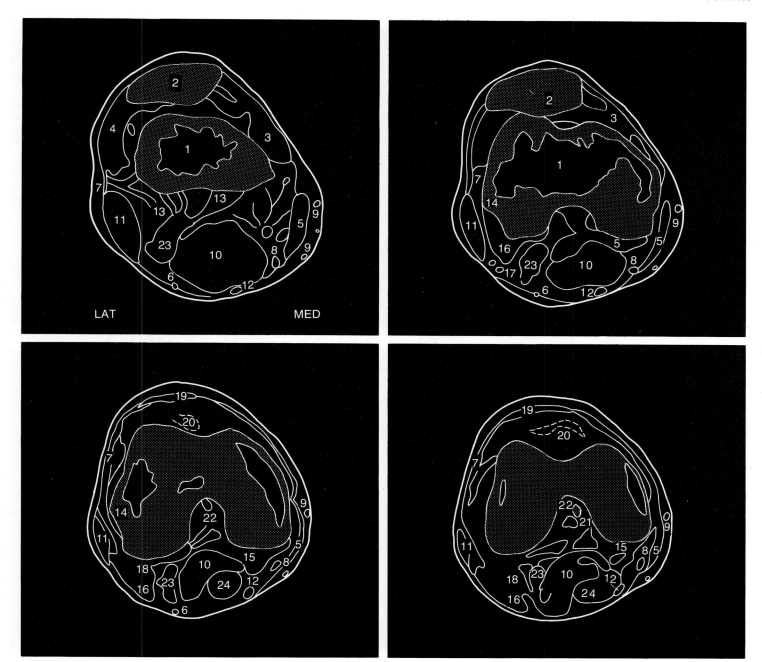

LAT MED

1	Femur	9	Long saphenous v.	17	Common peroneal n.
2	Patella	10	Semimembranosus m.	18	Plantaris m.
3	Vastus medialis m.	11	Biceps femoris m.	19	Ligamentum patellae
4	Vastus lateralis m.	12	Semitendinosus t.	20	Synovial cavity
5	Sartorius m.	13	Oblique popliteal lig.	21	Post. cruciate lig.
6	Short saphenous v.	14	Lat. epicondyle	22	Ant. cruciate lig.
7	Iliotibial tract	15	Gastrocnemius med. head	23	Popliteal vss.
8	Gracilis t.	16	Gastrocnemius lat. head	24	Baker's cyst

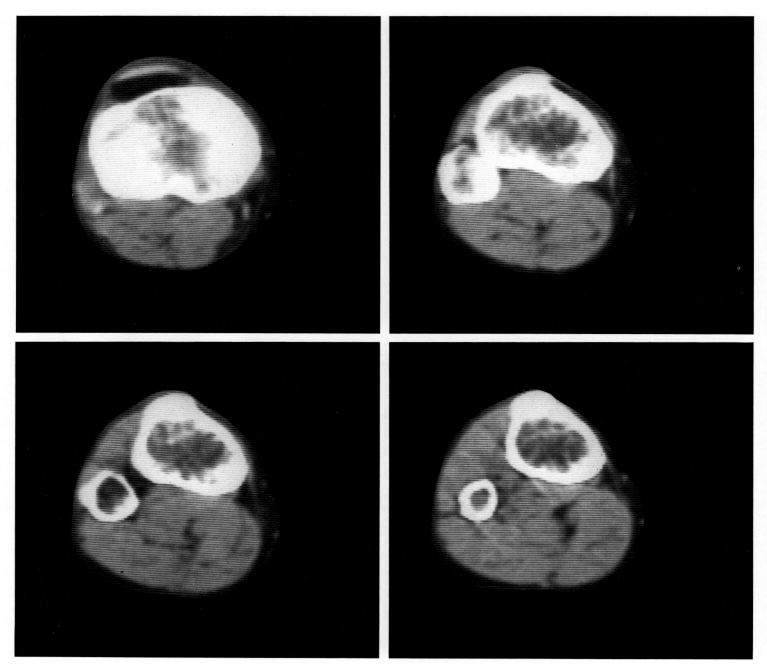

KNEE AND LOWER LEG: 2

The common peroneal nerve passes around the neck of the fibula, deep to the peroneus longus; it divides into the superficial and deep peroneal nerves. Compression of the common peroneal nerve may occur at the fibular neck. Prolonged driving with the leg resting against the gear lever has been known to cause this phenomenon! It should be noted that man is unique in having the big toe flexor (flexor hallucis longus) originating from the fibula. (Slice increments 10 and 20 mm)

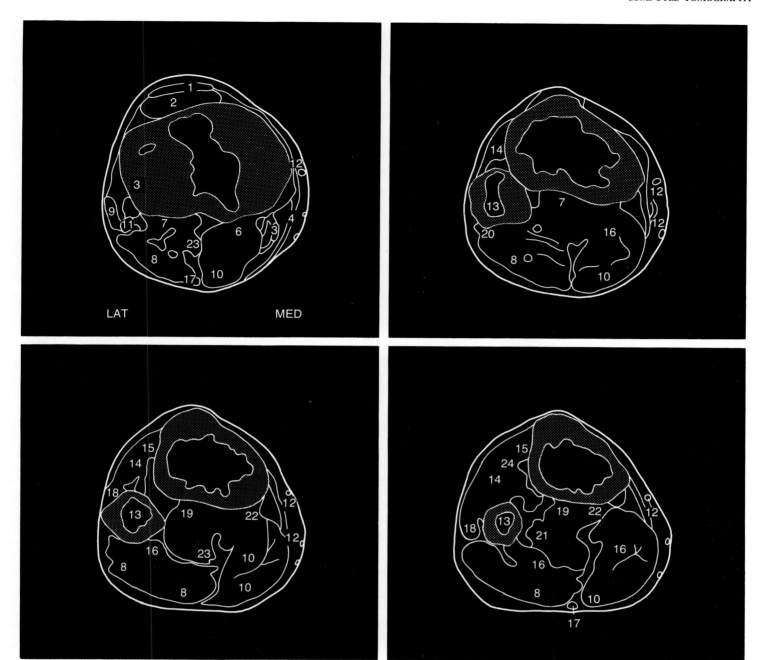

LAT MED

1 Ligamentum patellae	9 Biceps femoris m.	17 Short saphenous v.
2 Synovial cavity	10 Gastrocnemius med. head	18 Peroneus long. m.
3 Lat. tibial condyle	11 Fibular collateral lig.	19 Tibialis post. m.
4 Sartorius t.	12 Long saphenous v.	20 Common peroneal n.
5 Gracilis t.	13 Fibula	21 Fl. hallucis long. m.
6 Semimembranosus m.	14 Ext. digitorum long. m.	22 Fl. digitorum long. m.
7 Popliteus m.	15 Tibialis ant. m.	23 Popliteal vss.
8 Gastrocnemius lat. head	16 Soleus m.	24 Ext. hallucis long. m.

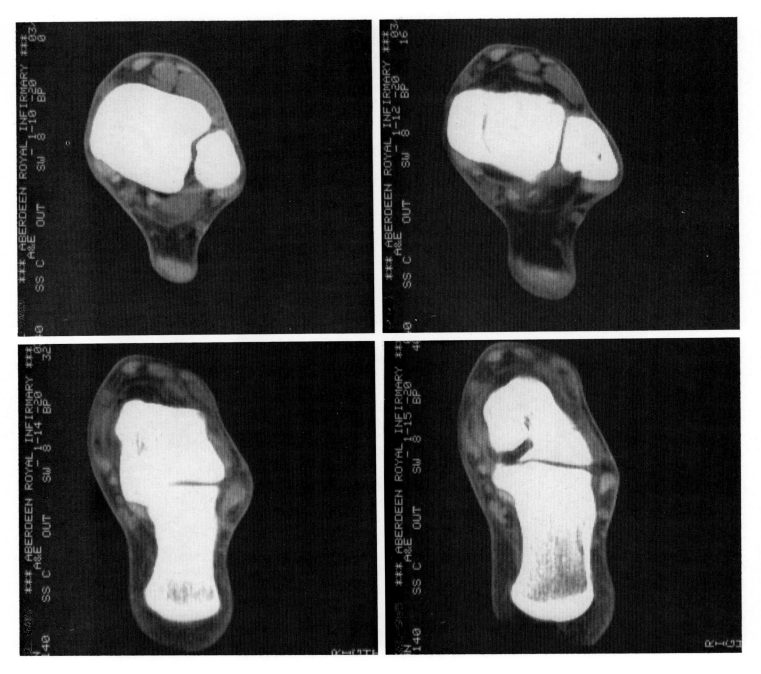

ANKLE AND FOOT

These four sections are through a left ankle and foot with increments of 16 mm.

The tendo calcaneus is the common tendon of the gastrocnemius and soleus and is inserted into the posterior surface of the calcaneum, with a bursa between it and the upper aspect of the bone.

The flexor hallucis longus tendon passes under the sustentaculum tali and uses it as a lever.

CT has a role to play in the investigation of some ankle and foot abnormalities, including trauma, infection and arthropathy, when conventional radiography may not provide sufficient information. (Slice increments 8 and 16 mm)

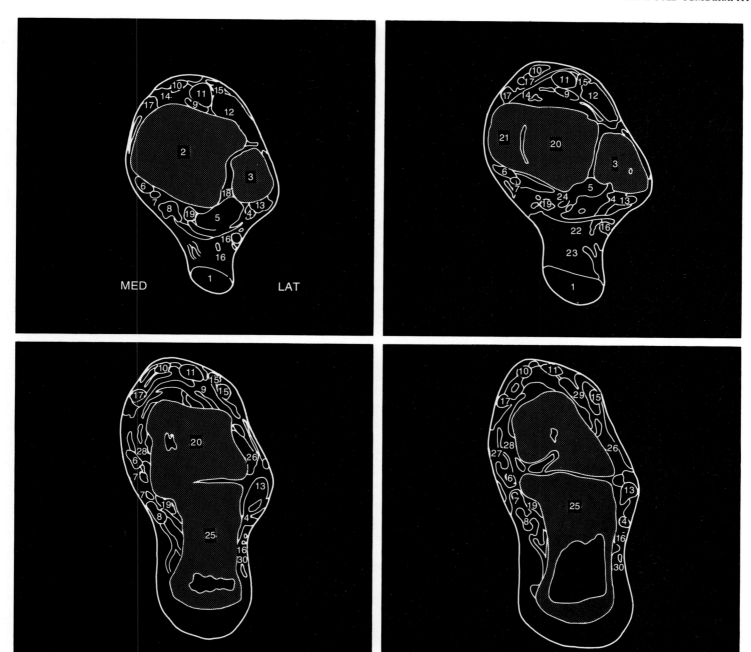

1	Tendo calcaneus	
2	Tibia	
3	Fibula	
4	Peroneus long. m.	
5	Fl. hallucis long. m.	
6	Tibialis post. t.	
7	Fl. digitorum long. m.	
8	Post. tibial vss. and n.	
9	Ant. tibial vss. and n.	
10	Tibialis ant. t.	

11	Ext. hallucis long. m.
12	Ext. digitorum long. m.
13	Peroneus brev. m.
14	Ext. retinaculum
15	Ext. digitorum long. t.
16	Short saphenous v.
17	Long saphenous v.
18	Post. tibiofibular lig.
19	Fl. hallucis long. t.
20	Talus

21	Med. malleolus
22	Fl. retinaculum
23	Fat pad
24	Tibial n.
25	Calcaneus
26	Ant. talofibular lig.
27	Plantar calcaneonavicular (spring) lig.
28	Deltoid lig.
29	Ext. hallucis brev. m.
30	Sural n.

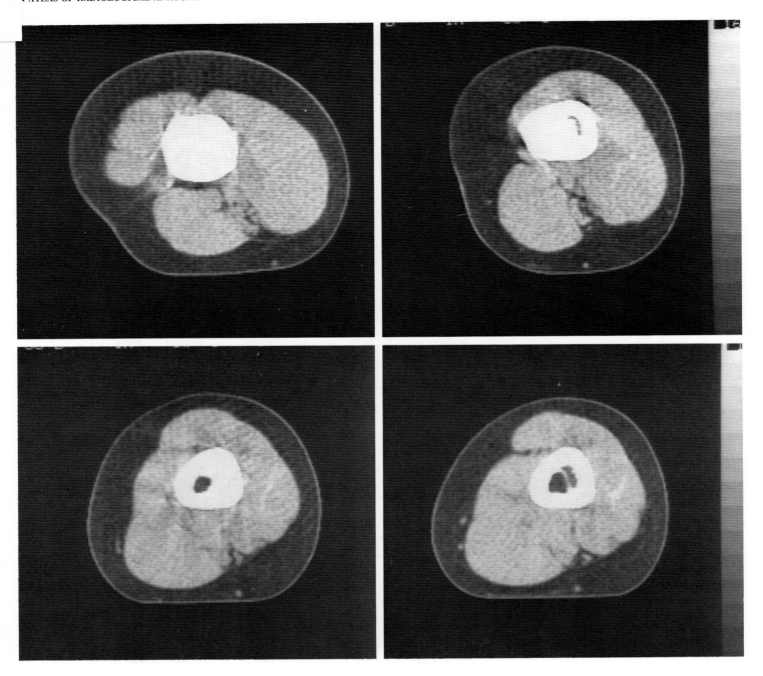

UPPER ARM

These sections are through a left upper arm at 30 mm increments. Despite the subject being obese, as shown by the amount of subcutaneous fat, muscle definition is poor, particularly in the forearm sections which follow. This is in contradistinction to the leg, where muscles have fat-laden fascial planes and are hence well demonstrated by CT. The reason for this lack of intermuscular fat in the upper limbs is unclear. (Slice increments 20 mm)

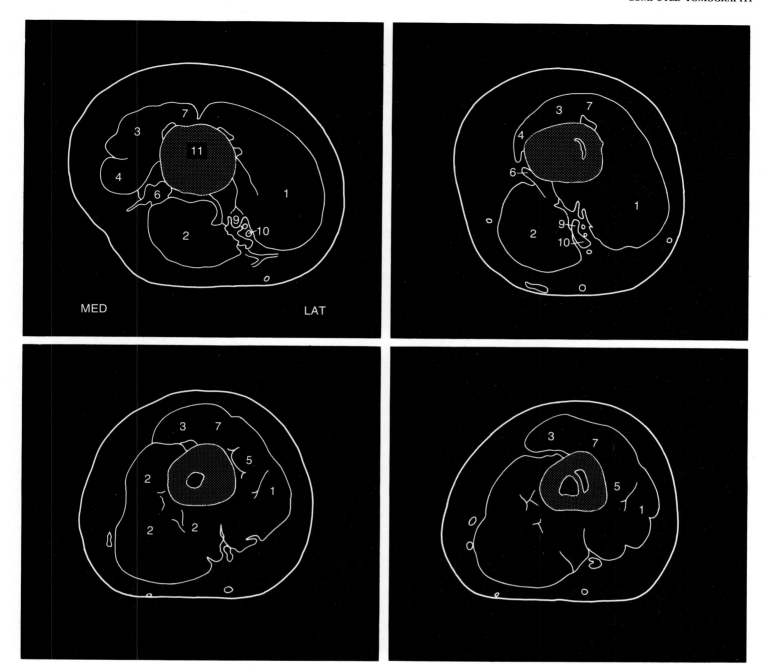

1   Deltoid m.

2   Triceps m.

3   Biceps m. (short head)

4   Coracobrachialis m.

5   Brachialis m.

6   Brachial vss.

7   Biceps m. (long head)

8   Axillary n.

9   Profunda brachii vss.

10   Radial n.

11   Humerus

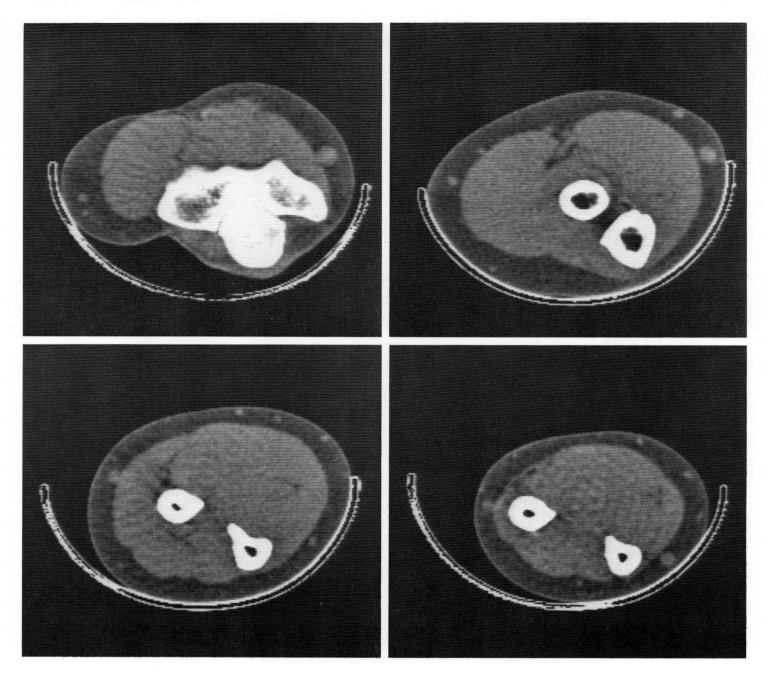

FOREARM AND WRIST: 1

This group and the next show a right forearm with sections at intervals of 50 mm. The radial nerve is the largest branch of the brachial plexus, with originating fibres from C5, 6, 7, 8 and T1 nerves. It lies between the brachialis and brachioradialis muscles, on the anterior aspect of the lateral epicondyles of the humerus. In the lower forearm, the nerve passes deep to the brachioradialis tendon and winds around the lateral side of the radius to give rise to the dorsal digital nerves. (Slice increments 20 mm)

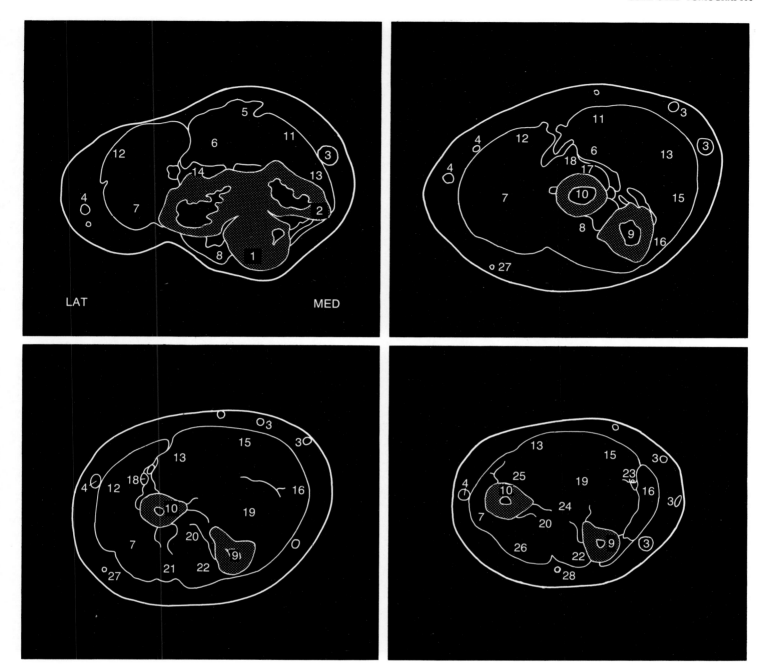

1 Olecranon	11 Pronator teres m.
2 Med. epicondyle	12 Brachioradialis m.
3 Basilic v.	13 Fl. carpi radialis m.
4 Cephalic v.	14 Radial n.
5 Biceps t.	15 Fl. digitorum superficialis m.
6 Brachialis m.	16 Fl. carpi ulnaris m.
7 Ext. carpi radialis long. m.	17 Supinator m.
8 Anconeus m.	18 Radial vss.
9 Ulna	19 Fl. digitorum profundus m.
10 Radius	

20 Ext. pollicis long. m.
21 Ext. digitorum m.
22 Ext. carpi ulnaris m.
23 Ulnar a.
24 Pronator quadratus m.
25 Fl. pollicis long. m.
26 Ext. indicis m.
27 Lat. cutaneous n. of forearm
28 Superficial radial n.

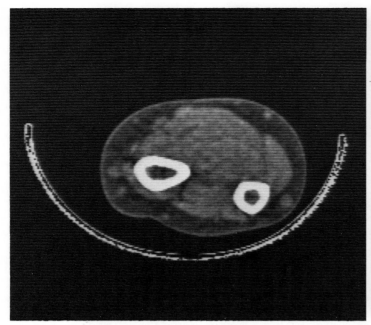 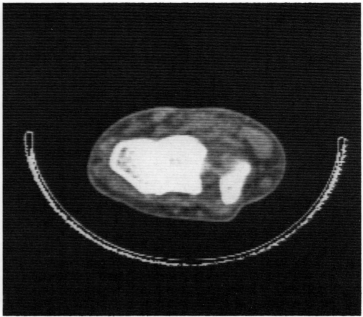

FOREARM AND WRIST: 2

Two synovial sheaths envelop the flexor tendons as they pass through the carpal tunnel. One contains the flexor digitorum superficialis and profundus tendons, and the other the tendon of flexor pollicis longus. There is also a synovial sheath surrounding flexor carpi radialis. The flexor carpi ulnaris inserts into the pisi- form bone. The anatomical snuffbox is formed by the tendons of extensor pollicis longus medially and abductor pollicis longus and extensor pollicis brevis laterally. The radial artery lies in its base, overlying the scaphoid bone. (Slice increments 20 mm)

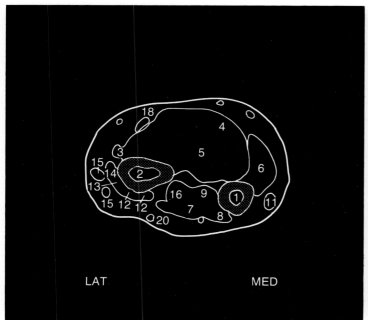
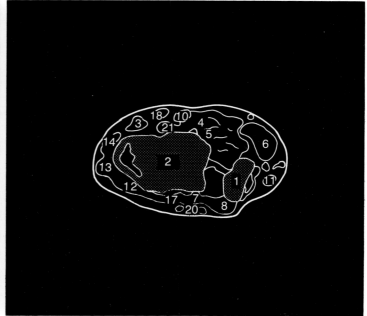

1	Ulna	8	Ext. carpi ulnaris m.	15	Cephalic v.
2	Radius	9	Pronator quadratus m.	16	Ext. indicis m.
3	Radial a.	10	Median n.	17	Ext. pollicis long. m.
4	Fl. digitorum superficialis m.	11	Basilic v.	18	Fl. carpi radialis t.
5	Fl. digitorum profundus m.	12	Ext. carpi radialis long. and brev. tt.	19	Distal radioulnar joint
6	Fl. carpi ulnaris m.	13	Ext. pollicis brev. m.	20	Superficial radial n.
7	Ext. digitorum m.	14	Abductor pollicis long. m.	21	Fl. pollicis long. m.

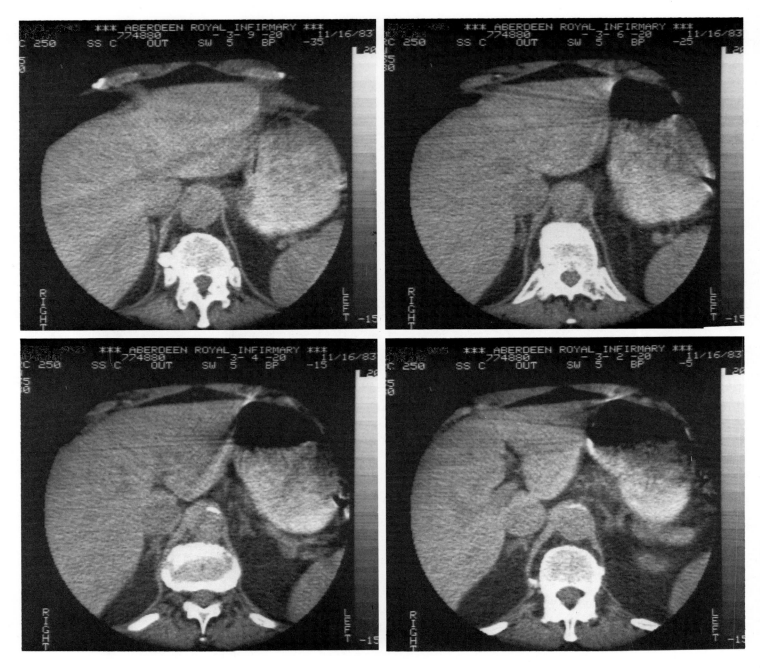

ADRENAL VIEWS

These sections are at 10 mm increments. The right adrenal gland lies immediately behind the inferior vena cava, between the right crus of the diaphragm medially and the liver laterally. It comprises a small body and two long limbs, the medial limb being most prominently seen, and may extend to 4 cm in length. The right adrenal gland is more pyramidal in shape, commonly taking the form of an inverted Y. It lies between the left crus of the diaphragm medially, the upper pole of the kidney posterolaterally, the stomach anterolaterally and the tail of the pancreas and splenic vessels anteriorly. Adequate fat helps visualization of the adrenal glands, with oral contrast to distend the stomach. Intravenous contrast to enhance the inferior vena cava may be necessary to delineate small adrenal masses. (Slice increments 10 mm)

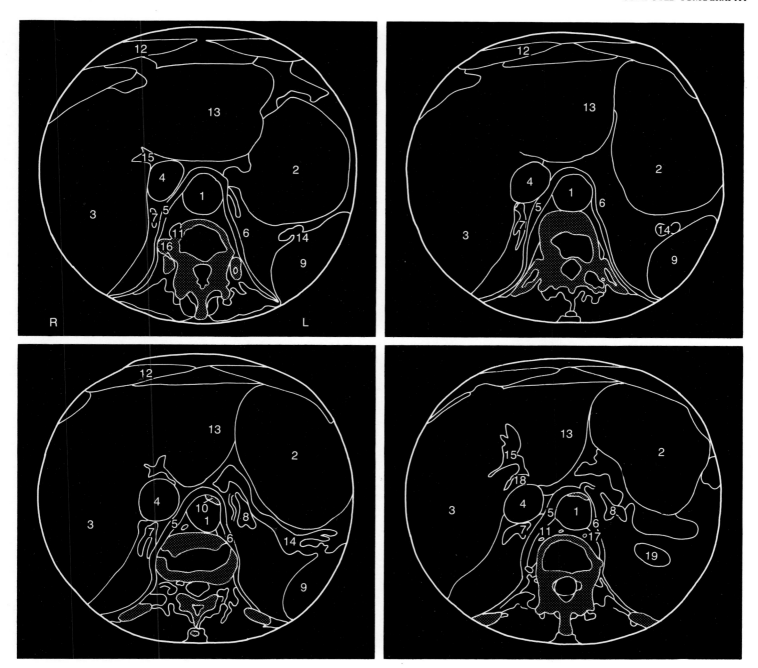

1	Aorta	8	L. adrenal gland	14	Splenic a.
2	Stomach	9	Spleen	15	Porta hepatis
3	R. lobe of liver	10	Calcium in aorta	16	Osteophyte
4	Inf. vena cava	11	Azygos v.	17	Hemiazygos v.
5	R. crus of diaphragm	12	Rectus abdominis m.	18	Liver, caudate lobe
6	L. crus of diaphragm	13	L. lobe of liver	19	Upper pole of l. kidney
7	R. adrenal gland				

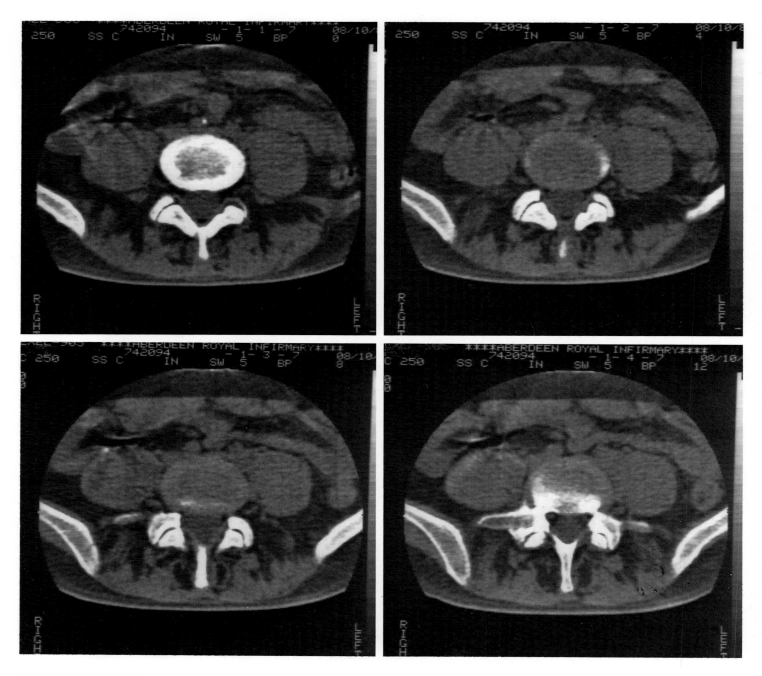

L4/5 NERVE ROOTS

These sections are taken through the L4/5 disc at 4 mm increments. The exact angulation of the scan plane is adjusted from an initial lateral planar view (or scanogram), to provide sections parallel to the disc. Different angles of scan tilt are required for different disc spaces depending on the degree of kyphosis or lordosis present. High-resolution CT scanners producing multiple thin-section scans can demonstrate prolapsed intervertebral discs without the need for thecal contrast.

CT is also extremely valuable in assessing spinal fractures, particularly 'burst' or 'crush' injuries. Bony definition is clearly seen, and small fragments of bone may be shown in the spinal canal. (Slice increments 4 mm)

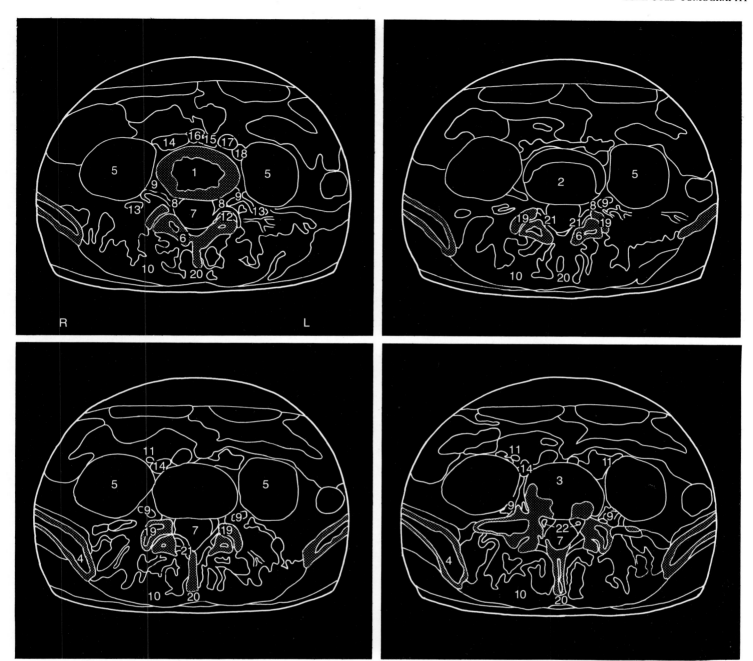

1	L4 body	9	Dorsal root ganglion	16	R. common iliac a.
2	Intervertebral disc L4/5	10	Erector spinae m.	17	L. common iliac a.
3	L5 body	11	Ureter	18	Inf. mesenteric v.
4	Ilium	12	Articular facet	19	Sup. articular process
5	Psoas major m.	13	Lumbar plexus	20	Spinous process
6	Lamina	14	R. common iliac v.	21	Ligamentum flavum
7	Cauda equina	15	L. common iliac v.	22	Nerve root sheath
8	Intervertebral foramen				

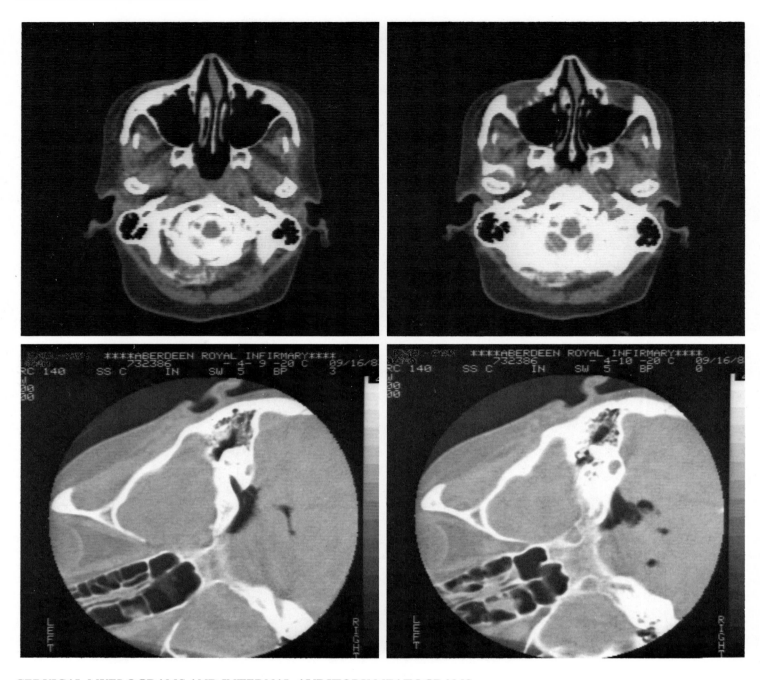

CERVICAL MYELOGRAMS AND INTERNAL AUDITORY MEATOGRAMS

The upper two sections are 3 mm apart and were recorded after cervical myelography. The vertebral arteries ascend in the foramina of the upper six cervical vertebrae to enter the skull through the foramen magnum. The cerebellar tonsils are seen in their normal positions in these sections. In the Arnold–Chiari malformation there is tonsillar herniation with frequent abnormalities of the cerebellum, enlargement of the foramen magnum and spina bifida of the upper cervical vertebrae.

The lower two sections are also 3 mm apart, and were taken after the patient had had air injected into the subarachnoid space and the head positioned to allow air to outline the contents of the cerebellopontine angle. The additional air contrast allows greater definition of the structures, and small acoustic neuromas may be diagnosed before any changes occur which are visible on plain films. (Slice increments 3 mm)

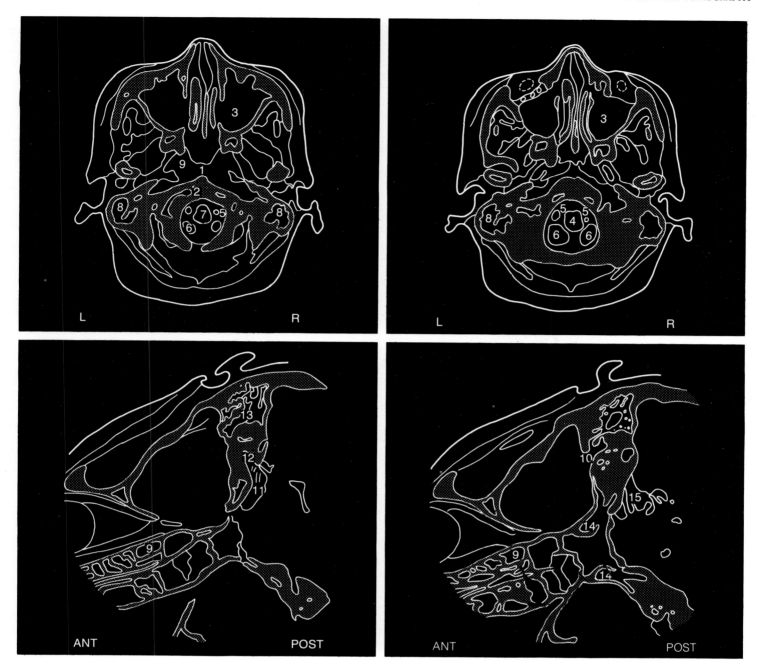

1	Basilar part of occipital bone	6	Cerebellar tonsils	11	Pontine cistern
2	Hypoglossal canal	7	Spinal cord	12	Internal auditory meatus
3	Maxillary sinus	8	Mastoid air cells	13	Mastoid antrum
4	Medulla	9	Ethmoidal air sinus	14	Carotid canal
5	Vertebral a.	10	Ossicles	15	Facial and vestibulocochlear nn.

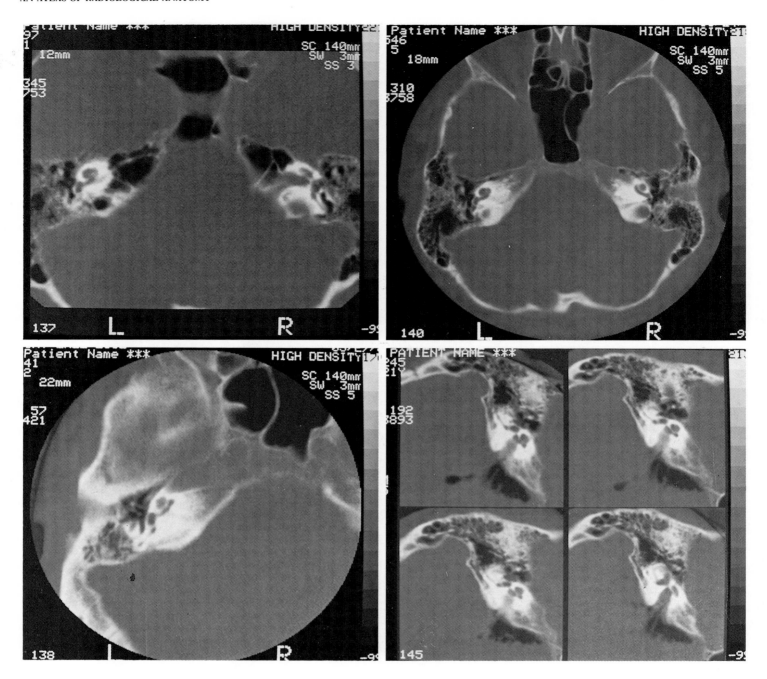

INTERNAL AUDITORY MEATOGRAMS

The internal auditory meatus transmits the vestibulocochlear nerve, the motor and sensory roots of the facial nerve and the internal auditory vessels. The middle ear ossicles—the malleus, incus and stapes—can be seen with high-resolution CT scanners, as can the detail of the internal ear. (Slice increments 3 mm)

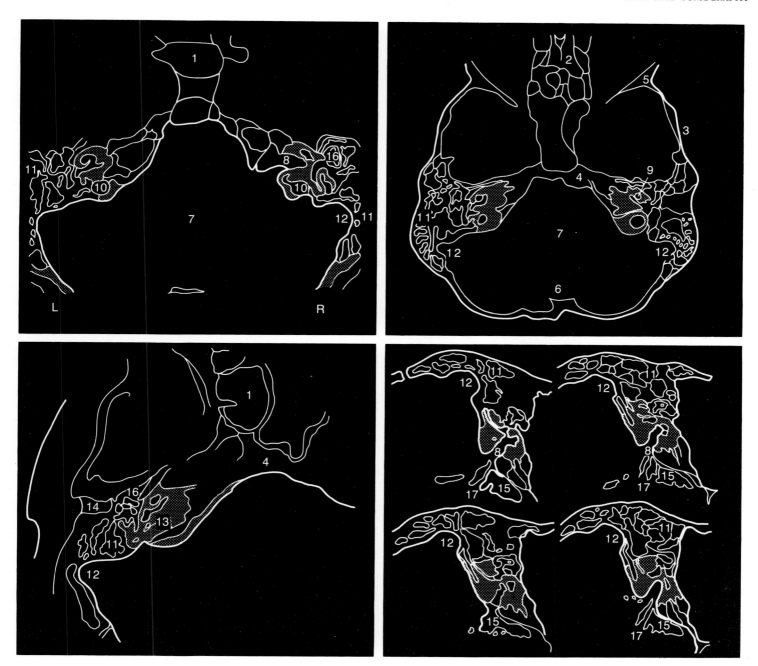

1	Sphenoid air sinus	
2	Ethmoid air sinus	
3	Squamous temporal bone	
4	Petrous temporal bone	
5	Greater wing of sphenoid bone	
6	Occipital bone	

7	Cerebellum
8	Internal auditory meatus
9	Cochlea
10	Jugular fossa
11	Mastoid air cells
12	Sulcus of sigmoid venous sinus

13	Semicircular canals
14	External auditory meatus
15	Air in cerebellopontine angle
16	Internal ossicles
17	VIIth and VIIIth cranial nn.

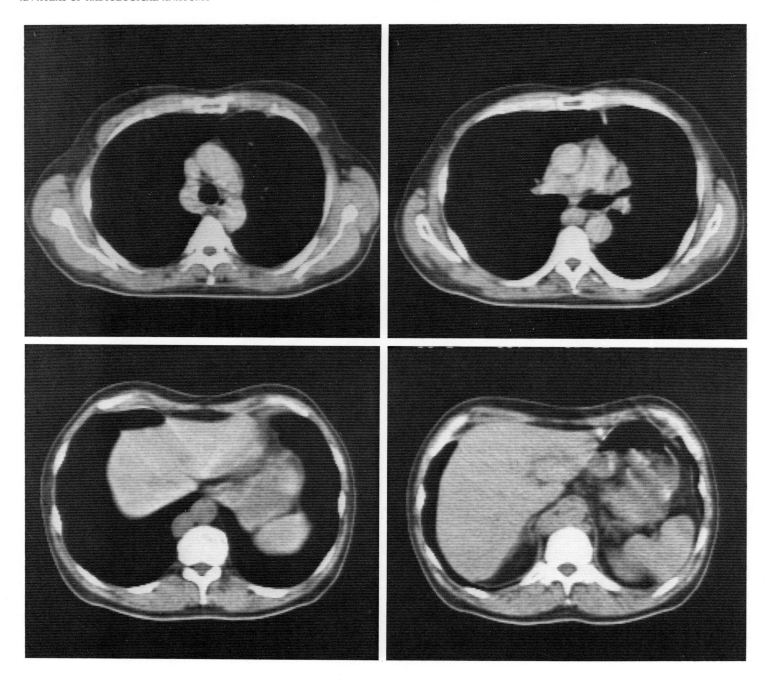

ABSENT INFERIOR VENA CAVA

The development of the inferior vena cava (IVC) is complicated and anomalies are common. In the fetus the posterior cardinal vein disappears on the left side, but on the right side its end persists as the terminal portion of the azygos vein. The cephalic end of the right subcardinal vein is partly incorporated in the IVC. The right supracardinal vein forms the postrenal segment of the IVC. The right azygos vein persists into adult life and, in the absence of the upper IVC, drains the abdomen, pelvis and lower limbs. The left azygos line forms the hemiazygos system.

The IVC is thus formed from below by the following veins: the right supracardinal vein; an anastomosis of the right supra- and subcardinal veins; the right subcardinal vein; an anastomosis between the right subcardinal and common hepatic veins and the common hepatic vein proper. (Varying slice increments)

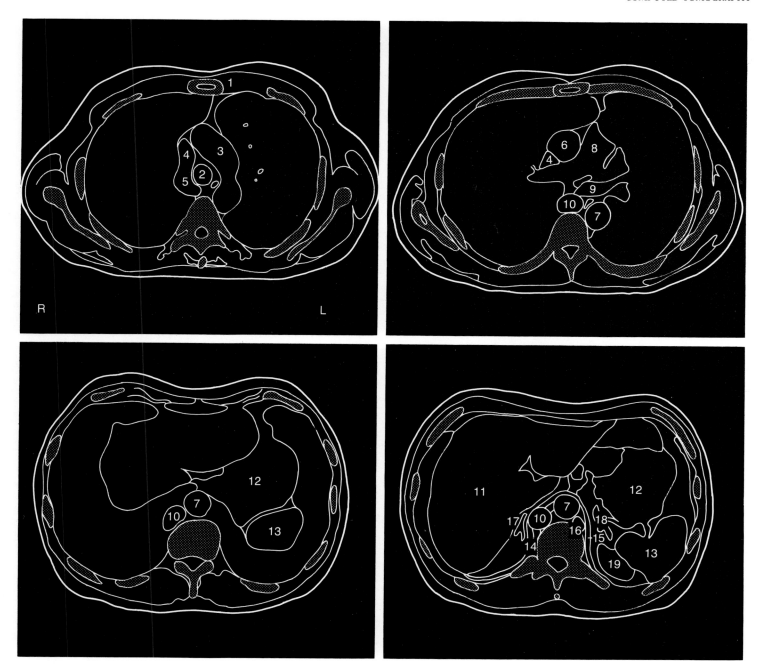

1	Sternum	8	Pulmonary trunk	14	R. crus of diaphragm
2	Trachea	9	L. main bronchus	15	L. crus of diaphragm
3	Aortic arch	10	Enlarged azygos v.	16	Hemiazygos v.
4	Sup. vena cava	11	Liver	17	R. adrenal gland
5	Azygos arch	12	Stomach	18	L. adrenal gland
6	Ascending aorta	13	Spleen	19	L. kidney
7	Descending aorta				

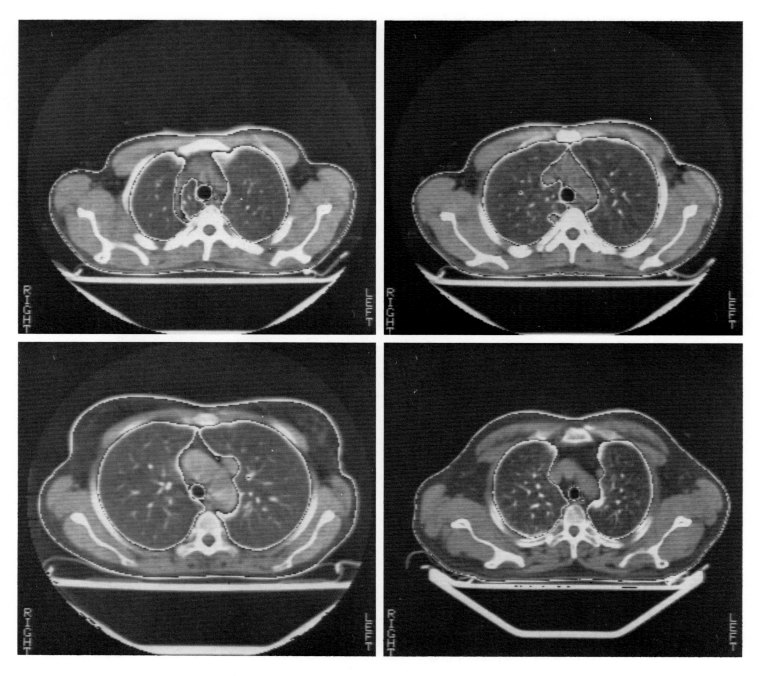

AZYGOS LOBE AND FISSURE, AND SUPERIOR VENA CAVA ANOMALIES

The upper two sections show a common congenital anomaly of an azygos fissure and lobe. This anomaly is present in approximately 1% of the population and occurs when the apex of the developing right lung meets the azygos arch and is cleft by it. Thereby, the right lung apex comes to lie either side of the arch. The azygos fissure demonstrated is thus composed of four layers of pleura, two visceral and two parietal, with the vein lying at the free edge. (Slice increment 15 mm)

The lower two sections demonstrate two patients with anomalies of the superior vena cava (SVC). The upper part of the SVC is formed by the right anterior cardinal vein and the lower part by the right duct of Cuvier. Below the left brachiocephalic vein, the left anterior cardinal vein and the left duct of Cuvier atrophy. If this atrophy does not occur then a double SVC results, shown on the right above. If the right-sided veins atrophy then a left SVC occurs, shown on the left above.

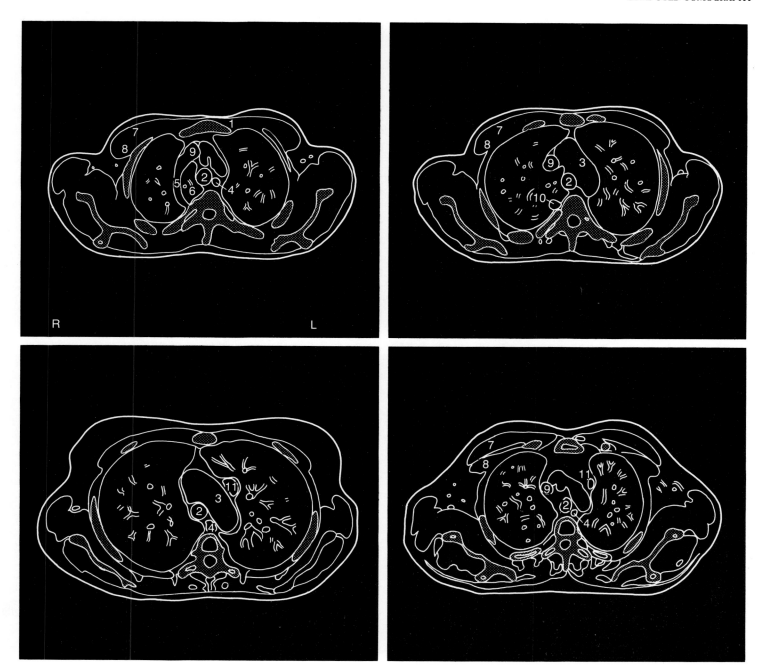

1	Manubrium	5	Azygos fissure	9	Sup. vena cava
2	Trachea	6	Azygos lobe	10	Azygos v.
3	Aortic arch	7	Pectoralis major m.	11	L.-sided sup. vena cava
4	Oesophagus	8	Pectoralis minor m.		

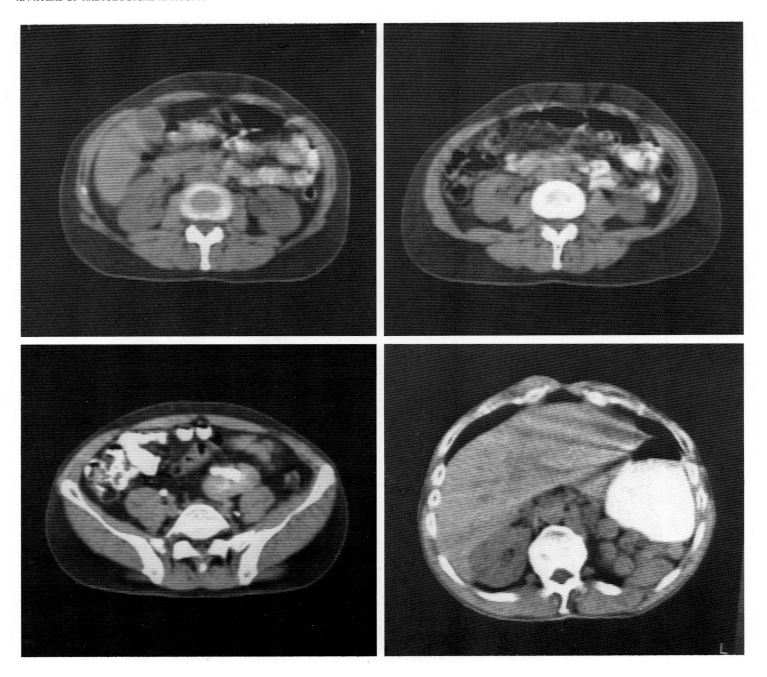

DUPLICATION OF INFERIOR VENA CAVA, PELVIC KIDNEY AND MULTIPLE SPLENUNCULI

A double inferior vena cava is shown in the upper two sections—a well-recognized and usually accidental finding. The veins often unite before draining normally into the right atrium. They should not be confused with para-aortic lymph nodes, and contrast enhancement will differentiate the two conditions. (Slice increment 30 mm)

The lower left section demonstrates a pelvic kidney. When the rudiment of the kidney first appears in the fetus, it lies in the pelvis, being supplied by local arteries, the median sacral and common iliac. As growth progresses, cranial movement occurs until the kidney comes to lie at the level of the second lumbar vertebra. The definitive renal artery arises from the lowest suprarenal artery, originally a persistent mesonephric artery. If cranial movement does not occur, a pelvic kidney is formed and it retains its local blood supply. The lower right section is from a patient with polysplenia. This may be an isolated condition, or be combined with multiple defects including right atrial isomerism and other cardiorespiratory anomalies.

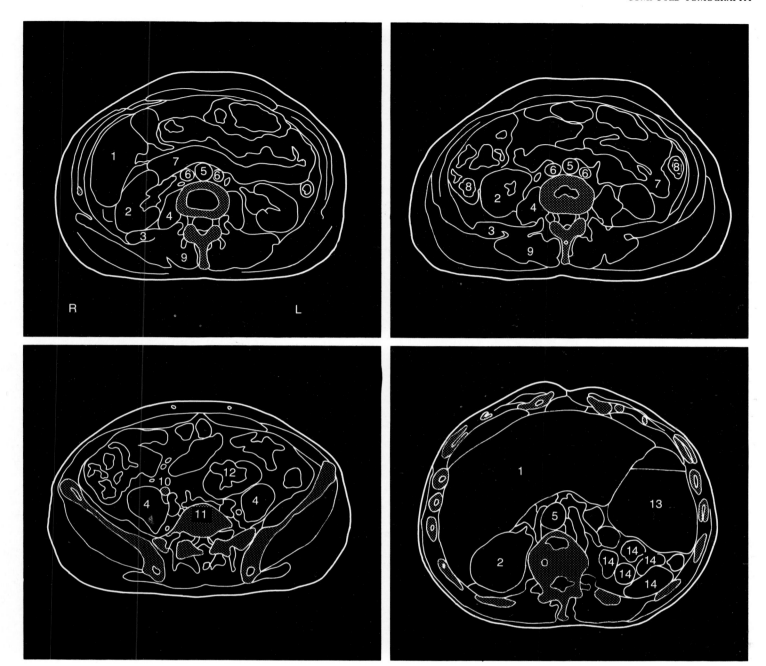

1 Liver	6 Inf. vena cava	11 Sacral promontory
2 Kidney	7 Duodenum	12 Pelvic kidney
3 Quadratus lumborum m.	8 Colon	13 Stomach
4 Psoas major m.	9 Erector spinae m.	14 Splenunculi
5 Aorta	10 Ureter	

ULTRASOUND

This section is included to clarify and enhance certain anatomical areas. The neonatal brain is shown in considerable detail as this technique is now widely available and is essentially operator dependent. Detailed knowledge of the normal appearances is necessary for those physicians involved in neonatal work.

Sections through the abdomen and pelvis, both male and female, show certain anatomical details not seen elsewhere. Standard echocardiographic projections and a scan through the eye are also demonstrated.

319

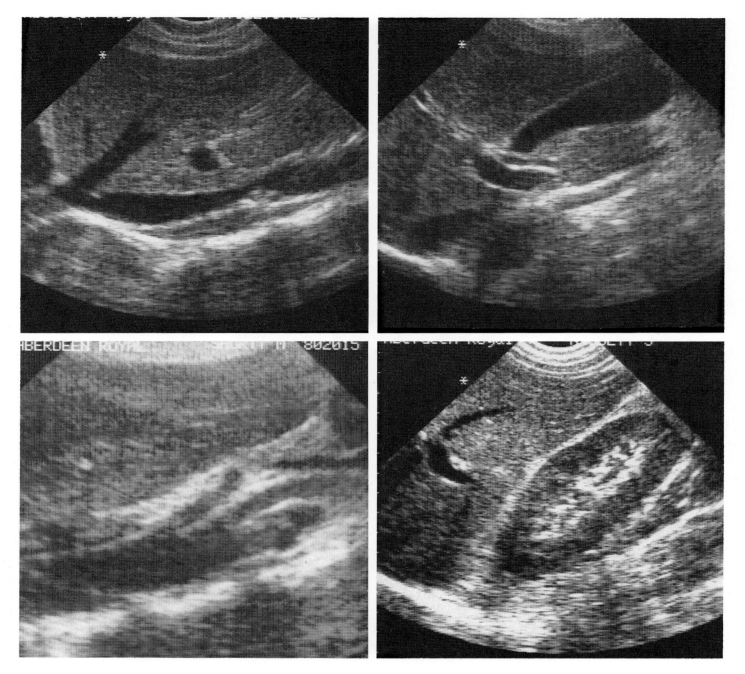

ABDOMEN

The echo pattern of the normal liver consists of diffusely scattered echoes of even size and intensity. The portal veins differ from the hepatic veins in being surrounded by echogenic structures giving a white edge effect. The walls of the hepatic veins do not show this appearance. On longitudinal scans, the portal vein and common hepatic duct are closely related, with the vein lying posterior to the duct.

Attenuation is also affected by the type of biological medium the sound wave passes through. In obese patients considerable attenuation occurs in the fat, and the structure to be visualized lies further from the transducer when compared to a lean patient. The quality of the image is thus reduced. In CT the position is reversed, obesity being helpful because of the low x-ray density of fat, and there is thus an increase in contrast resolution.

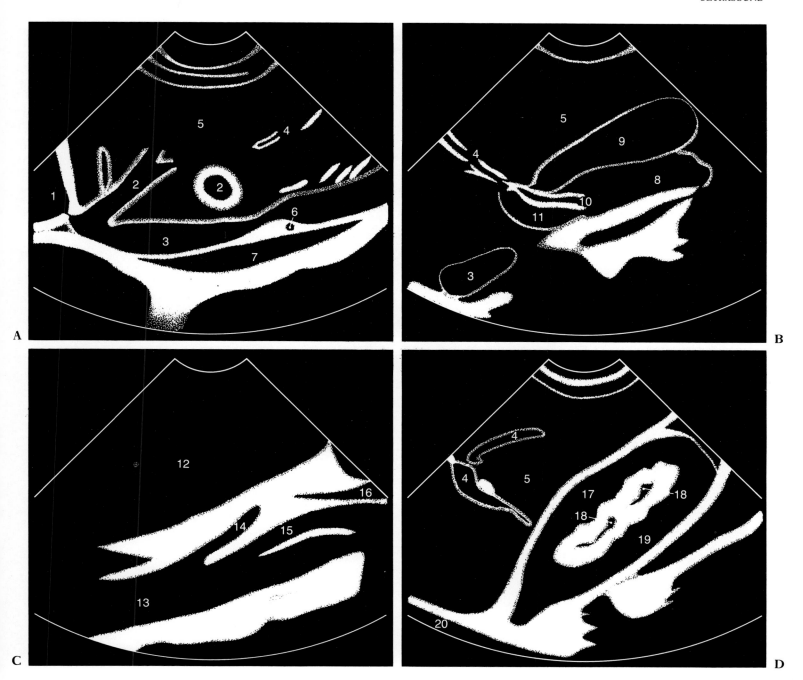

A	Parasagittal: 2 cm to right of midline	1	R. atrium	11	Portal v.
B	Parasagittal: 10 cm to right of midline	2	Hepatic vv.	12	L. lobe of liver
		3	Inf. vena cava	13	Aorta
C	Parasagittal: 1 cm to left of midline	4	Branch of portal v.	14	Coeliac axis
D	Oblique: long axis of right kidney	5	R. lobe of liver	15	Sup. mesenteric a.
		6	R. renal a.	16	Sup. mesenteric v.
		7	Prevertebral muscles	17	R. kidney
		8	Head of pancreas	18	Renal calyces
		9	Gall bladder	19	Renal sinus fat
		10	Common bile duct		

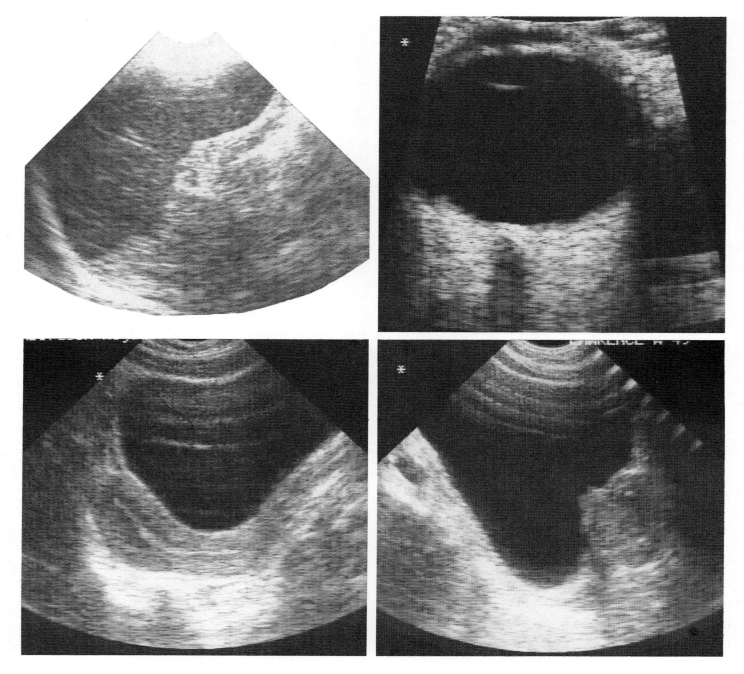

SPLEEN, EYE AND PELVIS

General abdominal ultrasonic scanning is performed with a 3.5 MHz transducer.

The eye scan above was recorded with a 7.5 MHz probe. As the frequency is increased, resolution increases but depth decreases. Thus superficial structures require high frequencies and deep structures low frequencies. In a normal eye the optic nerve is seen as a black notch, indenting the retro-orbital fat. Ultrasound will clearly show retinal detachment, small 1–2 mm retinal tumours and vitreous abnormalities. It is particularly useful in assessing the eye when the lens or vitreous is opaque and direct vision is not possible. Examination of the retro-orbital area is better performed using CT or NMR.

In the bladder scans prostatic definition is increased when a specialized rectal probe is used. Bladder carcinoma can also be accurately staged with ultrasound.

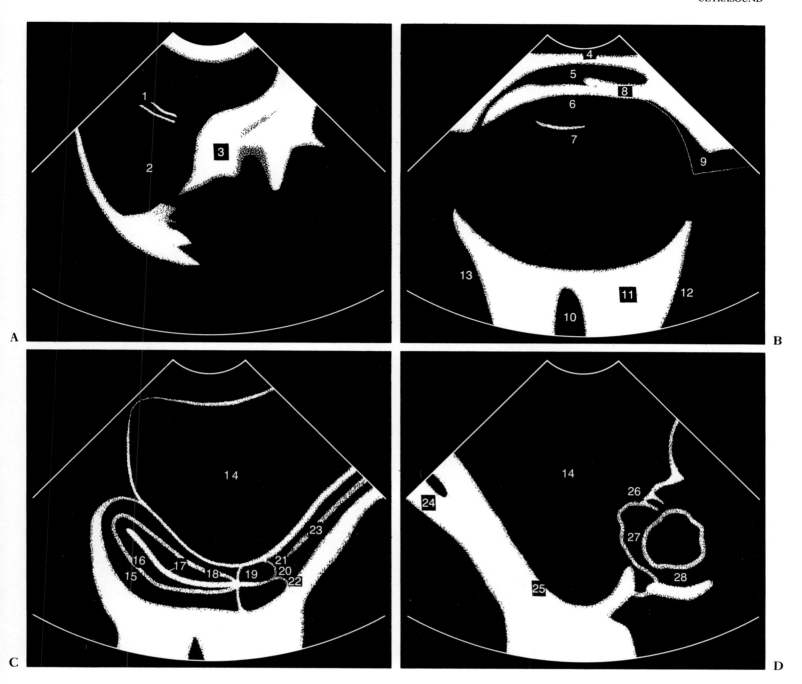

A	Coronal: long axis of spleen	6	Ant. aspect of lens	18	Internal os (endocervix)
B	Transverse axial: midline through eye	7	Post. aspect of lens	19	Cervix
		8	Edge of iris	20	External os (exocervix)
C	Sagittal: midline through bladder and uterus	9	Layers of the globe	21	Ant. fornix of vagina
		10	Optic nerve	22	Post. fornix of vagina
D	Sagittal: midline through bladder and prostate	11	Retro-orbital fat	23	Vaginal cavity
		12	Med. rectus m.	24	R. common iliac a.
		13	Lat. rectus m.	25	Bladder wall
1	Branch of splenic a.	14	Urinary bladder	26	Urethral orifice
2	Spleen parenchyma	15	Myometrium	27	Median lobe of prostate (hypertrophied)
3	Splenic hilum	16	Endometrium		
4	Eyelid and cornea	17	Uterine cavity	28	Post. lobe of prostate
5	Ant. chamber				

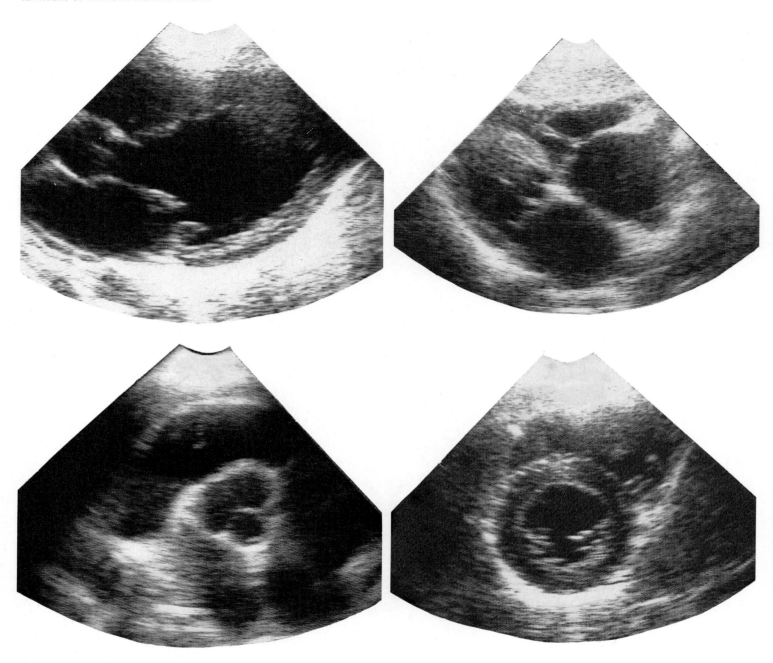

HEART

Four standard views of the heart are demonstrated. The concentric nature of the left ventricle is seen on the short axis view, with the right ventricle curving anteriorly around it. In normal subjects the interventricular septum forms part of left ventricular contraction. The sinuses of Valsalva show their relationship to the surrounding structures in the other short axis view; it is easy to appreciate from this view the complications which may arise if an aneurysm of a sinus develops. The commonest site is the right coronary sinus, which dissects into the right ventricular outflow tract; the non-coronary sinus is affected nearly as frequently and dissects into the septal wall of the right atrium. The rarest form involves the left coronary sinus, which will rupture into the pericardium or left ventricle. The four-chamber subcostal view demonstrates the relationship of the atrioventricular valves and is the single most useful view in assessing infants and children with congenital heart defects.

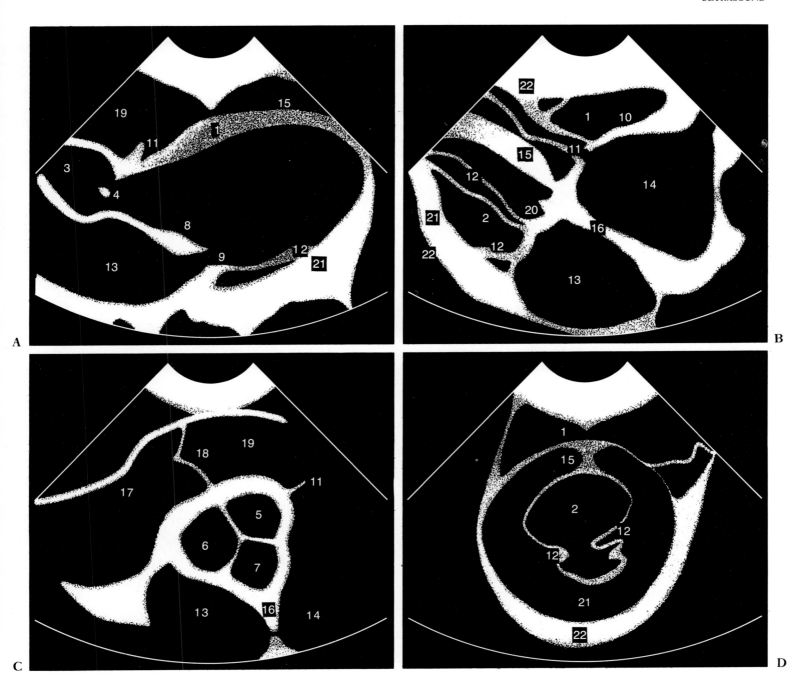

A	Long axis parasternal view of left heart	1	R. ventricle	12	Papillary mm.
B	Subcostal four-chamber view	2	L. ventricle	13	L. atrium
C	Short axis parasternal view of aorta and pulmonary artery	3	Aorta	14	R. atrium
		4	Aortic valve	15	Interventricular septum
D	Short axis parasternal view of left ventricle	5	R. coronary cusp	16	Interatrial septum
		6	L. coronary cusp	17	Pulmonary a.
		7	Non-coronary cusp	18	Pulmonary valve
		8	Ant. mitral leaflet	19	R. ventricular outflow tract
		9	Post. mitral leaflet	20	Mitral apparatus
		10	Ant. tricuspid leaflet	21	L. ventricular myocardium
		11	Septal tricuspid leaflet	22	Pericardium

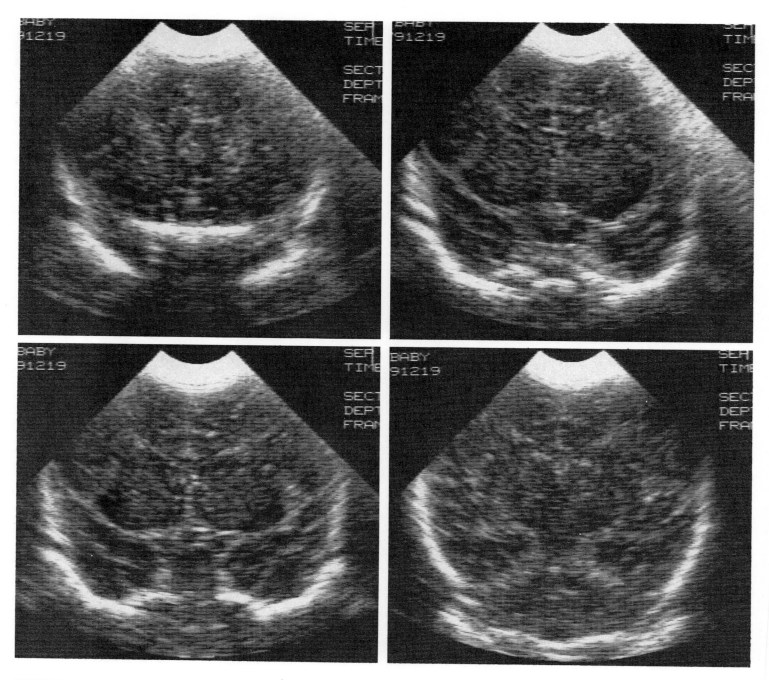

NEONATAL BRAIN: 1

This and the next group of sections are through the anterior fontanelle of a normal neonate.

Five coronal and three sagittal planes are demonstrated. The coronal sections begin through the anterior horn of the lateral ventricles, with strong echoes from the greater and lesser wings of the sphenoid. The interhemispheric fissure produces a prominent landmark, and pulsations of the anterior cerebral artery may be seen within it. The next two sections are taken through the fissures of Sylvius. Between the lateral ventricles lies the echo-dense septum pellucidum. Occasionally an echo-free cavum

septum pellucidum is visible.

The last coronal section on this page is dominated by the C-shaped echoes reflected from the parahippocampal gyri and the medial gyri of the temporal lobes. The foramen of Monro is just anterior to this section. The choroid plexuses within the ventricles are echogenic and some low level echoes are reflected from the thalamus. A large proportion of the internal cerebral echoes are due to collagen within vascular sheaths and ependyma. The brain substance itself is a poor reflector of sound.

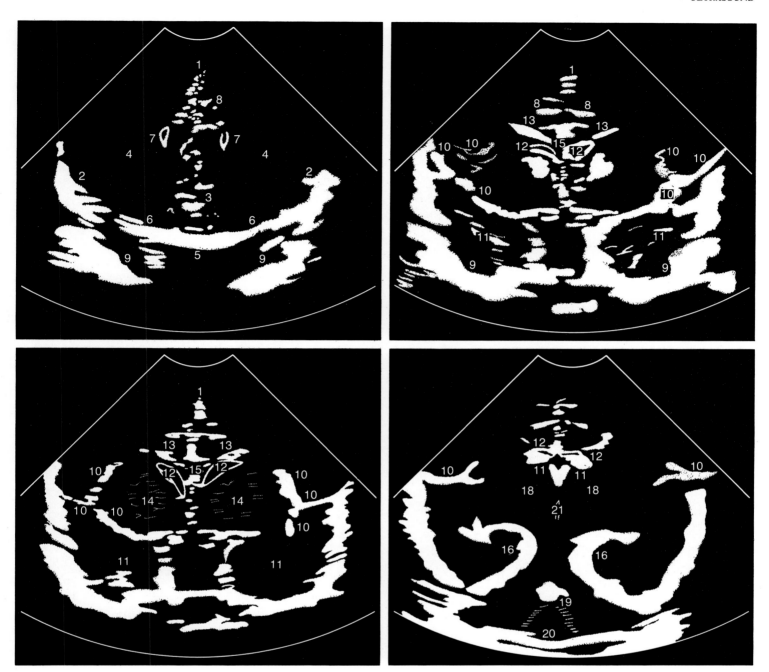

1   Interhemispheric fissure

2   Floor of ant. fossa or orbital roof

3   Ethmoid complex

4   Frontal lobe

5   Planum sphenoidale

6   Lesser wing of sphenoid

7   Ant. horn of lat. ventricle

8   Cingulate sulcus

9   Greater wing of sphenoid

10 Sylvian fissure

11 Temporal pole

12 Lat. ventricle

13 Corpus callosum

14 Caudate nucleus, adjoining
    internal capsule and lenticular
    nucleus complex

15 Septum pellucidum

16 Parahippocampal gyri and med.
    gyrus of temporal lobe

17 Choroid plexus

18 Thalamus

19 Pons

20 Cerebellum

21 Third ventricle

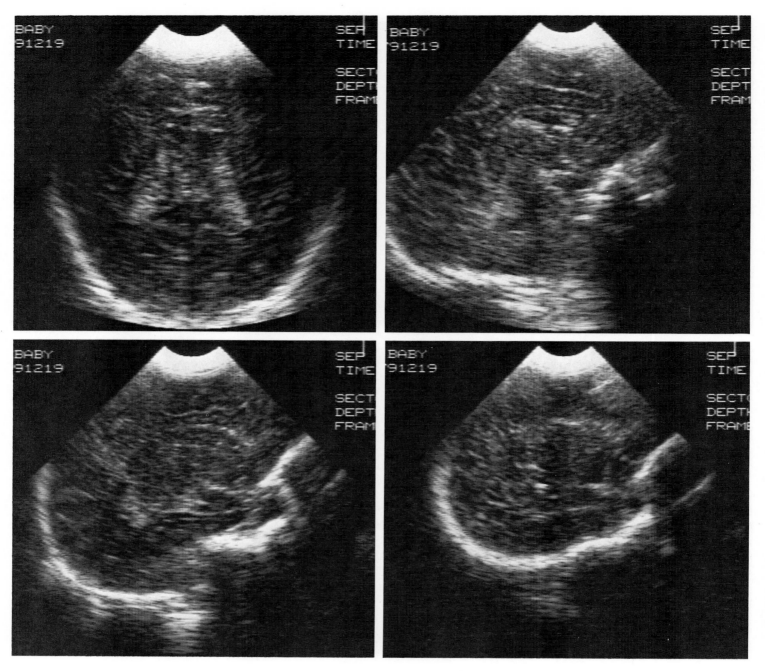

NEONATAL BRAIN: 2

The most posterior coronal plane demonstrates the echogenic choroid plexuses—the medium level echoes are from the cerebellum. The three sagittal planes are: upper right—midline; bottom left—15°; bottom right—30°. The ventricles are better appreciated if there is dilatation. The third and fourth ventricles are shown here, the fourth being roofed by the cerebellum, and anteriorly echoes are reflected from the pons, medulla and clivus.

In the 15° scan the lateral ventricle curves around the caudate nucleus and thalamus. The caudothalamic groove lies at the junction of caudate nucleus and the thalamus—it is a common site for cerebral haemorrhage.

The 30° scan is lateral to any normal ventricle. Pulsations may be seen from the middle cerebral artery within the sylvian fissure. By term, the vascular neural tissue of the germinal matrix has involuted and is situated subependymally. In premature babies, however, it is these areas of the germinal matrix which are prone to haemorrhage. Commonly affected sites include the caudothalamic groove, the region of the foramen of Monro, the head of the caudate nucleus and in the vascular choroid plexus.

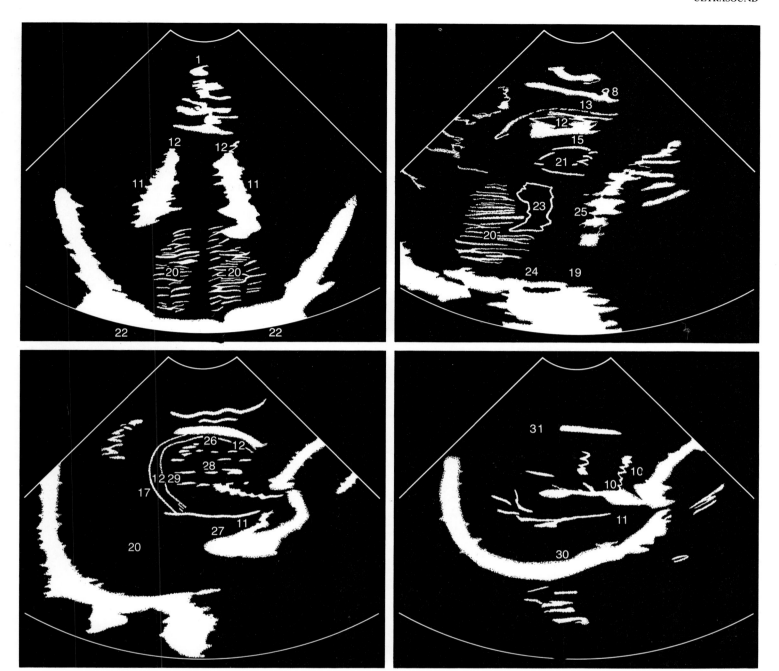

1	Interhemispheric fissure	
2	Floor of ant. fossa or orbital roof	
3	Ethmoid complex	
4	Frontal lobe	
5	Planum sphenoidale	
6	Lesser wing of sphenoid	
7	Ant. horn of lat. ventricle	
8	Cingulate sulcus	
9	Greater wing of sphenoid	
10	Sylvian fissure	
11	Temporal pole	

12	Lat. ventricle
13	Corpus callosum
14	Caudate nucleus, adjoining internal capsule and lenticular nucleus complex
15	Septum pellucidum
16	Parahippocampal gyri and med. gyrus of temporal lobe
17	Choroid plexus
18	Thalamus
19	Pons
20	Cerebellum

21	Third ventricle
22	Occipital bone
23	Fourth ventricle
24	Cisterna magna
25	Clivus
26	Caudothalamic groove
27	Floor of middle fossa
28	Caudate nucleus
29	Thalamus
30	Calvaria
31	Parietal lobe

NUCLEAR MAGNETIC RESONANCE

This last section demonstrates the adult brain in axial, coronal and sagittal sections, and the spinal cord. There is also a short section on the heart and the female pelvis.

The physical principles involved in nuclear magnetic resonance (NMR) are well documented and we suggest that the reader consult a specialized textbook; a note of such is given in the 'Further reading'. Before interpreting NMR anatomy, the basic principles in the production of the image should be studied.

As this Atlas is designed for the interpretation of normal anatomy only, the different images obtainable by NMR have not been included.

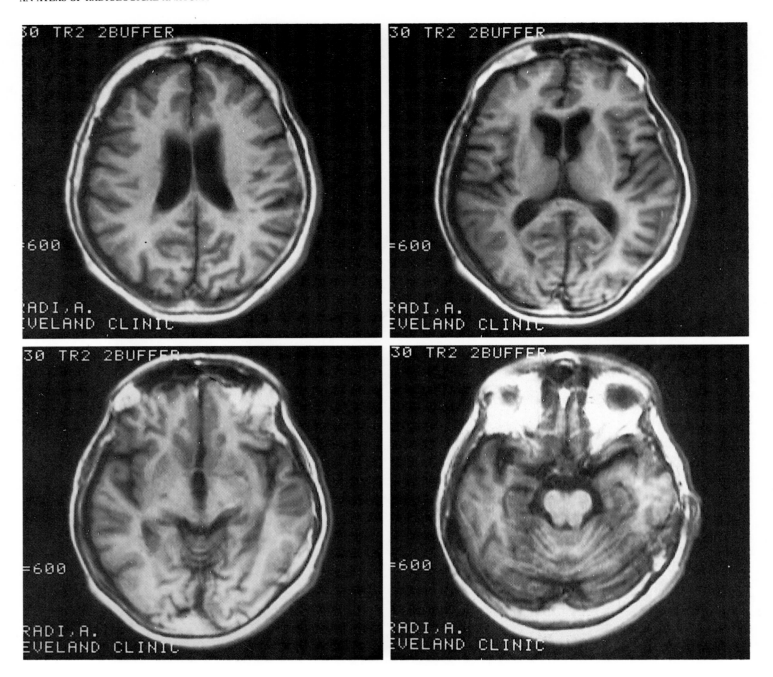

BRAIN: 1

This and the following three groups deal with the nuclear magnetic resonance (NMR) images of the brain in axial coronal and sagittal planes. NMR has several advantages over CT: bone artefacts are not a problem, direct coronal and sagittal scans can be performed and there is a high level of contrast between grey and white matter. NMR images depend on four basic parameters: proton density, T 1, T 2 and flow and diffusion effects. Partial saturation (PS) images largely reflect proton density, with areas of high proton density showing white and areas of low proton density dark. The partial saturation images also depend on T 1, and cerebrospinal fluid, despite a high proton density, will appear dark on these images. Inversion recovery (IR) images show good contrast resolution: white matter with a short T 1 appears white, grey matter with a longer T 1 appears grey and cerebrospinal fluid with a very long T 1 appears black. The four axial scans on this page are IR images.

The spin echo (SE) shows a low level of grey and white matter contrast and appear similar to CT images.

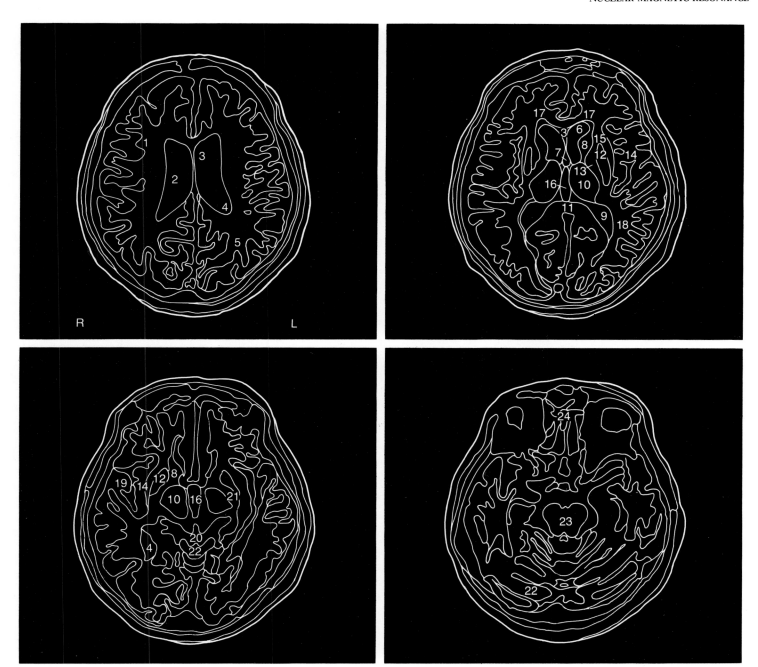

1	**Central sulcus**	9
2	**Body of lat. ventricle**	10
3	**Septum pellucidum**	11
4	**Occipital horn of lat. ventricle**	12
5	**Parieto-occipital sulcus**	13
6	**Frontal horn of lat. ventricle**	14
7	**Fornix**	15
8	**Head of caudate nucleus**	16

1 **Central sulcus**

2 **Body of lat. ventricle**

3 **Septum pellucidum**

4 **Occipital horn of lat. ventricle**

5 **Parieto-occipital sulcus**

6 **Frontal horn of lat. ventricle**

7 **Fornix**

8 **Head of caudate nucleus**

9 **Trigone of lat. ventricle**

10 **Thalamus**

11 **Splenium of corpus callosum**

12 **Putamen**

13 **Genu of internal capsule**

14 **Insula**

15 **External capsule**

16 **Third ventricle**

17 **Genu of corpus callosum**

18 **Optic radiations**

19 **Lat. sulcus**

20 **Ambient cistern**

21 **Globus pallidus**

22 **Cerebellum**

23 **Midbrain**

24 **Crista galli**

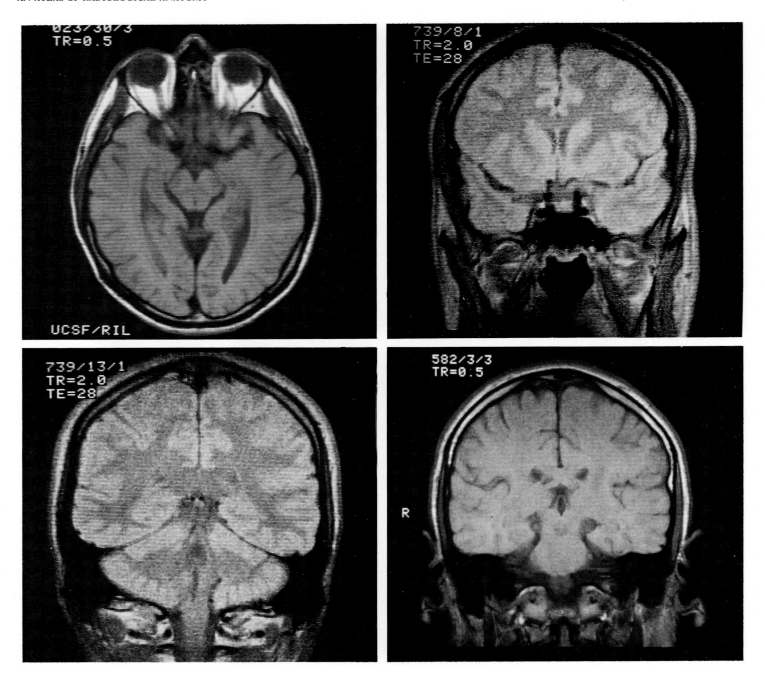

BRAIN: 2

The T 2 of grey and white matter is similar, with cerebrospinal fluid having a long T 2.

Many conditions, such as oedema and infarction, produce an increase in both T 1 and T 2 with less change in proton density. Occasionally a reduced T 1 may be seen in some tumours, but the majority show an increase. The plaques of demyelination in multiple sclerosis are best shown on the spine echo sequences and there is a much greater sensitivity with this technique than with CT. The upper left section is axial, the remaining three are coronal.

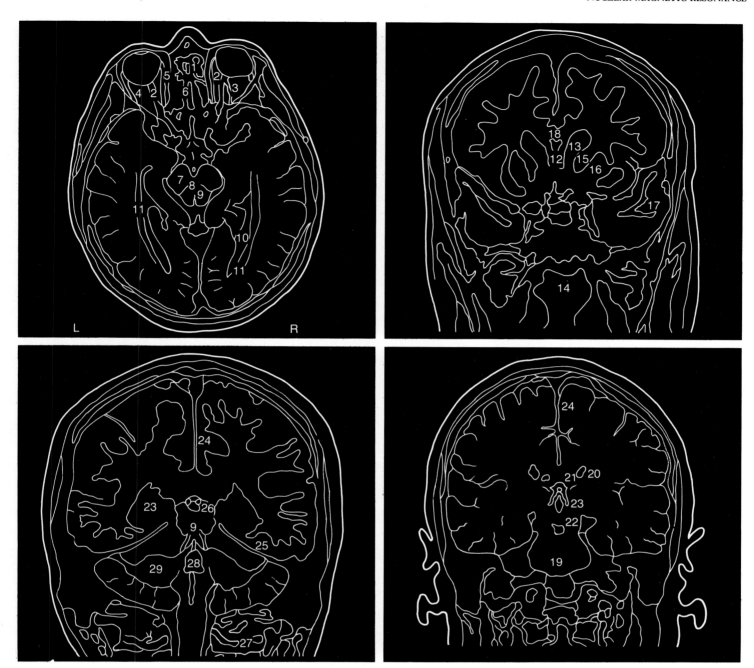

1	Ethmoid sinus	11	Optic radiation
2	Optic n.	12	Septum pellucidum
3	Ophthalmic a.	13	Caudate nucleus
4	Lat. rectus m.	14	Pharynx
5	Sup. oblique m.	15	Internal capsule
6	Olfactory n.	16	Putamen
7	Crus cerebri	17	Lat. sulcus
8	Cerebral aqueduct	18	Corpus callosum
9	Sup. colliculus	19	Pons
10	Inf. horn of lat. ventricle	20	Lat. ventricle

21	Fornix
22	Red nucleus
23	Thalamus
24	Falx cerebri
25	Tentorium cerebelli
26	Pineal body
27	Vertebral a.
28	Fourth ventricle
29	Cerebellum

BRAIN: 3

This sagittal scan, with a zoom projection below, demonstrates the normal anatomy of the brain stem and pituitary gland. It provides excellent anatomical information not obtainable by any other imaging technique. Higher magnetic fields increase the T 1 relaxation time and, at 1.5 tesla, T 1 for brain tissue is double that at 0.3 tesla. Using a high field strength image as shown above, the hypophyseal stalk and pituitary gland are clearly seen. An abnormal gland can be identified on NMR imaging by a change in its size and shape and by tissue characterization. It has recently been shown that it is possible to diagnose small adenomas within normal sized glands.

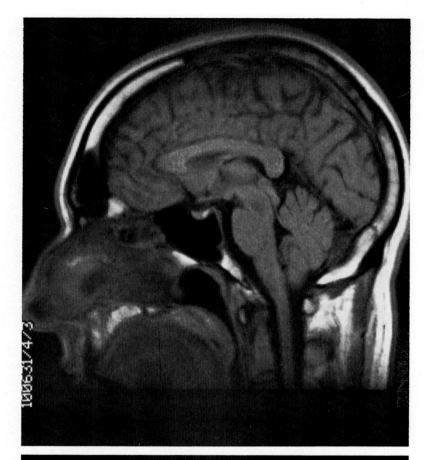

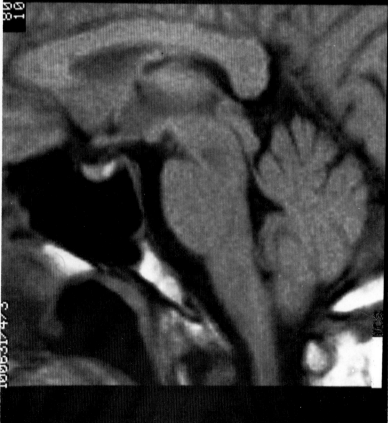

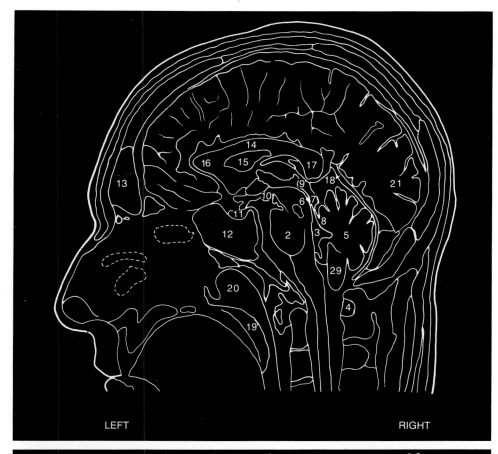

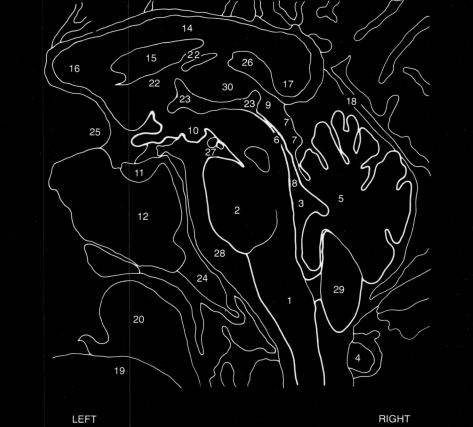

1   Medulla oblongata
2   Pons
3   Fourth ventricle
4   Post. arch of atlas
5   Cerebellum
6   Cerebral aqueduct
7   Colliculi
8   Sup. medullary velum
9   Pineal body
10 Mamillary body
11 Pituitary fossa
12 Sphenoid air sinus
13 Frontal air sinus
14 Corpus callosum
15 Lat. ventricle
16 Genu of corpus callosum
17 Splenium of corpus callosum
18 Tentorium cerebelli
19 Soft palate
20 Nasopharynx
21 Calcarine sulcus
22 Fornix
23 Third ventricle
24 Clivus
25 Subcallosal area
26 Suprapineal recess
27 Oculomotor n.
28 Pontine cistern
29 Cerebellar tonsil
30 Massa intermedia

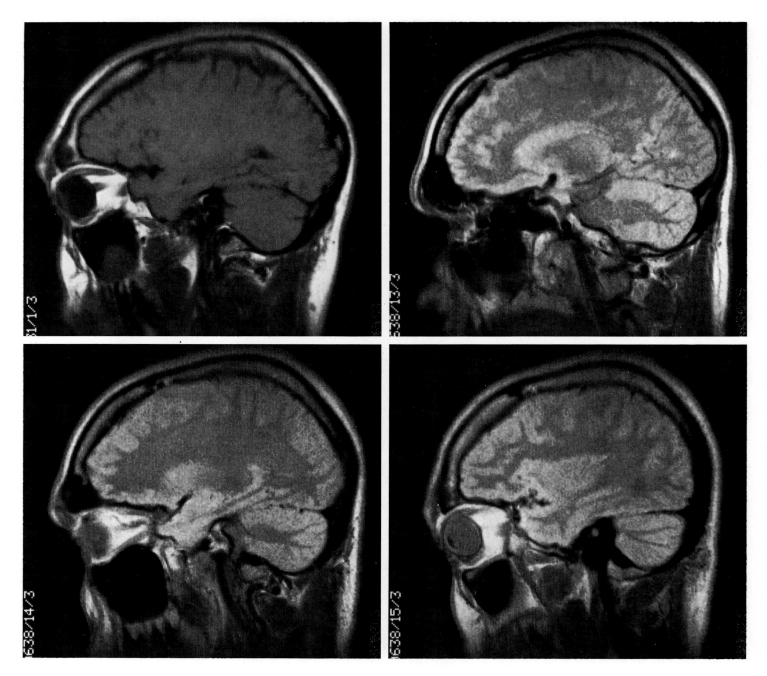

BRAIN: 4

These are parasagittal sections through the brain. A small poly-poidal area of mucosal thickening is present in the floor of the maxillary antrum. Contrast agents such as gadolinium–DTPA, a chelating substance, enhance contrast resolution and tissue differ-entiation. Their toxicity precludes their widespread use, but other paramagnetic elements are under production, including specifi-cally labelled monoclonal antibodies.

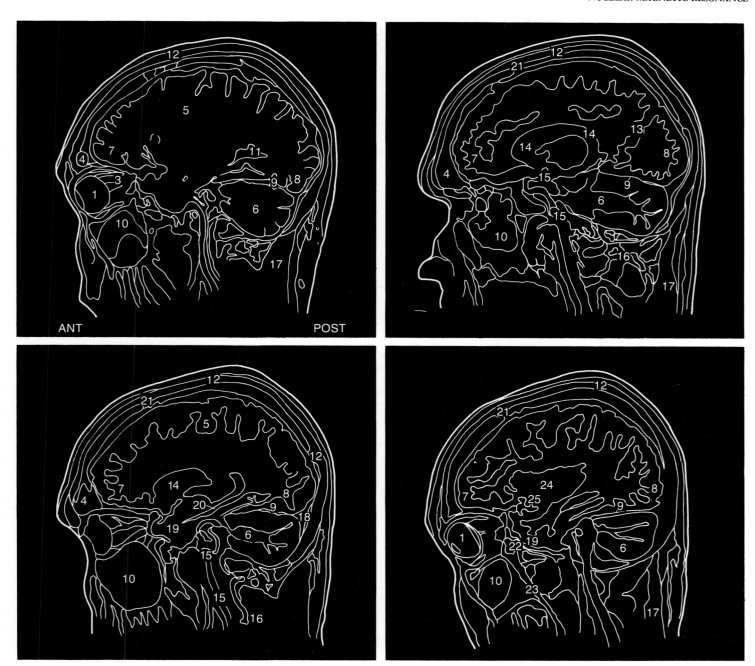

1	Globe	10	Maxillary air sinus	18	Transverse dural venous sinus
2	Levator palpebrae superioris m.	11	Lat. ventricle	19	Temporal lobe
3	Sup. rectus m.	12	Diploic bone	20	Temporal sulcus
4	Frontal air sinus	13	Parieto-occipital sulcus	21	Arachnoid granulations
5	Cerebral hemisphere	14	Corpus callosum	22	Pterygopalatine ganglion
6	Cerebellum	15	Carotid a. (syphon)	23	Pterygomaxillary fissure
7	Frontal lobe	16	Vertebral a.	24	Insula
8	Occipital lobe	17	Ligamentum nuchae	25	Lat. sulcus
9	Tentorium cerebelli				

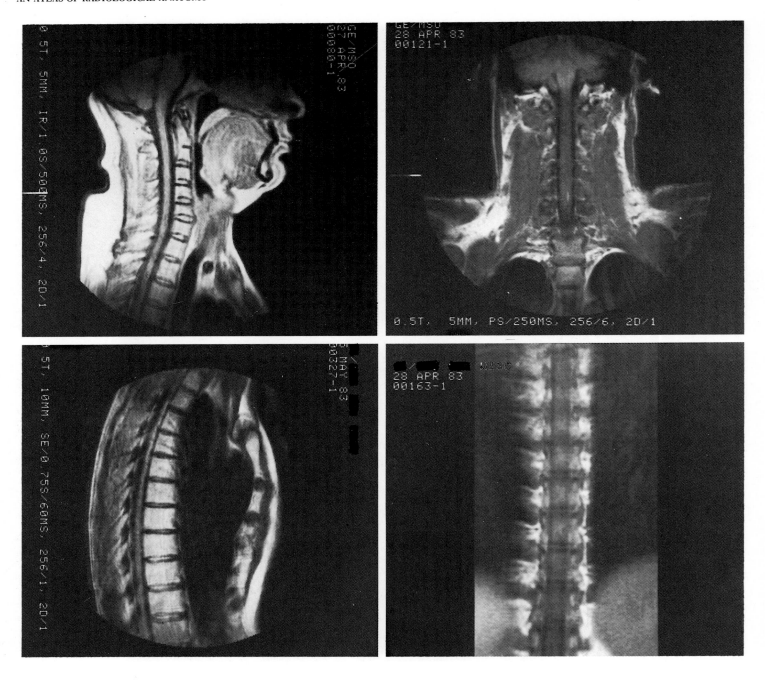

SPINAL CORD

These are sagittal and coronal views of the cervical and thoracic spine. The entire spinal cord is seen as a structure with intermediate signal activity surrounded by a low-intensity cerebrospinal fluid. The filum terminale is difficult to visualize clearly and individual nerve fibres are not resolved clearly.

Although inversion-recovery images detect and separate the grey and white matter well in the brain, it is not possible to obtain this differentiation in the spinal cord.

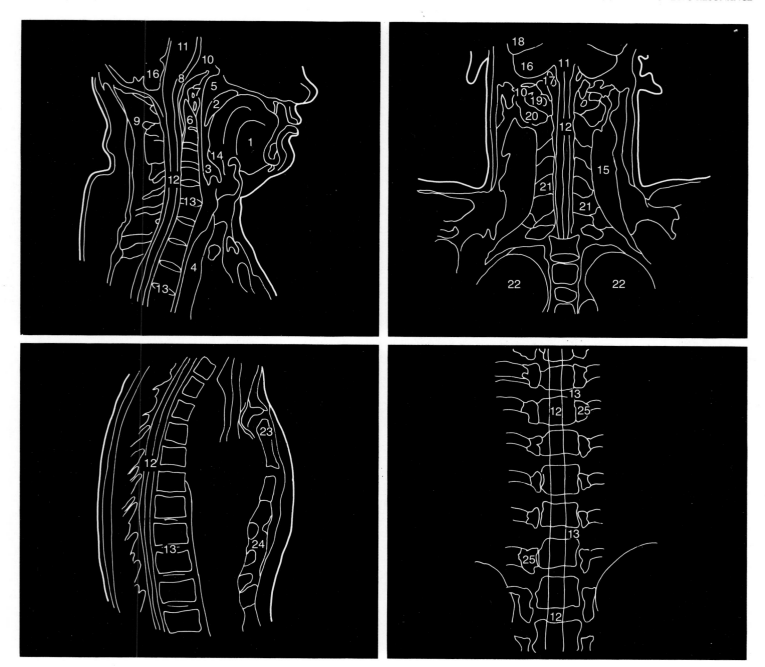

1	Tongue	10	Basiocciput	18	Tentorium cerebelli
2	Soft palate	11	Medulla oblongata	19	Vertebral a.
3	Laryngopharynx (hypopharynx)	12	Spinal cord	20	Inf. oblique m.
4	Trachea	13	Intervertebral disc	21	Cervical spinal n.
5	Nasopharynx	14	Epiglottis	22	Apex of lung
6	Odontoid peg (dens) of axis	15	Semispinalis capitis m.	23	Manubrium
7	Ant. longitudinal lig.	16	Cerebellum	24	Sternal body
8	Membrana tectoria	17	Cerebral tonsils	25	Costal articulations
9	Ligamentum nuchae				

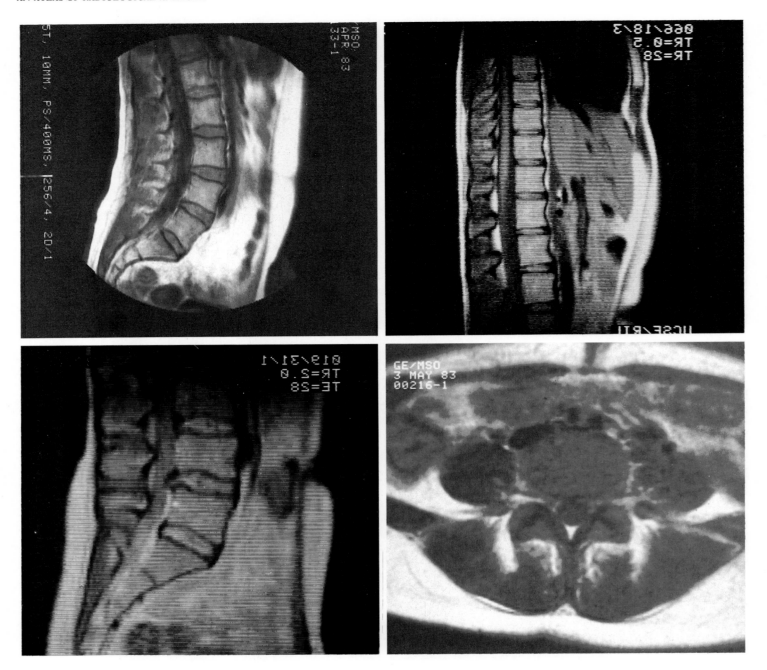

SPINAL CORD AND CAUDA EQUINA

The marrow-containing cancellous bone in the vertebral bodies shows mid to high signal intensity, whilst the compact cortical bone is of low signal intensity. The nucleus pulposus is of mid intensity and will appear as bright as cancellous bone. There is a high-intensity signal pattern to extra dorsal fat and this may be seen in the lower thoracic and lumbar regions around the theca.

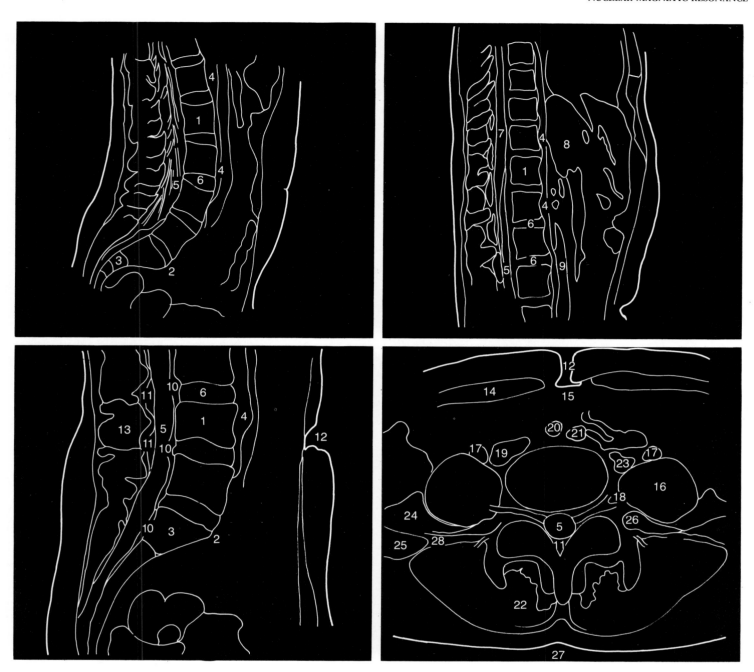

1	Lumbar vertebrae	11	Ligamentum flavum	20	R. common iliac a.
2	Sacral promontory	12	Umbilicus	21	L. common iliac a.
3	Sacrum	13	Spinous process	22	Erector spinae m.
4	Ant. longitudinal lig.	14	Rectus abdominis m.	23	Gonadal vss.
5	Cauda equina	15	Linea alba	24	Ilium
6	Intervertebral disc	16	Psoas major m.	25	Gluteus maximus m.
7	Spinal cord	17	Ureter	26	Lumbosacral trunk
8	Liver	18	Lumbar spinal n.	27	Supraspinous lig.
9	Aorta	19	Bifurcation of inf. vena cava	28	Lumbar fascia
10	Post. longitudinal lig.				

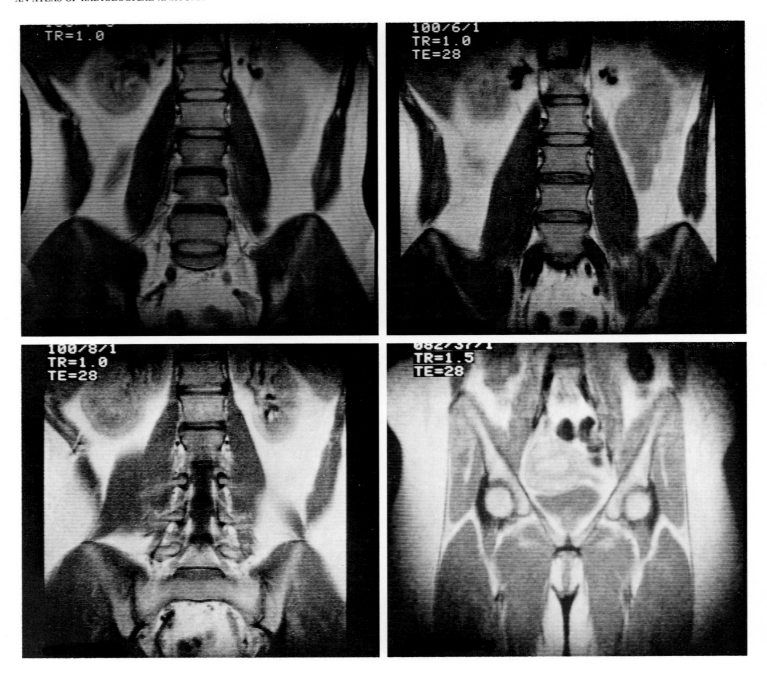

FEMALE ABDOMEN AND PELVIS

The ability of NMR to obtain any reconstruction plane is of immense value and has advantages over axial CT, even if computer reconstruction is used. NMR imaging of the female pelvis allows differentiation of uterine structure, with a high-intensity signal from the endometrium separated from the myometrium by a low-intensity band which some workers believe to be the stratum basale. The definition of the uterus and any uterine or cervical mass is better shown by NMT than by CT. CT will not differentiate the uterine tissues. The levator ani is best seen in the coronal section, separating the floor of the pelvis from the perineum.

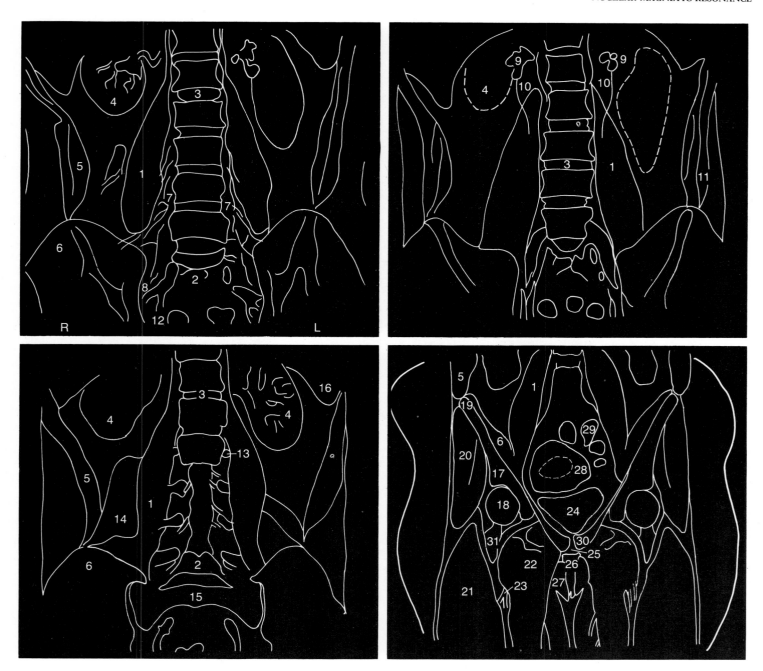

1	Psoas major m.	12	Internal iliac a.	22	Adductor m.
2	Sacral promontory	13	Lumbar vv.	23	Femoral vss.
3	Intervertebral disc	14	Quadratus lumborum m.	24	Bladder
4	Kidney	15	Sacrum	25	Vagina
5	Abdominal wall mm.	16	Spleen	26	Introitus
6	Iliacus m.	17	Innominate bone	27	Labia
7	Lumbar plexus	18	Femoral head	28	Uterus
8	External iliac a.	19	Iliac crest	29	Sigmoid colon
9	Pelvis of kidney	20	Gluteal m.	30	Levator ani m.
10	Ureter	21	Quadriceps m.	31	Rectus femoris m.
11	External abdominal oblique m.				

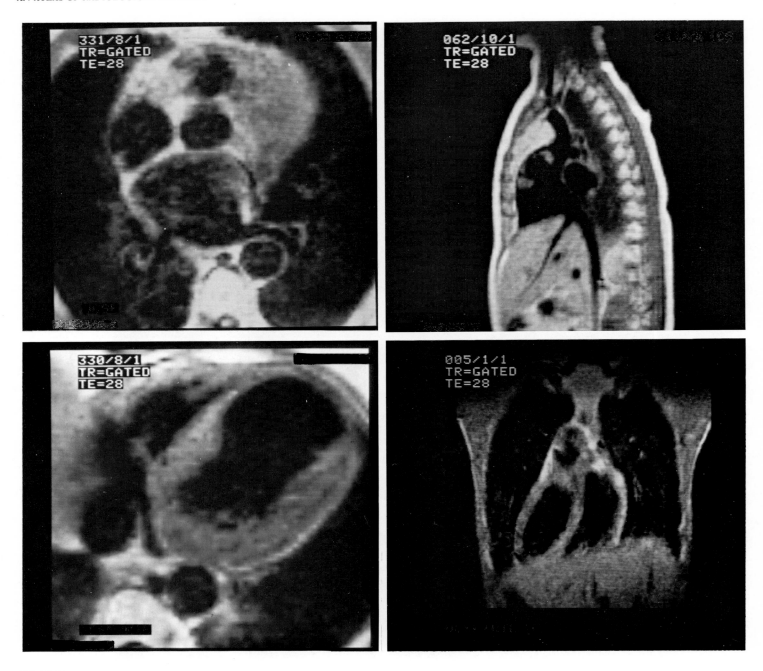

HEART

To obtain satisfactory cardiac scans, ECG gating is required, with an acquisition time of approximately 5 minutes.

The scans shown are in the sagittal, coronal and axial planes. The patient has an abnormality seen on the axial view through the left ventricle where there is thinning and bulging of the anterior wall due to a myocardial infarct.

High-resolution superconducting magnets producing 2 tesla or more have demonstrated serial changes in the myocardium following infarction and can be used to monitor progress. Serial dynamic NMR scanning with blood flow analysis has also been successful in assessing the anatomical and physiological changes formed in congential heart disease.

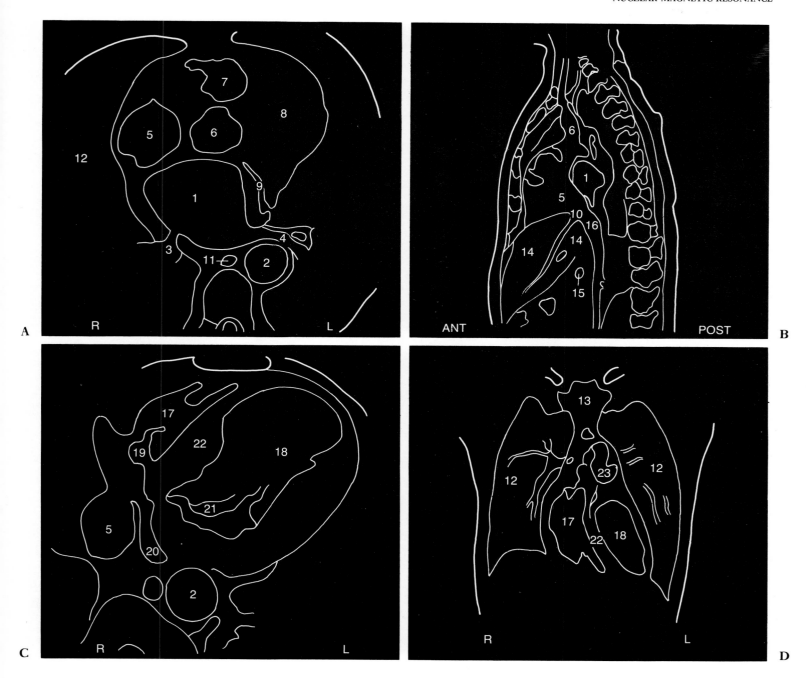

1	L. atrium	9	Circumflex a.	17	R. ventricle
2	Descending aorta	10	Hepatic v.	18	L. ventricle
3	R. pulmonary v.	11	Azygos v.	19	Tricuspid valve
4	L. pulmonary v.	12	Lungs	20	Coronary sinus
5	R. atrium	13	Manubrium	21	Mitral apparatus
6	Ascending aorta	14	Liver	22	Intraventricular septum
7	Pulmonary a.	15	Portal v.	23	R. ventricular outflow tract
8	Myocardium	16	Inf. vena cava		

A, axial; B, sagittal; C, axial; D, coronal.

FURTHER READING

ANATOMY

Abrahams P, Thatcher M 1981 Pocket Examiner in Regional and Clinical Anatomy. Pitman, London

Abrahams P H, Webb, P J 1981 Clinical Anatomy of Practical Procedures. Pitman, London

Basmajian J V 1979 Grant's Method of Anatomy, 10th edn. Williams & Wilkins, Baltimore

Brock R C 1954 The Anatomy of the Bronchial Tree. Oxford University Press, London

Cahill D, Orland M 1984 Atlas of Human Cross-sectional anatomy. Lea & Febiger, Philadelphia

Ellis H 1983 Clinical Anatomy: a revision and applied anatomy for clinical students, 7th edn. Blackwell Scientific, Oxford

Frazer J E 1965 The Anatomy of the Human Skeleton, 6th edn. Churchill Livingstone, London

Gardner E, Gray D J, O'Rahilly R 1975 Anatomy: a regional study of human structure, 4th edn. Saunders, Philadelphia

Ger R, Abrahams P 1985 Essentials of Clinical Anatomy. Pitman, London

Grant J C B 1982 Grant's Atlas of Anatomy, 8th edn. Williams & Wilkins, Baltimore

Hollinshead W H 1974 Textbook of Anatomy, 3rd edn. Harper & Row, Hagerstown, Maryland.

McAlpine W A 1975 Heart and Coronary Arteries. Springer-Verlag, New York

Netter F H 1983 Ciba Collection of Medical Illustrations, vols 1–7. Ciba-Geigy, New York

Romanes G J 1981 Cunningham's Textbook of Anatomy, 12th edn. Oxford University Press, London

Stephens R B, Stilwell D L 1969 Arteries and Veins of the Human Brain. Thomas, Springfield, Illinois

Warwick R, Williams P L 1980 Gray's Anatomy, 36th British edn. Churchill Livingstone, Edinburgh

RADIOLOGY

Abrams H 1983 Angiography, vols I & II, 3rd edn. Little, Brown, Boston

de Roo T 1975 Atlas of Lymphography. Lippincott, Philadelphia

Di Chiro G 1971 An Atlas of Detailed Normal Pneumoencephalographic Anatomy, 2nd edn. Thomas, Springfield, Illinois

Etter L E 1972 Roentgenography and Roentgenology of the Temporal Bone, Middle Ear and Mastoid Process, 2nd edn. Thomas, Springfield, Illinois

Hamilton W J, Simon G 1958 Surface and Radiological Anatomy for Students and General Practitioners, 4th edn. Heffer, Cambridge

Keats T E 1984 An Atlas of Normal Roentgen Variants that may Simulate Disease, 3rd edn. Year Book Medical, Chicago

Kinmonth J B 1982 The Lymphatics: surgery, lymphography and diseases of the chyle and lymph systems, 2nd edn. Edward Arnold, London

Lloyd G A S 1975 Radiology of the Orbit. Saunders, London

Meschan I 1975 An Atlas of Anatomy Basic to Radiology. Saunders, Philadelphia

Netter F H 1983 Ciba Collection of Medical Illustrations, vols 1–7. Ciba-Geigy, New York

Ross P, du Boulay G H 1976 Atlas of Normal Vertebral Angiograms. Butterworths, London

COMPUTED TOMOGRAPHY

Lee J K T (ed.) 1983 Computed Body Tomography. Raven Press, New York

Maue-Dickson W 1983 Computed Tomographic Atlas of the Head and Neck. Little, Brown, Boston

Shipps F C 1978 Anatomical Exercises in Computerized Body Scanning. Thomas, Springfield, Illinois

NUCLEAR MAGNETIC RESONANCE

Newton T H, Potts D G (eds.) 1983 Modern Neuroradiology, vol. 2, Advanced Imaging Techniques. Clavadel Press

ULTRASOUND

Cosgrove D O, McCready V R 1982 Ultrasound Imaging: liver, spleen and pancreas. Wiley, Chichester

Meire H B, Farrant P 1982 Basic Clinical Ultrasound, BIR teaching series no. 4. British Institute of Radiology, London

Meire H B, Dewbury K C, Cosgrove D O 1983 Ultrasound Teaching Cases. London Ultrasound Publishing, London

Weir J, Pridie R B 1984 An Atlas of Clinical Echocardiography. Pitman, London

INDEX